Guidelines for Nurse Practitioners in Gynecologic Settings

Eighth Edition

Joellen W. Hawkins, RNC, PhD, FAAN, is a professor in the William F. Connell School of Nursing where she is responsible for the women's health nurse practitioner tract. Her research focuses on the evolution of WHNPs and on intimate partner violence and child witness to violence. She also is a nurse practitioner at Sidney Borum Community Health Center in Boston and teaches a prenatal class at Pine Street Inn to homeless pregnant women. She is the author or editor of 33 books and over 100 articles in professional journals and edits *Clinical Excellence for Nurse Practitioners: International Journal of NPACE* published by Springer.

Diane Roberto-Nichols, BS, APRNC, is an OB/GYN nurse practitioner. She has been employed at Ellington OB/GYN, a solo physician practice, for the last 12 years. Her focus has been women's health, starting as coordinator of the Women's Health Clinic at the University of Connecticut where she was instrumental in making contraception and confidential health care available to female students. She also codeveloped a protocol and implemented an assault crisis service for sexually and physically abused students at the University of Connecticut. Throughout the years, she has continued to conduct outreach programs for the student population and community.

Lynn Stanley-Haney, MA, APRN, has been a nurse practitioner since 1980. She has organized and implemented school-based health centers, worked in a college student health center, and in a community women's health and private gynecology setting. Stanley-Haney has a long history as a women's health advocate with a special interest in teens and issues facing young women. In addition to her gynecology practice, she also maintains a private psychotherapy practice.

Guidelines for Nurse Practitioners in Gynecologic Settings

Eighth Edition

Joellen W. Hawkins, RNC, PhD, FAAN
Diane M. Roberto-Nichols, BS, APRN-C
J. Lynn Stanley-Haney, MA, APRN-C

 Springer Publishing Company

Springer Publishing Company, Inc.
536 Broadway
New York, NY 10012-3955

Acquisitions Editor: Ruth Chasek
Production Editor: Sara Yoo
Cover design by Joanne Honigman

04 05 06 07 08 / 5 4 3 2 1

RG105
, H368
2004
c 0826116264

Library of Congress Cataloging-in-Publication Data

Hawkins, Joellen Watson.
    Guidelines for nurse practitioners in gynecologic settings / Joellen
W. Hawkins, Diane M. Roberto-Nichols, J. Lynn Stanley-Haney.—8th ed.
        p. ; cm.
    Rev. ed. of: Protocols for nurse practitioners in gynecologic settings.
7th ed. Tiresias Press, c2000.
    Includes bibliographical references and index.
    ISBN 0-8261-1626-4
    1. Gynecologic nursing.   2. Nursing care plans.
    [DNLM: 1. Genital Diseases, Female—nursing.   2. Nurse Practitioners.
3. Nursing Care—methods.   4. Patient Care Planning.   WY 156.7 H393g
2004]   I. Hawkins, Joellen Watson. Protocols for nurse practitioners in
gynecologic settings.   II. Roberto-Nichols, Diane M.   III. Stanley-Haney,
J. Lynn.   IV. Title
RG105 .H368 2004
618.1'0231—dc22

                                                            2003066534

Printed in the United States of America by Sheridan Books.

Table of Contents in Brief

Table of Contents in Depth

PART II: APPENDIXES

Preface to the Eighth Edition

This extensively revised and updated edition of *Guidelines for Nurse Practitioners in Gynecologic Settings* is designed to be used to guide nursing management of the common gynecological conditions women present with in community-based or ambulatory settings. These include concerns such as vaginitis, vaginosis and sexually transmitted diseases, fear of HIV exposure, contraceptive needs across the reproductive life span, life transitions including menarche and menopause, preconception care and desire for pregnancy, mental and emotional health, sexuality, sexual assault, and intimate partner violence. The guidelines and patient materials were originally prepared for the Women's Clinic at the Student Health Services of the University of Connecticut, Storrs. Those guidelines and patient materials still form the core of this ever-evolving book.

The three principal authors are nurse practitioners practicing in women's health settings. All were actively involved in the original book's development and are responsible for its continual updating. Two guidelines, cervical cap and natural family planning, were developed by advanced practice nurses who were chosen for their expertise with those methods of fertility regulation.

This eighth edition has a number of special features to assist you in your practice. In addition to an up-to-date bibliography for each guideline, it contains new information on contraceptive methods, the latest CDC guidelines for management of STDs, vaginitis, vaginosis, and miscellaneous conditions affecting the genital area, smoking cessation, assessing risk of heart disease, osteoporosis assessment and prevention, management of abnormal Pap smears including Bethesda 2001 and the 2002 Guidelines for Pap Smear Management, hepatitis, hormone therapy, breast conditions and breast cancer risk, and emergency contraception. The new guidelines are weight management, mental health and emotional issues appropriate for assessment and treatment in women's health settings, polycystic ovary syndrome, and all the new contraceptive methods. The new patient materials include polycystic ovary syndrome, the contraceptive ring, FemCap, and the contraceptive patch.

As we go to press, several promising new contraceptives are on the horizon. These include oral contraceptives with a new progestin, two new implants, a progestin-only injectable with microspheres or microcapsules in 1, 3, and 6 month formulations, transdermal cream and a frameless and a threadless IUD. New barrier and spermicidal methods for contraception include Ove's cap and a sponge already available in Canada for the past several years. The Today sponge is poised to return to the market. A selective tubal occlusion device promises a new option for reversible sterilization. Male methods under investigation include incapacitators targeting sperm-producing cells, hormones to decrease sperm counts, implants to release hormones, antifertility vaccines, and a nonlatex condom eZ-on. Vaginal microbicides show promise in decreasing risks of STDs.

The book is designed for ease of use in your practice settings. Web sites are included for your use and that of your patients.

—Joellen W. Hawkins
Diane M. Roberto-Nichols
J. Lynn Stanley-Haney

Acknowledgments

The authors wish to express their gratitude to colleagues who, over the years, have worked with them to develop, evaluate, and rewrite the protocols as they are being tested in clinical practice. Gratitude is also due to the many graduate students who have worked with the protocols and teaching materials and offered important suggestions. Our clients, too, have been very helpful in suggesting changes for the educational materials and in expressing a need for information that led to the development of some of the materials.

Special thanks go to Eleanor S. Tabeek, Nancy Keaveney and Mary Finnigan for materials on natural family planning, R. Mimi Clarke Secor for information on the cervical cap, Kathleen K. Furniss and Jacqueline Campbell for consultation on the sexual assault domestic violence materials, Richard Ferri for the HIV/AIDS Risk Self-Assessment, and Martha Sternberg who coauthored the urinary tract infection guideline.

And finally, we wish to thank the late Dorothy Lewis for her belief in this project through seven editions and the late Helen Behnke for her intelligent and skillful editing of the original manuscript of this book.

Introduction

Nurse practitioners in any area of practice need to consider the issues sur-rounding the use of guidelines. Many states mandate that nurse practitioners practice underwritten protocols or guidelines. There is growing support for such legislation; some agencies and institutions already require the use of clinical guidelines by nurse practitioners, and may even specify by whom these are to be developed. Furthermore, protocols or practice guidelines are being required in some states where nurse practitioners have prescription writing privileges in order for nurse practitioners to be approved to do so. Managed care systems, too, often mandate use of clinical guidelines by their practitioners.

Of course, controversy exists as to whether guidelines should be used at all. Opponents argue that guidelines are too rigid, that they stifle creativity and the development of problem-solving ability, and that they run counter to individu-alization of care. Some types of guidelines do not require the skills of an advanced practitioner of nursing, to be sure, and there are some who would protest that they prolong the dependency syndrome of nurse practitioners, par-ticularly when the guidelines are prepared by physicians and there is little or no nursing input. Guidelines can be unrealistic for some practitioners in some settings with some clients. If used as a measure of care from a legal perspective, such guidelines could open up the practice to malpractice charges.

Proponents argue that guidelines offer a wealth of research data for use in validating nursing management strategies. By providing a guide for stan-dardization of data collection, a record audit can be done to determine whether patient outcomes are beneficial. Guidelines can be written so as to build in problem solving, and can serve as recommendations rather than a rigid set of rules. They can be used with a record-keeping system such as Weed's prob-lem-oriented medical record system. Guidelines can facilitate continuity and coordination of care, as well as enhance documentation of the clinical deci-sion-making process. As such, they can prove extremely valuable in quality improvement programs and in measuring clinical outcomes. They can be developed to reflect the confidence level and needs of the nurse practitioners using them and delineate areas of competence and responsibility for the various health care professionals in a multidisciplinary setting.

The guidelines in this book were designed originally for a particular setting and thus take into account the common presenting problems in a women's clinic, who was going to use the guidelines (nurse practitioners), the setting in which they would be used (women's clinic in a student health service), the availability of physician colleagues and other health care professionals for consultation, the referral system already in place, the laboratory facilities available, the basis for nurse practitioner practice in the state, and the nurse practice act. The authors now practice in other settings, so the guidelines reflect those settings and the women's needs. As each guideline is now developed and tested in their clinical practices, the authors record ideas for the annual revision and updating of the material. A search of the literature is done for each guideline and is updated yearly as well.

The guidelines that appear in this book are the result of an ongoing effort at research, writing and rewriting and of testing in clinical practice by the authors, their colleagues, and graduate students. We hope they will be useful to you in your practice as you adapt, revise, and update them to meet the needs of your patients.

REFERENCES

Courtney, R. (1997). Working with protocols. *American Journal of Nursing, 97*(2), 16E–16F, 16H

Hawkins, J.W., & Roberto, D. (1984). Developing family planning nurse practitioner protocols. *Journal of Obstetric, Gynecologic, and Neonatal Nursing, 13*(3), 167–170.

Mahoney, D.F. (1992). Nurse practitioners as prescribers: Past research trends and future study needs. *The Nurse Practitioner, 17*(1), 44, 47–48, 50–51.

Moniz, D.M. (1992). The legal danger of written protocols and standards of practice. *The Nurse Practitioner, 17*(9), 58–60.

Pearson, L. (2003). Update: How each state stands on legislative issues affecting advanced nursing practice. *The Nurse Practitioner, 28*(1).

Stock, C.M. (1995). Ten tips for writing and using practice protocols. *Contemporary Nurse Practitioner, 2*(1), 51–52.

Weed, L.L. (1969). *Medical records, medical education, and patient care.* Chicago: Year Book Medical Publishers.

PART I. CLINICAL GUIDELINES

1

METHODS OF FAMILY PLANNING

HORMONAL CONTRACEPTION

I. TYPES OF HORMONAL CONTRACEPTION
A. ORAL CONTRACEPTIVES
1. Oral contraceptives (OC) (also known as birth control pills) are pills that when taken by mouth produce systemic changes that prevent conception. Types of Pills
   a. A combination of synthetic estrogen and progestin
   b. Progestin only (also known as mini-pills)
   c. See Table 1.1 (pages 13–16, for oral contraceptives marketed in the U.S.
2. Directions for use (combination):
   a. The pill is taken for 21 days, and an inert pill (or no pill) for 7 days, during which time withdrawal bleed should occur; some packets have 21 oral contraceptive pills only, so the woman then takes no pills for 7 days.
   b. A tri-cycle regimen is widely used in Europe and is becoming more widely used in the United States. This regimen, 3 packs or more of a monophasic pill used consecutively, may be considered in certain situations, including:
      1) headaches regularly occurring during withdrawal weeks
      2) heavy withdrawal bleeds
      3) endometriosis after work-up
   c. A regimen of 21 combination pills, 2 inert pills (days 22 and 23) and 5 days of ethinyl estradiol (days 24–28).
   d. A regimen of 84 combination pills. Packaged in an extended cycle dispenser containing a 3 month supply. This regimen reduces menses to 4 times per year.
3. Directions for use (progestin only):
   Progestin only pills are taken continuously.
   a. Indications for Using Progestin-only Pill:
      1) Is a good choice in situations when estrogen is contraindicated:
         a) Smokers
         b) Lactation
         c) History/current deep vein thrombosis/pulmonary embolism

3

        d) Surgery with immobilization
        e) Valvular heart disease
        f) Severe headaches including migraine without focal neurological symptoms
        g) Gallbladder disease
        h) Seizure disorders
     2) Elevated blood pressure $\geq$ 140/90

  b. Other considerations for progestin only methods (advantages may outweigh risks):
     1) Undiagnosed breast cancer
     2) Gallbladder disease while on combined method
     3) Diabetes without vascular involvement (Type 1 or 2)
     4) Diabetes with nephropathy, retinopathy, neuropathy
     5) History of current ischemic heart disease
     6) History of cerebrovascular accident
     7) Severe headaches, including migraines, with focal neurological symptoms
     8) Mild cirrhosis (uncompensated)
     9) Undiagnosed hypertension (not hypertension in pregnancy)

  c. Women who fit the above criteria after appropriate screening and physical exam may be candidates for progestin only, bearing in mind that irregular bleeding may present a major clinical problem. Since number of pills varies with manufacturer, carefully review instructions on use and pill pack.

4. Procedure for pill related bleeding problem, i.e., amenorrhea, scant menses, break-through bleeding
  a. Rule out the following:
     1) Faulty OC taking (review packet)
     2) Pregnancy
     3) Uterine or cervical pathology—leiomyomata, polyp, cancer
     4) Pelvic or vaginal infection
     5) Drug interference
     6) Gastrointestinal problems
     7) Endometriosis
  b. Based on information gained, treatment as follows:
     1) Amenorrhea or scant menses
        a) Reassure woman
        b) Consider method change
     2) Break-through bleeding
        a) During the first 3 months of hormone use, reassure only
        b) Consider method change

c) Consider adding exogenous estrogen (PO or transdermal) (20 mcg ethinyl estradiol, 1–2 mg estradiol, or 0.625 conjugated estrogen) beginning the first day of break-through bleed x 7 days regardless of where the woman is in her cycle

d) If treatment for a or b is unsuccessful and symptoms persist, consult with gynecologist.

3) For hormonal amenorrhea

a) Pregnancy test

b) If amenorrhea continues after six months, consider progestin agent to induce menses and if no withdrawal bleed, refer to amenorrhea protocol for work-up

4) If a woman is on any medications that decrease contraceptive effect, she should be offered the option of back-up contraception such as condoms and/or spermicidal protection. Decisions about hormonal contraceptive use with medications (see Table 1.2) should be individualized. If there is any question regarding drug interaction and interference of method with other drugs, consult with gynecologist or pharmacist.

5. Explanation of Method:

a. Ways in which oral contraceptives are taken

1) Start oral contraceptive on day 1 (first day of menses) or on Sunday of week menses start

2) Oral contraceptive must always be taken at the same time of day (within an hour either way)

3) Back-up contraception is necessary for 7 days (first cycle only)

4) Missed pills

a) One pill missed: woman to take pill when she remembers, and then take scheduled pill at regular time

b) Two pills missed in first 2 weeks: take 2 pills at regular time for 2 days. Use back-up contraception x 7 days

c) Two or more pills missed in third week, or 3 or more pills missed any time (and woman starts on Sundays), she should keep taking a pill each day until Sunday, then start a new packet that Sunday. Instruct woman to use a back-up method for 7 days. If woman does not start on Sundays, she should throw out pill pack and start a new pack that day. A back-up method of birth control should be used for the first 7 days of this new pill pack.

d) If 1 or more pills are missed and no back-up contraception is used and no withdrawal bleed, woman should be instructed to call to discuss possible pregnancy test

B. TRANSDERMAL CONTRACEPTIVE
   CONTRACEPTIVE PATCH ORTHO EVRA
   1. Definition and Use:
      The contraceptive patch is a 3 layer transdermal polyethylene/polyester device about the size of a matchbook, with an adhesive on one side. It is impregnated with norelgestromin (NGMN), a synthetic progestin, and ethinyl estradiol (EE), a synthetic estrogen, and releases 150 micrograms of NGMN and 20 micrograms of EE every 24 hours.
   2. Directions for Use:
      Patch is changed weekly for 3 weeks then off for 1 week
   3. Explanation of Method:
      a. Ways in which the patch is used
         1) Apply the patch on first day of menses or on the first Sunday after bleeding begins; postpartum nonnursing 4 weeks or with resumption of menses.
         2) Apply to clean, dry, healthy skin on buttocks, abdomen, upper outer arm, or upper torso. Patch should not be applied to breasts.
         3) Instruct woman not to use lotions, cosmetics, creams, powders or other topical products in area of patch or area where patch will be applied.
         4) Instruct the woman to press down firmly on patch for at least 10 seconds and then check that the edges adhere.
         5) Instruct woman to check patch daily.
         6) If patch detaches, instruct woman to immediately apply a new patch. Supplemental tapes or adhesives should not be used.
         7) Apply a new patch the same day of the week 7 days after first patch. Repeat this in week 3.
         8) No patch is applied in week 4.
         9) Begin a new cycle on the same day of the week for week one and repeat cycle of 3 weeks on and one week off.
         10) Withdrawal bleed will occur during 4th week.
         11) If the woman forgets to apply a new patch and less than 48 hours have passed, she can apply a new patch as soon as she remembers and then apply that next patch on the usual renewal day.
         12) If more than 48 hours have elapsed, the woman should stop the current cycle and immediately begin a new 4–week cycle by applying a new patch. The day for patch renewal will now change. Instruct her to use back up contraception for one week.
         13) If missed change day occurs at the end of the 4–week cycle,

instruct the woman to remove the patch and apply a new patch on the usual change day to begin a new cycle.

C. INTRAVAGINAL CONTRACEPTIVE
CONTRACEPTIVE VAGINAL RING NUVA RING
1. Definition and Use:
   The contraceptive vaginal ring is flexible, transparent, colorless, and about 2 inches in diameter. It is impregnated with etonogestrel, a synthetic progestin, and ethinyl estradiol (EE), a synthetic estrogen, and releases 120 micrograms of progestin and 15 micrograms of EE every 24 hours over a period of 3 weeks.
2. Explanation of method and way in which ring is used:
   a. Insert ring into vagina between day 1 and day 5 of menstrual cycle.
   b. Keep ring in place for 3 weeks in a row.
   c. Remove ring for one week for withdrawal bleeding.
   d. Insert new ring for 3 weeks, with one week out intervals.
   e. If ring is removed during the 3 weeks and is out for more than 3 hours, back up contraception is required for the next 7 days.

A. INTRAMUSCULAR CONTRACEPTIVE
CONTRACEPTIVE INJECTABLES (Depo-Provera®)
1. Definition:
   a. Synthetic hormonal substance in Depo-Provera (depot-medroxyprogesterone acetate or DMPA) that acts by blocking gonadotropin, thus preventing ovulation from occurring. This injectable decreases sperm penetration through cervical mucus, and causes endometrial atrophy preventing implantation. Injected intramuscularly every 12 weeks into the muscle of the upper arm or buttocks.
2. Explanation of use:
   a. Depo-Provera is injected intramuscularly (in gluteal or deltoid muscle) in the first 5 days of the menstrual cycle (after onset of menses), within 5 days postpartum, or, if breastfeeding, at 4–6 weeks postpartum.
   The injection consists of one 150–milligram dose every 12 weeks for as long as contraceptive effect is desired. If time between injections is greater than 13 weeks, do pregnancy test before administration.
   Inject with 1.5" up to 3" needle (depends upon size of woman since it needs to be deep intramuscular) and do not rub the site as rubbing breaks up the microcrystals and increases absorption. Available in

150 mg/ml prefilled syringes as well as single and multiple-dose vials.

Visit every 12 weeks for injection.

II. PHYSICAL CHANGES OCCURRING WITH HORMONAL CONTRACEPTION

A. Ovulation is suppressed
B. The endometrium becomes deciduous making it unreceptive to implantation
C. The cervical mucus is altered, so it is hostile to sperm
D. Transport of the ovum may be altered
E. Possible luteolysis
F. Possible inhibition of capacitation of sperm

III. EFFECTIVENESS

A. 99.6% effectiveness rate for combination pill
B. 97% effectiveness rate for progestin only pill
C. 98–99% effectiveness rate for vaginal contraceptive ring
D. 99% effectiveness for contraceptive patch
E. 99%+ effectiveness for contraceptive injectables

IV. CONTRAINDICATIONS

A. Absolute contraindications to hormonal contraception:
   1. Thromboembolic disorder (or history thereof) including postpartum deep vein thrombosis, pulmonary embolism or thromboembolism
   2. Thrombotic cerebrovascular accident (or history thereof)
   3. Coronary artery disease (or history thereof); current angina pectoris; structural heart disease complicated by pulmonary hypertension, atrial fibrillation, valvular heart disease with complication
   4. Known or suspected carcinoma of the breast
   5. Major surgery with prolonged immobility or any surgery on the legs
   6. Known impaired liver function at present time, liver problems, hepatic adenoma, liver cancer or history of active viral hepatitis, severe cirrhosis; benign or malignant liver tumor with prior OC use or other estrogen product
   7. Known or suspected estrogen dependent neoplasm (or history thereof) including endometrial carcinoma
   8. Over 35 and currently a smoker
   9. Triglyceride level greater than 350 mg/dl; hypercholesterolemia (type II hyperlipidemia)
   10. Known or suspected pregnancy

11. Chronic hypertension and smoking or uncontrolled hypertension
12. Weight ≥ 198 lbs (90 kg) > weight decreases efficacy
13. Undiagnosed abnormal vaginal/uterine bleeding
14. History of OC-related cholestasis or cholestatic jaundice of pregnancy
15. Leiden factor V mutation
16. Allergic reaction to any components of the ring, patch or Depo-Provera or any of its ingredients (check allergic reaction to local anesthetics for dental or other procedures—the carrier substance is the same for local anesthetics and Depo-Provera)

B. Relative contraindications
   1. Severe headaches or common migraines, which start or worsen with initiation of pill use
   2. Hypertension with resting diastolic BP of 90 or more, or resting systolic BP of 140 or more on 3 or more separate visits, or an accurate measurement of 110 diastolic BP or more on a single visit
   3. Impaired liver function (i.e., mononucleosis, acute phase, medication induced changes)
   4. Hypertriglyceridemia; worrisome LDL:HDL ratio
   5. Gallbladder disease: medically treated, current biliary tract disease

D. Other considerations (advantages of hormone contraception generally outweigh disadvantages):
   1. Diabetes: without vascular disease
   2. Congenital hyperbilirubinemia (Gilbert's disease)
   3. Failure to have established regular menstrual cycle (without prior work-up) [See amenorrhea guideline]
   4. Conditions likely to make it difficult for woman to take OCs correctly and consistently (learning disability, major psychiatric problems, alcoholism or other drug abuse, history of repeatedly taking oral contraceptives or other medications incorrectly)
   5. Major surgery with no prolonged immobilization
   6. Undiagnosed breast mass
   7. Cervical cancer awaiting treatment; CIN
   8. Use of drugs affecting liver enzymes (altering absorption of medication), eliphenytoin, carbamazapine, barbiturates, topiramate, primidone, rifampin, rifabutin, griseofulvin
   9. Under 35 and heavy smoker (>15/day)
   10. Use in breast feeding not yet approved for Nuva Ring and Ortho Evra
   11. Skin disorder that may predispose to application site reactions

V. ADVERSE DRUG INTERACTIONS

Management of hormonal contraceptive drug interaction (see Table 1.2, pp. 17–20)

A. All women prior to starting hormonal contraception and on a yearly follow-up basis should review and re-sign informed consent for method of choice—emphasizing drug interaction and knowledge of danger signs.

B. If a woman is on any medications that decrease contraceptive effect, she should be offered the option of back-up contraception such as condoms and/or spermicidal protection. Decisions about hormonal contraceptive use with medications (see Table 1.2) should be individualized. If there is any question regarding drug interaction and interference of method with other drugs, consult with gynecologist or pharmacist.

VI. LABORATORY

A. Lipid screen
   1. Lipid screen prior to using hormonal contraception
   Significant immediate family history
      a. Under age 50— stroke, coronary, or sudden death
      Do lipid screen. If levels abnormal, consult with MD before starting hormonal contraception. If normal levels, start hormonal contraception and repeat test in 2 years.
   2. Lipid screen strongly advised if parents or siblings have hypertension, vascular disease, myocardial infarction, arteriosclerotic heart disease, and/or hyperlipidemia before age 50 or are on medication for hypertension.

B. Monitor carefully any prediabetic and diabetic women using hormonal contraception. Consider screening with fasting blood sugar and/or 2 hour postprandial blood sugar if parents or siblings are diabetic or woman is otherwise at increased risk for developing diabetes.

C. Liver profile if woman has had mononucleosis or mono-like illness within past year or if patient has history of hepatitis or other liver disease or drug or alcohol history.

D. In combination hormonal methods, Leiden factor V for women with personal or family history of venous thromboembolism.

VII. FOLLOW UP

A. For all methods of hormonal contraception:
   1. Blood pressure check as needed
   2. Smoking cessation counseling
   3. Review of side effects and danger signs

B. For injectables:

1. Depo-Provera
   a. Revisit every 12 weeks
   b. If greater than 13 weeks since last injection, use very sensitive pregnancy test prior to injection.

See Appendix D for consent form and informational handout on oral contraceptives for patients. See Bibliography.

NOTE

Tables 1.1 and 1.2 (pages 13–20) provide guidelines on possible drug interactions/interferences with oral contraceptives and information on contraceptives currently marketed in the United States.

Evaluation of Headaches Occurring While on Oral Contraceptives*

Current pill Used _____ Length of Time on Pill _____
Name _____ ID _____ Date _____
Subjective Findings (to be filled out by patient, interviewer, or clinician)

	Yes	No	Don't Know
1. Have your headaches been worse in the past 48 hours?	___	___	___
2. Have you started having headaches or have your headaches become worse since you started taking birth control pills?	___	___	___
3. Do you have light headedness, dizziness, or nausea at the same time as you have headaches?	___	___	___
4. Do you ever vomit at the time of your headaches?	___	___	___
5. Have you ever been told you have high blood pressure (hypertension)?	___	___	___
6. Do you have spots in front of your eyes, double or blurred vision when you have your headaches?	___	___	___
7. Do you ever lose your vision, that is, become blind or partially blind?	___	___	___
8. Do your headaches usually occur on just one side of your head?	___	___	___
9. Do you note watering of one or both eyes at the time of your headaches?	___	___	___

	Yes	No	Don't Know
10. Have you ever been told you had migraine headaches?	—	—	—
11. Does anyone in your family have a history of migraine headaches?	—	—	—
12. Are your headaches throbbing headaches?	—	—	—
13. If you use aspirin or an aspirin substitute, do your headaches continue even after you take the aspirin or aspirin substitute?	—	—	—
14. Do any foods seems to bring on headaches?	—	—	—
15. Do alcohol (such as red wine), caffeine, and/or any drugs worsen or cause headaches?	—	—	—
16. Do you have a history of or have sinusitis?	—	—	—
17. Do you have a history of or do you now have postnasal drip?	—	—	—
18. Have you ever seen a physician for your headaches? If so, what were the results?	—	—	—
19. Allergies	—	—	—
20. Have you ever had numbness or tingling of face or extremities (arms, legs, feet, hands) associated with headaches?	—	—	—
21. What bothers you most about your headaches?	—	—	—

Objective Findings: B/P ___/___ Fundi: _____

Other Findings: _____

Localized Tenderness: _____

Assessment: _____

Plan: _____

Nurse Practitioner: _____

*Adapted from Emory University Family Planning Program. Used with permission.

Table 1.1 Oral Contraceptives Marketed in the United States: Formula and Dosage

*Progestin Content

	Norethindrone Estrogenic Effect 1.0 Androgenic Effect 1.0	Drospirenone	Ethynodiol Diacetate Estrogenic Effect 3.4 Androgenic Effect 0.6	Norethindrone Acetate Estrogenic Effect 1.5 Androgenic Effect 1.6	Norgestrel Estrogenic Effect 0 Androgenic Effect 4.2	Norgestimate Estrogenic Effect 0 Androgenic Effect 1.9	Levonorgestrel Estrogenic Effect 0 Androgenic Effect 8.3	Desogestrel Estrogenic Effect 0 Androgenic Effect 3.4	Mestranol µg	Ethinyl Estradiol µg	Number of Hormonal Pills	Number of Other Pills
Alesse 28 (LevLite,† Aviane 21, Lessina 28 same)							0.10			20	21	7 Inert
Brevicon-21 & 28	0.5									35	21	7 Inert
Demulen 1/35-21 & 28			1.0							35	21	7 Inert
Zovia 1/35/28			1.0							50	21	7 Inert
Demulen-21 & 28										30	21	7 Inert
Desogen Apri (same)								0.15		35	21	7 Inert
Genora 0.5/35	0.5									35	21	7 Inert
Genora 1/35-21 & 28	1.0									50	21	7 Inert
Genora 1/50-21 & 28	1.0									30	21	7 Inert
Levlen							0.15			35	21	7 Inert
Levora							0.15			35	21	7 Inert
Jenest 28	0.5 mg(7) 1.0 mg(14)									35	21	7 Inert
Loestrin FE 1/20**				1.0						20	21	7 Iron
Loestrin FE 1.5/30				1.5						30	21	7 Iron
Lo/Ovral-21 & 28 (Cryselle & Low-Ogestrel 0.3/0.030 same)					0.3					30	21	7 Inert

*Gestodene is on the market in Europe but has not yet been approved in the U.S.

**Also available as Loestrin 1/20 and 1.5/30 with 7 Inert.

From *Nurse Practitioner's Drug Handbook*. (2003); Wilson, B. A., Shannon, M. T., & Stang, C. L. *Nurses Drug Guide*. (2002). Upper Saddle River, NJ: Prentice-Hall.

Table 1.1 (*continued*)

	*Progestin Content								Estrogen Content			
	Norethindrone (Estrogenic Effect 1.0 / Androgenic Effect 1.0)	Drospirenone	Ethynodiol Diacetate (Estrogenic Effect 3.4 / Androgenic Effect 0.6)	Norethindrone Acetate (Estrogenic Effect 1.5 / Androgenic Effect 1.6)	Norgestrel (Estrogenic Effect 0 / Androgenic Effect 4.2)	Norgestimate (Estrogenic Effect 0 / Androgenic Effect 1.9)	Levonorgestrel (Estrogenic Effect 0 / Androgenic Effect 8.3)	Desogestrel (Estrogenic Effect 0 / Androgenic Effect 3.4)	Mestranol μg	Ethinyl Estradiol μg	Number of Hormonal Pills	Number of Other Pills
Wodicon-21 & 28 (Necon .05/35 same)												
Nelova 1/35E	1.0									35	21	7 Inert
Necon 1/35 same										35	21	7 Inert
Nelova 0.5/35E	0.5									35	21	7 Inert
Nelova 1/50M	1.0								50		21	7 Inert
Nelova 10/11 (NEE	1.0(10 days)									35	10	7 Inert
10/11 same)	0.5(11 days)									25	11	
Norcept E 1/35	1.0									35	21	7 Inert
Nordette 21 & 28 (Levora, Portia and LevLen same)							1.5			30	21	7 Inert
Norethin 1/35E	1.0									35	21	7 Inert
Norethin 1/50M	1.0								50		21	7 Inert
Necon 1/50M same											21	7 Inert
NEE 0.5/35	0.5									35	21	7 Inert
NEE 1/35	1.0									35	21	7 Inert
Norinyl 1/35	1.0									35	21	7 Inert
Norinyl 1+50/21 & 28	1.0								50		21	7 Inert
Necon 1/50 same											21	7 Inert
Norlestrin 2.5/50-21				2.5						50	21	
Norlestrin 2.5/50-FE				2.5						50	21	7 inert
Norlestrin 1/50-21 & 28				1.0						50	21	7 Inert
Norlestrin 1/50-FE				1.0						50	21	7 Inert
Ortho-Cept 21 & 28 (Apri same)								0.15		30	21	7 Inert

Table 1.1 *(continued)*

	Norethindrone (Estrogenic Effect 1.0, Androgenic Effect 1.0)	Drospirenone	Ethynodiol Diacetate (Estrogenic Effect 3.4, Androgenic Effect 0.6)	Norethindrone Acetate (Estrogenic Effect 1.5, Androgenic Effect 1.6)	Norgestrel (Estrogenic Effect 0, Androgenic Effect 4.2)	Norgestimate (Estrogenic Effect 0, Androgenic Effect 1.9)	Levonorgestrel (Estrogenic Effect 0, Androgenic Effect 8.3)	Desogestrel (Estrogenic Effect 0, Androgenic Effect 3.4)	Mestranol µg	Ethinyl Estradiol µg	Number of Hormonal Pills	Number of Other Pills
						← *Progestin Content* →				← *Estrogen Content* →		
Ortho-Cyclen 21 & 28 (Sprintec same)						0.250				35	21	7 Inert
Ortho-Novum 1/35										35	21	7 Inert
21 & 28 (Nortrel same)	1.0											
Ortho-Novum 10/11/21 & 28 Necon 10/11 same												
White tablets	0.5(10)											
Peach tablets	1.0(11)									35	21	7 Inert
Ortho-Novum 1/50-21 & 28	1.0								50		21	7 Inert
Ovcon-35	0.4									35	21	7 Inert
Ovcon-50	1.0									50	21	7 Inert
Ovral 21 & 28 (Ogestrel same)					0.5					50	21	7 Inert
Zovia 1/50			1.0							50	21	7 Inert
Mircette (Kariva same)								0.15		20(21) 10(5)	26	2 Inert
MINI (Progestin only)												
Micronor	0.35										28	
Nor-Q-D	0.35										42	
Ovrette					0.075						28	
Yasmin		3.0								30	21	7 Inert
TRIPHASICS												
Cyclessa								0.100(7) 0.125(7) 0.150(7)		25 25 25	21	7 Inert

Table 1.1 (*continued*)

	*Progestin Content — Norethindrone (Estrogenic Effect 1.0, Androgenic Effect 1.0)	Drospirenone	Ethynodiol Diacetate (Estrogenic Effect 3.4, Androgenic Effect 0.6)	Norethindrone Acetate (Estrogenic Effect 1.5, Androgenic Effect 1.6)	Norgestrel (Estrogenic Effect 0, Androgenic Effect 4.2)	Norgestimate (Estrogenic Effect 0, Androgenic Effect 1.9)	Levonorgestrel (Estrogenic Effect 0, Androgenic Effect 8.3)	Desogestrel (Estrogenic Effect 0, Androgenic Effect 3.4)	Estrogen Content — Mestranol µg	Ethinyl Estradiol µg	Number of Hormonal Pills	Number of Other Pills
Estrostep 21				1mg 1mg 1mg						20(5) 30(7) 35(9)	21	
Estrostep®FE				1mg						20(5) 30(7) 35(9)	21	75 mg Fe
Triphasil 21 & 28 (TriLevLen, Enpresse, Trivora, same)							0.050(6) 0.075(5) 0.125(10)			30(6) 40(5) 30(10)	21	7 Inert
Ortho-Novum 7/7/7/21 & 28 (Nortrel 7/7/7 same)	0.5(7) 0.75(7) 1.0(7)									35	21	7 Inert
Tri-Norinyl 21 & 28	0.5(7) 1.0(9) 0.5(5)									35	21	7 Inert
Tri-Cyclen						0.180(7) 0.215(7) 0.250(7)				35 35 35	21	7 Inert
OrthoTri-Cyclen Lo						0.180(7) 0.215(7) 0.250(7)				25	21	7 Inert

Tri-Cyclen is the only OC currently indicated to treat acne vulgaris in women 15 and older who have no contraindications to OC use, want contraception, have achieved menarche, and have not responded to topical antiacne medications.

Table 1.2 Possible Interactions Between Oral Contraceptives and Other Drugs

Interacting Drugs	Adverse Effects	Comments and Recommendations
When in doubt, consult with a pharmacist		
Antipyretics and analgesics Acetaminophen, aspirin, meperidine, antipyrine	Possible decrease in pain relief (increased metabolism)	Monitor pain-relief response; may have to adjust analgesic dosage
Alcohol	Possible increased effect of alcohol ($\downarrow$ metabolism)	Caution patient
Antibiotics Troleandomycin Cyclosporine	$\uparrow$ serum levels, risk to liver	Choose alternative method
Anticongulants (Oral)	Decreased anticoagulant effect ($\uparrow$ factor VII & X)	Use alternate contraceptive
Antidepressants Tricyclics amitriptyline, desipramine, imipramine, nortriptyline	Possible increased antidepressant effect ($\downarrow$ metabolism)	Monitor antidepressant effect
Anti-infectives: sulfonamides	Possible decreased contraceptive effect; possible breakthrough bleeding	Use back-up method during treatment
Barbiturates/Anticonvulsants (phenobarbital, primidone, carbamazepine, pheyntoin, topirimate, succimide)	Decreased contraceptive effect ($\uparrow$ metabolism)	Avoid simultaneous use; alternative contraceptives for long course of treatment; consider 50 mcg ethinyl estradiol OC
Benzodiazepine Tranquilizers such as: diazepam (Valium), nitrazepine, chlordiazepoxide (Librax, Librium), alprazolam (Xanax)	Possible increased or tranquilizer effects including psychomotor impairment and possibly impairs elimination due to $\downarrow$ clearance	Use with caution. Greatest impairment during menstrual pause in contraceptive dosage

Adapted from: R.A. Hatcher, J. Trussell, F. Stewart, W. Cates G.K. Stewart, F. Guest and D. Kowal (1998), *Contraceptive Technology* (17th ed.), New York: Ardent Media; R.P. Dickey (2002), *Managing Contraceptive Patients* (11th ed.), Durant, OK: Essential Medical Information Systems (EMIS); *Nurse Practitioner's Drug Handbook* (2003), Springhouse, PA: Springhouse; L.A. Eisenhauer & M.A. Murphy (1998). *Pharmacotherapeutics and Advanced Nursing Practice*. New York: McGraw-Hill.

Table 1.2 Possible Interactions Between Oral Contraceptives and Other Drugs *(continued)*

Interacting Drugs	Adverse Effects	Comments and Recommendations
Beta-blockers such as: propranolol (Inderal) atenolol (Tenormin) metoprolol (Lopressor) pindolol (Visken) Nadolol (Corgard)	Possible increased blocker effect (↓ metabolism)	Monitor cardiovascular status; ↓ drug dosage if necessary
Betamimetics: isoproterenol (Isuprel, Aerolone, Vaso-Iso)	↓ response due to ee	Adjust drug dose, monitor closely
Cholesterol Lowering Agents: clofiborate, gemtibrozil	↑ clearance rate	May need to ↑ dose, monitor lipid profile
Corticosteroids (cortisone, prednisone)	Possible increased corticosteroid toxicity (may impair elimination of drug)	Possibly need to ↓ dosage
Griseofulvin (Fulvicin, Grisactin Grifulvin, others)	Decreased contraceptive effect (↑ metabolism)	Use alternative contraceptive
Guanethidine (Ismelin)	Decreased guanethidine effect (mechanism not established)	Avoid simultaneous use
Methyldopa (Adoril, Aldomet, Amodopa, Dopamet, Apomethyldopa, Novomedopa)	Decreased hypertensive effect	Avoid simultaneous use
Oral Antidiabetics such as: chlonopropamide (Diabinese), glipizide (Glucotrol), tolazamide (Tolinase), tolbutamide (Tolinase)	Possible decreased hypoglycemic effect	Monitor blood glucose using low dose estrogen & progestin; consider other birth control
Penicillins	Decreased contraceptive effect possible; breakthrough bleeding	Low but unpredictable incidence; use alternative contraceptive during treatment

Table 1.2 Possible Interactions Between Oral Contraceptives and Other Drugs *(continued)*

Interacting Drugs	Adverse Effects	Comments and Recommendations
Phenytoin (Mesantoin); mephenytoin. (Dilantin) phenytoin sodium (Di-Phen, Diphenylan)	Decreased contraceptive effect; possible decreased phenytoin effect	Use alternative contraceptive; 50 mEq. ethinyl estradiol; monitor phenytoin concentration
Rifampin (Rifadin, Rimactane)	Decreased contraceptive effect (↑ metabolism of progestins)	Use alternative contraceptive
Tetracycline/ ampicillin short-term<10 days	Decreased contraceptive effect	Use back-up contraceptive during and then x 7 days after treatment.
Theophyllines (Aerodate, Bronkodyl, Slo-bid, Slo-Phyllin, Theobid, Theolair, Theophyl, Theo-Dur, others)	Increased theophylline effect (↓ clearance by 30–40%)	Monitor theophylline concentration; use with caution
Troleandomycin (TAO)	↑ risk of hepatotoxicity ↑ effects of TAO	Avoid simultaneous use
Vitamins C, B_1 B_2 B_6 B_{12} folic acid, calcium, magnesium, zinc	Decreased serum concentration, ↑ serum concentration of estrogen with ≥ 1 gm vitamin C/day	Adjust dietary sources ↑
Vitamin A, copper, iron	Decreased serum concentration	Adjust dietary sources; use supplements with caution

Individual practitioner evaluation is important to assure that women can choose the best contraceptive method and avoid adverse effects.

Diaphragm*

I. Definition/Mechanism of Action

A diaphragm is a shallow rubber or silicone cap with a flexible rim which is placed in the vagina so as to cover the cervix. It serves as both a mechanical barrier and a receptacle for (contraceptive) spermicidal cream or jelly which must be used to insure effectiveness.

II. Effectiveness and Benefits

A. Method: 97% effectiveness rate
B. User: 80–85% effectiveness rate
C. May be inserted up to four hours prior to intercourse
D. May have some protective effect against transmission of certain sexually transmitted diseases
E. Effective form of contraception for women who have infrequent intercourse or in whom there are contraindications for other methods

III. Side Effects and Complications

A. Allergic reaction of patient or her partner to rubber or to the spermicidal agent (a silicone diaphragm is available)
B. Inability to achieve satisfactory fitting
C. Inability of patient to learn correct insertion and/or removal technique
D. Use may be associated with an increased incidence of urinary tract infection due to upward pressure of the rim of the diaphragm against the urethra
E. Pelvic discomfort, cramps, pressure on the bladder or rectum can occur if
   1. Diaphragm is too large
   2. Patient has chronic constipation
F. Toxic shock syndrome: severe cases occurring immediately after use have been reported in diaphragm users during menses (although these appear to be related to damage to vaginal walls during scanty flow by tampon use rather than diaphragm use per se)
G. Foul-smelling vaginal discharge may occur if the diaphragm is left in too long

IV. Types (Representative of Several Manufacturers)

A. Arcing spring
   1. Sturdy rim with firm spring strength (spiral, coiled spring)

---

*See also appendix on Femcap®.

2. Firm construction allows diaphragm to be kept in place despite recto-cele, cystocele, mild pelvic relaxation, uterine retroversion
3. Folds in an arc-shape
B. Coil spring
   1. Spring in rim is spiral, coiled, and sturdy
   2. Best suited for women with good vaginal tone and no uterine displace-ment
   3. Folds flat for insertion
C. Wide-seal
   1. Cuff inside rim
   2. Available in arcing and coil spring; also in silicone

V. Fitting
A. Most diaphragms are available in sizes ranging from 50 or 55 millimeters to 95 or 100 millimeters (available sizes in 5 millimeter gradations)
B. Fit should be snug between the posterior fornix, pubic symphysis and lateral vaginal walls, but should cause no pressure or discomfort
C. The patient may review and sign informed consent form (see Appendix D)
D. After a diaphragm has been fitted, instructions have been given, and the patient has demonstrated her ability to insert and remove it, she may be given an appointment for a follow-up visit in one week. During this week the patient is instructed to practice wearing the diaphragm for at least 8–hour intervals. (In many settings, one-week follow-up may be unrealistic, so diaphragm fitting and use will be taught at one visit and the patient given the prescription or kit.) It is helpful for the patient to be given a phone number and times to call about any concerns or problems.
E. At optional follow-up appointment
   1. Diaphragm is checked for fit and proper insertion
   2. Instructions are again reviewed and patient is given an opportunity to ask questions
F. If above criteria are met, patient is then given prescription for diaphragm
G. Yearly diaphragm check is recommended, but the patient should return for recheck sooner if she
   1. Gains or loses 10–15 pounds (although some sources query the neces-sity of this and suggest return if diaphragm does not seem to fit well or can be displaced)
   2. Has any pelvic surgery
   3. Has miscarriage, abortion, or wishes to resume using diaphragm after giving birth
   4. Is having problems with use

Appendix D may be photocopied and used as an informational handout on the diaphragm, as well as a consent form, for your patients. See Bibliography.

Intrauterine Devices (IUDs)

I. Definition/Mechanism of Action

A. A sterile foreign body placed in the uterus to prevent pregnancy. This is accomplished through several mechanisms:

   1. A local sterile inflammatory response to the foreign body (IUD) causes a change in the cellular makeup of the endometrium; with the copper devices there is an effect on the endometrium of interfering with the enzyme systems, and with the progesterone device, an effect over time of a less well-developed endometrium

   2. A possible increase in the local production of prostaglandins that may increase endometrial activity

   3. Alteration in uterine and tubal transport

   4. IUDs probably exert an antifertility effect beyond the uterus and interfere with fertility before an ovum reaches the uterus

   5. Alteration of cervical mucus causing a barrier to sperm penetration (progesterone IUD)

   6. Ovulation suppression first year with levonorgestrel intrauterine system (LNG IUS) Mirena®. Releases 20 mcg/day of levonorgestrel.

B. The exact mechanisms of action are not completely understood. One thing that has become clear is that the IUD does not act as an abortifacient.

C. Different types of IUDs use varying mechanisms of action to prevent pregnancy

II. Effectiveness

A. Theoretically: 92.0–99.9% effectiveness rate

B. User: 92–99% effectiveness rate
The range is close since the patient's participation is low and therefore there is little possibility of patient error.

III. Contraindications

A. Absolute contraindications

   1. Active pelvic infection (acute or subacute), including known or suspected gonorrhea or chlamydia

2. Known or suspected pregnancy
3. Recent or recurrent pelvic infection; postpartum endometritis, post-abortion infection (past 3 months)
4. Purulent cervicitis; untreated acute cervicitis or vaginitis
5. Undiagnosed genital bleeding
6. Distorted uterine cavity (bicornuate; severely flexed)
7. History of ectopic pregnancy
8. Allergy to copper (known or suspected) or diagnosed Wilson's Disease (ParaGard only); hypersensitivity to any part of Mirena®.
9. Abnormal Pap smear; cervical or uterine malignancy or premalignancy (endometrial hyperplasia, cervical intraepithelial neoplasia or cancer)
10. Impaired responses to infection (diabetes, steroid treatment, immuno-compromised patients)
11. Presence of previously inserted IUD
12. Genital actinomycosis
13. Acute liver disease or liver tumor (Mirena®)
14. Known or suspected breast cancer (Mirena®)

B. Relative contraindications (benefits usually outweigh risks)
1. Multiple sexual partners or partner has multiple partners
2. Emergency treatment difficult to obtain should complications occur; this would primarily be a problem in very rural areas or developing countries
3. Cervical stenosis
4. Impaired coagulation response (ITP anticoagulant therapy, etc.)
5. Uterus sounding less than 6 cm or more than 10 cm
6. Endometriosis
7. Leiomyomata
8. Endometrial polyps
9. Severe dysmenorrhea (Mirena® may be therapeutic).
10. Heavy or prolonged menstrual bleeding without clinical anemia; consider oral iron or nutritional alterations to prevent with IUD (Mirena® may be therapeutic)
11. Impaired ability to check for danger signals
12. Inability to check for IUD string
13. Concerns for future fertility
14. History of PID; with subsequent intrauterine pregnancy risk decreased
15. Valvular heart disease (potentially making woman susceptible to subacute bacterial endocarditis); for insertion and removal woman needs to receive:

      a. Oral: Amoxicillin 2 grams 1 hour before procedure

      b. Parenteral: Ampicillin 2 grams IM or IV within 30 minutes before the procedure; Gentamicin (Garamycin, and others) 1.5 mg/kg (120 mg max) IM or IV 30 minutes before the procedure

      c. Penicillin allergy: Vancomycin (Vancocin, and others) 1 gram IV infused slowly over 1 hour beginning 1 hour before the procedure; Gentamicin 1.5 mg/kg (120 mg. max) IM or IV 30 minutes before procedure

  16. Diabetes: monitor for blood glucose (Mirena®)

IV. Insertion Technique

A. Procedure

  1. Woman is scheduled for appointment for insertion only during menses or within 7 days of onset of menses (Mirena®) and after

      a. Negative Papanicolaou smear (within 6 months)

      b. Negative gonorrhea/Chlamydia testing

      c. Appropriate medical and menstrual history is obtained

  2. Patient should be instructed to eat before coming to an appointment

  3. Take oral analgesic or nonsteroidal anti-inflammatory 30–60 minutes before procedure

  4. IUD consent form (see Appendix D) and minor surgical consent form must be reviewed and signed at the time of an IUD consultation and evaluation, after discussion of

      a. Procedure

      b. Mechanism of the device

      c. Side effects and complications

      d. Relationship to woman's needs

  5. Atropine 0.5 mg should be available at the time of insertion for severe vasovagal response

  6. Anxious woman, or woman for whom it is deemed necessary to perform a paracervical block and/or use IV atropine (to decrease likelihood of vasovagal reaction), should be referred to a gynecologist for insertion

  7. Insertion under sterile technique

      a. Bimanual examination to determine uterine position and size; insert warmed speculum

      b. Cleanse the vagina, cervix, and endocervical canal with iodine solution (unless allergic to iodine)

      c. Xylocaine gel or hurricane spray could be used to decrease discomfort of tenaculum

    d. Use tenaculum to straighten the uterine body and cervical canal

    e. Sound the uterus (depth less than 6 cm. or more than 10 cm. is contraindication)

    f. Insert specific IUD as instructed by manufacturer

    g. Spasm of the internal cervical os may occur; it is usually relieved by simply waiting. *Never* force entry of the sound or applicator

    h. After insertion, observe the patient for weakness, pallor, diaphoresis, either bradycardia or tachycardia, hypotension and syncope which may occur (check blood pressure several times following insertion)

    i. If patient has mild cramping, the following may be used:
       1) Nonaspirin analgesic 650 mg every 4 hours, or
       2) A prostaglandin inhibitor (NSAID) such as Motrin® 400 mg p.o., qid

    j. Explain to patient that the IUD is effective immediately. In some settings it is recommended that the patient abstain x 1 day due to disruption of cervical mucus barrier

    k. Instruct patient to check for presence of IUD string post menstruation or after unusual cramping prior to relying on device for continued contraception effect

    l. Follow-up with appointment in 6 weeks to 3 months; at that time be sure the woman can feel the IUD strings

V. Complications Following Insertion and What to Do About Them

A. Immediate, severe vasovagal response
    1. Notify physician
    2. Place patient in shock position
    3. Monitor pulse and blood pressure until stable
    4. Administer oxygen as needed
    5. Atropine 0.4 mg subcutaneously or intramuscularly may be administered if appropriate

B. Severe immediate cramping: remove IUD

C. Excessive pain or bleeding is often a sign of perforation (fundal); physician consult for management

D. Side effects or later complications
    1. Two or more missed periods: recommend a serum pregnancy test. (Paragard®). With Mirena®, irregular, little or no bleeding is normal. Missed menses: 2 of 10 women no menses after 1 year of Mirena®. Pregnancy is rare but when this happens, there is a 50% chance of miscarriage. If IUD is removed, this drops to 25%
    2. Pregnancy occurring while IUD is in place: it is now recommended

that, due to risk of infection, the IUD should be removed at the time of diagnosis whether the pregnancy is continued or terminated. There should be consultation with a gynecologist prior to removal of the IUD by the gynecologist or nurse practitioner

3. Break-through bleeding related to IUD: use the following guidelines for removal:
   a. Bleeding is associated with endometritis
   b. Hematocrit falls 5 points
   c. There is a hematocrit of 30–32% or lower
   d. The IUD is partially expelled
   e. The patient wants the IUD removed
4. Cramping and pelvic pain
   a. Rule out ectopic pregnancy
      1) Obtain a serum pregnancy test
      2) Consider ultrasound and surgical consult (physician consult)
   b. Pain or cramping caused by or associated with
      1) Partial expulsion of IUD
         a) Remove IUD
      2) Pelvic inflammatory disease (a long-standing foul-smelling discharge in an IUD wearer is presumed to be PID until proven otherwise)
         a) Remove IUD
         b) Treat infection; culture and sensitivity at time of removal and adjust treatment as indicated
         c) Consult a physician prior to inserting another IUD (some sources advise waiting a year)
      3) Spontaneous abortion
5. Migraine headache
   1) First time or focal migraine with asymmetrical vision loss or other symptoms of transient cerebral ischemia
   2) Exceptionally severe headache
   a) Remove IUD
6. Expulsion
   a. Objective findings when the cervix is visualized
      1) The IUD is seen at the cervical os or in the vagina
      2) The IUD string is lengthened (partial expulsion)
      3) The IUD string is absent (complete expulsion)
      4) The IUD cannot be located using various methods of probing (physician consult)
      5) The IUD is absent on ultrasound of abdomen
   b. Removal and reinsertion of IUD

1) If partial expulsion occurs, IUD should be removed. IUD may be reinserted immediately if there is no infection or possibility of pregnancy, or with the next menses

2) If completely expelled, a new IUD may be reinserted as outlined above

7. Lost IUD strings

   a. Referrals for locating IUD include

      1) Exploration of canal with gentle probing; if not found, then

      2) Ultrasound

      3) Flat plate of abdomen

      4) Hysterosalpingogram

8. Difficulty in removing IUD

The following techniques may help in the removal of IUDs

   a. Remove only during menses

   b. Employ gentle, steady traction, remove IUD slowly. If IUD does not come out easily, physician consult is in order

   c. If IUD strings are not visible, nurse practitioner may probe for them in the cervical canal with narrow forceps

9. Uterine perforation (fundal or cervical), embedding of the IUD

   a. Objective findings include

      1) Absence of IUD string

      2) Inability to withdraw IUD if string is still present

      3) Demonstration of displaced IUD by ultrasound, hysteroscopy or x-ray

   b. If perforation or embedding is suspected, referral to physician is in order

   c. Reinforcement of education that multiple partners increase the risk of infection, including HIV infection

VI. Follow-up

A. Yearly Papanicolaou test and pelvic examination with removal and reinsertion as the particular IUD requires (Mirena® 5 years; ParaGard T 380A® (10 years)

B. As needed for any of above-mentioned complications with physician consultation as necessary.

Appendix D may be photocopied for your patients as an informational handout as well as a consent form for using an IUD. See Bibliography.

Web sites: www.paragardiud.com   www.Mirena.com/dtp

Contraceptive Spermicides and Condoms

Spermicides

I. Definition

Spermicides are substances used alone or with a vaginal barrier to prevent sperm from reaching the uterus. All contain an inert base or carrier substance and an active ingredient, most commonly the surfactant nonoxynol-9, which disrupts the integrity of the sperm cell membrane.

II. Effectiveness and Benefits

A. Method: 96% effectiveness rate
B. User: 60% effectiveness rate
C. Inexpensive and readily available

III. Side Effects and Disadvantages

A. Local irritation from spermicide or allergy to spermicide or carrier substance
B. Can necessitate interruption of lovemaking for application
C. Emotional reaction to touching one's own body

IV. Types*

A. Creams, jellies, gels
B. Foams
C. Foaming tablets
D. Suppositories
E. Vaginal contraceptive film
F. Bioadhesive gel
G. Water soluble lubricant with spermicide

V. How to Use

A. Instructions should be read carefully prior to using any spermicide. Method of insertion, time of effectiveness, time needed prior to intercourse, etc., vary with each type
B. A new insertion of spermicide is needed before each act of intercourse
C. Wash the applicator with soap and water after each use

---

*Koromex® cream and Ortho Gynol® have Octoxynol as the spermicide. Concentration of spermicide varies from 1–12.5% depending on the product. Some spermicides are flavored and some are colored. Protectaid sponge has nonoxynol-9, sodium cholate, and benzalkonium chloride—available OTC in Canada.

D. When the woman uses a spermicide alone, the partner should always use a condom

E. Frequent use of Nonoxynol 9 can cause genital and rectal lesions and increase the risk of HIV and other STDs*

VI. Follow-up

Yearly physical examination including Papanicolaou smear is recommended.

See Appendix A for patient handout on spermicides and condoms and Bibliography for references.

Condoms

I. Definition

Condoms are thin sheaths, most commonly made of latex but also made of sheep intestine or polyurethane, which prevent the transmission of sperm from the penis to the vagina. The female condom (vaginal pouch) is made of polyurethane.

II. Effectiveness

A. Method: 97–98% effectiveness rate

B. User: 70–94% effectiveness rate; 85% for female condom (range 74.0– 91.1%)

C. Inexpensive and readily available

D. Offer protection against the sexually transmitted diseases, including the AIDS virus (HIV)

E. Encourage male participation with birth control (conventional male condom)

F. Female condom is polyurethane (fewer allergic reactions as compared with latex)

III. Side Effects and Disadvantages

A. Allergic reactions to latex (rare) or lubricant or spermicide on products with either of these in place

B. Use necessitates interruption of lovemaking for application

C. May decrease tactile sensation

D. Psychological impotency may occur

E. Only latex condoms can be considered effective protection against

---

*Per CDC guidelines, 2002.

the AIDS virus (HIV); the polyurethane vaginal pouch (female condom) is twice as thick as latex and viral permeability may be less than latex

F. Polyurethane male condoms are more likely than latex to break or slip off, but they are useful for persons who don't like latex condoms or are latex sensitive

Use of both vaginal spermicides and condoms has an effectiveness rate in the high nineties when both methods are used correctly.

IV. Types

Condoms (male) vary in color, texture (smooth, studded, or ribbed), shape, size, and price. They come lubricated or non lubricated, impregnated with spermicide* or plain. Some are extra strength, some are sheerer and thinner, and some are uniquely shaped or scented.

V.A. How to Use the Male Condom

A. The male condom should always be put on an erect penis before there is any sexual contact, and used in every act of intercourse

B. The male condom should not be pulled tightly over the end of the penis; about one inch should be left for ejaculation fluid and to avoid breakage; some condoms have a reservoir tip

C. The penis should be withdrawn before it becomes limp, and the open end of the male condom should be held tightly while withdrawing to prevent spilling the contents

D. The partner should always use a contraceptive spermicide when a male condom is used

E. Condoms should be used only once

V.B. How to Use the Female Condom (comes prelubricated)

A. Pinch ring at closed end of pouch and insert like a diaphragm, covering the cervix; adding 1 or 2 drops of additional lubricant makes insertion easier and decreases or eliminates squeaking noise and dislocation during intercourse

B. Adjust other ring over labia

C. Can be inserted several minutes to 8 hours prior to intercourse

D. Remove after intercourse before standing up by squeezing and twisting the outer ring and pulling out gently

---

*Should not be used for STD prevention or for anal intercourse per CDC 2002 guidelines.

VI. Follow-up

A. Annual examination, Papanicolaou smear, mammogram as appropriate to age.

NOTE: Clinicians should remind patients that if a condom breaks or slips off, emergency contraception is available.

Appendix A has information on contraceptive spermicides and condoms that you may wish to photocopy for distribution to your patients. See Bibliography.

Cervical Cap*

I. Definition

The cervical cap is a thimble-shaped, deep-domed barrier device that fits over the cervix, and is used in combination with a spermicidal preparation (See Figure 1.1). The cervical cap is FDA approved for general use as a birth control method in the United States.

II. Effectiveness and Benefits

A. Current use effectiveness rates range from 92–96%
B. May be inserted up to 12 hours before intercourse and kept in place for several days, and additional spermicide is not necessary with repeated lovemaking (intercourse with ejaculations)
C. Possible option for women unable/not desiring to use other methods of contraception
D. Increased comfort and reduced risk of cystitis as compared to the diaphragm
E. Less disruption of sexual response compared to diaphragm

III. Side Effects and Complications of Use

A. Inability to achieve satisfactory fitting due to anatomic abnormalities, normal variations of cervix or vagina, and limited sizes and designs of caps (only 50–70% of women can be fit)
B. Inability of patient to learn correct insertion and/or removal techniques (rare)
C. Partner's or woman's complaints of discomfort (rare)
D. Allergic reaction to rubber or spermicidal agent (very uncommon)
E. Lack of trained practitioner to fit cap

*This guideline was developed by R. Mimi Clarke Secor, R.N., C.S., F.N.P., M.Ed., M.S., Certified Family Nurse Practitioner. Used with her permission.

Figure 1.1 Cervical Cap

IV. Types
A. Prentif Cavity Rim Cervical Cap, imported from England; four sizes: 22, 25, 28, and 31 mm (inner diameter)
B. Additional styles have been developed and are being researched currently including a silicone cap

V. Fitting
A. Review of medical history
   1. Allergies (including spermicidal agents)
   2. Current medications
   3. Past or present illness/medical condition
   4. Past surgery
   5. Review of systems, noting especially history of constipation, which may lead to cap dislodgement
B. Review of gynecologic history
   1. Menstrual history (cap should be fitted when woman is not menstruating)
   2. Contraceptive history, past and present (reasons for choosing or changing methods)
   3. Papanicolaou smear history (most recent Pap should be normal for cap fitting to occur)
   4. Past/current genitourinary infections (resolve before cap fitting or use)
   5. History of toxic shock or other serious infections, especially any associated with hospitalization
   6. Sexual history (especially vaginal/digital foreplay, as this may cause cap dislodgement)
   7. Pregnancy history, including if currently breast feeding. (After vaginal delivery, woman should wait 6–8 weeks for initial cap fitting or refitting; should be refit after breast feeding is discontinued as size may have changed)

8. Vaginal health: self-care habits such as douching, use of tampons or pads

C. Informed consent

Since FDA approval of the cap, an informed consent statement is optional but recommended. This consent statement should include: explanation of the current status of the cap and its effectiveness, potential side effects, contraindications, and recommended guidelines for use and follow-up care. A statement regarding willingness to use a back-up method of birth control the first 1–3 months is also recommended. Some sources suggest back-up birth control only the first six times the cap is used. There are no clear guidelines on this issue; it is suggested that each clinician examine the data and reach a consensus among clinicians with whom she/he practices.

D. Pelvic examination

1. Speculum examination
   a. Observe for vaginal or cervical abnormalities/infections
   b. Observe cervical characteristics, including size, shape, position, length and color, and characteristics of the cervical os
   c. Think about suitability for cap and consider which size cap might be appropriate

2. Bimanual examination
   a. Note any uterine or adnexal pathology
   b. Note position of cervix relative to the vaginal axis (parallel, oblique, perpendicular*)
   c. Note any vaginal abnormality such as a partial septum
   d. Evaluate vaginal tone and muscle supports, presence of cystocele or rectocele, uterine prolapse, or extreme vaginal laxity
   e. Estimate the length and diameter of the cervix and the vagina (note if cervix is proximal or distal to the vaginal introitus)
   f. Again consider suitability for cap and which size might be appropriate
   g. Note any rectal condition such as hemorrhoids, fissures, constipation

E. Cap assessment: criteria for suitable cap fitting

1. Cervical characteristics

Parallel: cervix and os angled toward the vaginal opening
Oblique: cervix angled down toward the floor of the vagina
Perpendicular: cervix and os angled toward the tailbone/rectum at 90-degree right angle to vaginal axis.

      a. Cervical length of at least 1.5 cm (there are certain exceptions to this, but such cases should be reserved for the experienced cap fitter)

      b. Cervical width of at least 1.0 cm and no more than 3.0 cm

      c. Cervical angle should be as nearly parallel to the axis of the vagina as possible (parallel, best angle; oblique, usually acceptable; perpendicular, relative contraindication)*

      d. Other cervical characteristics (or abnormalities)

  2. Vaginal characteristics

      a. The general tone of the vaginal tissues determines, in part, the quality of the cap fit, affecting the degree of suction present

      b. In addition, a vagina tapering toward the cervix provides better cap suction and therefore is a desirable characteristic (this anatomical feature requires experience to evaluate properly)

      c. The vaginal walls should be free of lesions or structural abnormalities such as septal wall defects. (Vaginal infections are a temporary contraindication and should be resolved before a cap fitting is attempted)

      d. Vaginal length should be adequate to ensure that the cervix is distal enough from the introitus to prevent dislodgement or partner complaints (this requires experience to evaluate properly)

  3. General considerations

      a. The candidate should be in good health at the time of the fitting and be free of genitourinary infection or abnormal conditions (such as abnormal Papanicolaou smear)

      b. The candidate should be comfortable touching her body, especially her cervix and vagina. As needed, preteaching and counseling are recommended prior to the cap fitting appointment

      c. The more a candidate is involved in the cap fitting process and gains experience in using the cap, the greater the effectiveness is likely to be

      d. There is no correlation between the size diaphragm a woman wears and the size cap she will wear

F. Fitting of cervical cap

  1. In order to fit a cervical cap a provider must be trained in the proper technique.

Appendix A contains information on the cervical cap which you may wish to photocopy for distribution to your patients. See Bibliography.

---

*However, fitters disagree regarding this recommendation.

Natural Family Planning*

I. Definition
Natural family planing is an umbrella term for methods that use naturally occurring fertility signs to determine the fertile and infertile days of the menstrual cycle.

II. Etiology
Effects of hormones on basal body temperature, cervical mucus, the position of the cervix, the cyclical nature of the ovulatory and endometrial cycles, and the physical process of the release of an egg make possible knowledge of occurrence of ovulation.

III. Background for Electing the Method
A. What the patient presents with
  1. Motivation to learn natural signs and symptoms of ovulation for purposes of fertility regulation
  2. Often a history of previous use of other methods of family planning
  3. Failure, dissatisfaction, or lack of harmony in values with other methods
  4. Cultural, ethnic, religious values and personal beliefs harmonious with natural family planning
  5. Medical contraindications to the use of one or more other methods
B. Additional background information to be obtained from the patient
  1. Medical/surgical history
  2. Obstetrical history
  3. Gynecological history including menstrual history
  4. Family planning method currently being used
  5. The patient's knowledge about the female human body, especially the ovulation cycle
  6. Family history

IV. Physical Examination
A. Vital signs
  1. Temperature   2. Pulse   3. Blood pressure
B. Complete physical examination
C. External examination of genitalia

---

*This guideline was developed by the late Eleanor Tabeek, RN, PhD, CNM, and is used with her permission and that of her family. Updates by Nancy Keaveney, RN, BS, and Mary Finnigan, BA, MA.

D. Vaginal examination utilizing a speculum
   Position of cervix; observation of mucus
E. Bimanual examination, noting
   1. Adnexal pain   2. Masses   3. Tenderness

V. Laboratory Test
A. Papanicolaou smear if none within past year; cultures, wet mount as appropriate or per protocol
B. Mammography as recommended

VI. Differential Diagnosis
Preference for other method

VII. Teaching About Natural Family Planning
See Appendix A, Natural Family Planning
A. Fertility awareness
B. General introduction to natural family planning
C. Basic information about natural family planning and methods
   1. Ovulation method
   2. Temperature method (BBT)
   3. Fertile and infertile periods
   4. Cervical palpation
   5. Symptothermal methods
   6. Keeping and interpreting a chart
D. Aspects of method having to do with interpersonal and intimate relationships

VIII. Complications
A. Inability of patient to interpret signs and symptoms
B. Lack of acceptability of method to partner
C. Unplanned pregnancy

IX. Consultation/Referral
To specialist or program for teaching of natural family planning

X. Follow-up
A. Annual examination and Papanicolaou smear
B. Evaluation of effectiveness of the method
C. Evaluation of patient satisfaction

See Appendix A. See Bibliography. See www.cyclebeads.com

Emergency Contraception

I. Definition
Emergency contraception (EC), often known as the "morning after pill,"* is pharmacologic or mechanical intervention after exposure to the possibility of conception with no or uncertain contraceptive protection. Such intervention is based on inhibiting fertilization or implantation. The means for intervention are either mechanical (an intrauterine device) or hormonal (high dose, short-term oral contraceptives or progestational agents).

II. Etiology
Disruption of fertilization or of implantation beginning within 72 hours after unprotected intercourse is based on several theoretical premises:
A. Progestational agents will change or interfere with sperm migration or the capacity of a sperm to penetrate the egg
B. Progestational agents are thought to inhibit motility of the fallopian tubes; also to affect follicle growth and development of the corpus luteum
C. Estrogen, specifically ethinyl estradiol, is thought to reduce plasma level of progesterone and may, therefore, interfere with the function of the corpus luteum or possibly the function of luteinizing hormone, thereby disrupting ovulation
D. Progestational agents and estrogen (estradiol) are known to shorten the luteal phase of the cycle
E. IUDs, specifically copper bearing devices, are thought to interfere with the enzyme systems of the endometrium and perhaps alter the permeability of the endometrial microvasculature, perhaps interfering with implantation

III. Effectiveness
Used within 72 hours, hormonal emergency contraception reduces risk of pregnancy by 75% for those women who would have become pregnant (8 of 100), so 2 of 100 will become pregnant.

IV. History
A. What the patient presents with
    1. Last act of unprotected intercourse within the past 72** hours
    2. Desire to inhibit fertilization or implantation

---

*The FDA has approved labeling of some oral contraceptives for emergency contraception use.
**Some new data indicate up to 120 hours.

B. Additional information to be obtained
1. Cycle history and any previous use of contraceptives
2. Estimated day(s) of exposure to sperm without any protection or with known method failure (i.e., condom broke, slipped off; IUD expelled; cervical cap or diaphragm displaced; missed 7 or more combination birth control pills in past 2 weeks, or missed 2 or more progestin only pills)
3. Contraindications to hormone or IUD use
4. Circumstance of unprotected exposure—rape, possible STD exposure; teratogen exposure
5. Other acts of unprotected intercourse during this cycle

V. Physical Examination
A. Pelvic exam—speculum and bimanual—if appropriate
B. Collect specimens following rape/sexual assault guideline (pages 187–198) as necessary/desired by woman; complete the assessment for evidence

VI. Laboratory Diagnosis
A. Pregnancy test
B. STD testing as warranted by history

VII. Differential Diagnosis
A. Consider alternatives should woman desire to keep a pregnancy if one should occur
B. Sexual assault—consider rape counseling
C. Pregnancy already established prior to current exposure with unprotected intercourse

VIII. Treatment
A. Combined OCS (Yuzpe method) and progestin-only oral contraceptives must be initiated within 72 hours of exposure*
1. Ovral 2 white pills p.o. stat, followed by 2 white pills in 12 hours
2. Lo-Ovral 4 white pills p.o. stat, followed by 4 white pills in 12 hours
3. Nordette 4 light orange pills p.o. stat, followed by 4 light orange pills in 12 hours
4. Levlen 4 light orange pills p.o. stat, followed by 4 light orange pills in 12 hours
5. Triphasil 4 yellow pills p.o. stat, followed by 4 yellow pills in 12 hours.
6. Tri-levlen 4 yellow pills stat, followed by 4 yellow pills in 12 hours
7. Alesse 5 pink pills stat and 5 pink pills in 12 hours

---

*Some new data indicate up to 120 hours.

      8. LevLite 5 pink pills stat and 5 pink pills in 12 hours
      9. Levora 4 white pills stat and 4 white pills in 12 hours
     10. Trivora 4 pink pills stat and 4 pink pills in 12 hours
     11. Ovrette 20 yellow pills p.o. stat followed by 20 more yellow pills in 12 hours
  B. Preven*—2 light blue pills stat then 2 light blue pills in 12 hours (0.05 mg ethinyl estradiol and 0.25 mg levonorgestrel)
  C. Plan B (levonorgestrel): treatment must be initiated within 72 hours" (causes less nausea and vomiting) 1 white pill then 1 more white pill 12 hours later
  D. Mechanical agents
      1. Copper IUD insertion within 5–7 days of exposure with precautions for IUD use, STD exposure, risk factors for IUD use; some guidelines specify prophylactic antibiotics with insertion

IX. Explanation of Method
A. Education: for each woman specific for postcoital intervention method including side effects of intervention and danger signs; if IUD is inserted, instructions about IUD use, danger signs, and complications and potential for 10 years of protection against pregnancy
B. Education about resumption of menses: based on woman's cycle history, if hormones are taken during follicular phase, menses will follow about day 21; if during ovulation, around day 26, and if in luteal phase, about day 29

X. Complications and Side Effects
A. Pelvic infection with IUD use (see protocol for PID)
B. Ectopic pregnancy: possible increased risk with hormone use (up to 100% of pregnancies); copper IUD use won't inhibit tubal implantation (see information on ectopic pregnancy in the guideline "Acute Pelvic Pain")
C. Pregnancy
      1. Decision-making regarding continuation or termination of pregnancy
D. Nausea and vomiting
      1. Drink glass of milk or eat a snack with each oral dose to reduce risk of nausea and vomiting
      2. Compazine 25 mg rectal suppository q 12 hours or 10 mg p.o. qid
      3. Tigan, 200 mg suppository q 12 hours
      4. Meclizine hydrochloride (Antivert, Dramamine II) 25 mg 1 hour before EC pills

---

*Preven available in an emergency contraception kit.

5. Give extra tablets of oral contraceptives in event of vomiting dose; instruct woman to take repeat dose if vomiting within one hour after taking the dose and pills are visible in vomitus

XI. Consultation and Referral
A. For pregnancy exposure as the result of sexual assault/rape, refer to rape crisis center, rape counseling
B. For complications of postcoital intervention as necessary

XII. Follow-up
A. No menses within 3 weeks after intervention, return for evaluation for continued pregnancy (failure of emergency contraception or preexisting pregnancy); to rule out ectopic pregnancy
B. For a contraceptive method chosen by woman for use following the emergency contraception
  1. Immediate use: Condoms, diaphragm, spermicides.
  2. With next menses:
     OCs—Sunday start or first day start; injectible, contraceptive patch, vaginal ring,
     IUDs—insert with or after menses,
     NFP—initiate with menses,
  3. Sterilization anytime

The Emergency Contraceptive Hotline, 1-800-NOT-2-LATE, is a 24-hour toll-free service offered in English and Spanish. Callers can get names, phone numbers, and location of 3 local providers. Internet access: http://not-2-late.com, www.go2planB.com
See Appendix D and Bibliography.

Sterilization

I. Definition
Sterilization in women is the purposeful occlusion of the fallopian tubes by surgical disruption. Several methods are practiced through closed laparoscopy, open laparoscopy, or suprapubic mini-laparotomy. The method of tubal occlusion depends on the surgical route. These occlusion methods include excision of a portion of each tube and suturing of the ends; excision of the fimbriated end; excision of a portion and then suturing of the proximal end into the muscle of the uterus and the distal end in the broad ligament; banding with silastic bands (Falope rings, Yoon band) or clips (Hulka-Clem-

ens Clip, Filshie Clip); ligation of a loop of the tubes with nonabsorbable suture material; occlusion by bipolar cautery. A new method is transcervical to place Essure® tubal occlusion device.

II. Background for Electing Sterilization
Decision by the woman to seek permanent sterilization through tubal ligation as a means of fertility regulation

III. History
A. What the woman may present with:
   1. History of use of one or more methods of contraception
   2. Dissatisfaction with available methods and/or method failure
   3. Experiencing problems with one or more methods and decision not to have any more children
   4. Medical contraindications for use of one or more methods
   5. Psychosocial contraindications for use of one or more methods
   6. Desire to have no more children or no children; need/ desire for permanent method
   7. Premenopause, less than one year without a period
B. Additional information to be obtained
   1. Knowledge about all family planning methods used
   2. Psychosocial and cultural aspects: size of family desired, beliefs about sterilization, family attitudes
   3. Knowledge about the sterilization procedures available and beliefs about reversibility
   4. History of any previous pelvic surgery, partial or total hysterectomy, oophorectomy, salpingectomy, laparoscopy, plastic surgery such as tubal reconstruction (See Fig. 1.2)
   5. Medical/surgical history, present use of medications
   6. Type of anesthesia for previous surgeries; any untoward effects
   7. Gynecologic and obstetric history: pregnancies, live births, abortions, ectopic pregnancies, endometriosis, uterine anomalies, presence of adhesions, uterine Ieiomyomas (fibroids)
   8. Menstrual history to the present; last period; PMS; character of menses and menstrual cycle
   9. Contraceptive use to present and reasons discontinued

IV. Physical Examination
A. Vital signs
   1. Blood pressure   2. Pulse

B. General physical exam: lungs, heart, neck, abdomen, breasts, extremities, thyroid
C. Pelvic examination

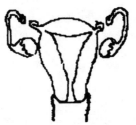

Figure 1.2 Tubal Ligation.

1. External: Skene's glands, Bartholin's glands, urethra
2. Vaginal examination: walls, discharge, cervix; inspect for cystocele, rectocele, urethrocele
3. Uterus: masses, tenderness, enlargement, possible pregnancy
4. Adnexa: masses, tenderness, palpable ovaries or tubes, enlargement

V. Laboratory (for preoperative work-up only or for symptoms of problem)
A. Urinalysis, culture if signs of urinary tract infection
B. Complete blood count
C. Pregnancy test
D. Gonorrhea culture
E. Chlamydia test
F. Papanicolaou smear

VI. Differential
None

VII. Treatment
Teaching
A. Methods of sterilization and possible failure
B. Chance of future reversal; choice of method of sterilization related to this
C. Information on informed consent
D. Risks and benefits
E. Discussion of regret
F. Information on waiting period
G. Postoperative implications, i.e., restrictions
H. Sexual adjustments following procedure
I. Information on possible post-tubal ligation syndrome

VIII. Complications
Conditions contraindicating procedure or choice of procedure such as previous surgery or extensive adhesions; allergy or untoward response to anesthesia

IX Consultation/Referral
To provider who does tubal ligations if the procedure is not offered in the practice setting

X. Follow-up
A. Postoperative care

  See Bibliography.

Sterilization: Postoperative Care

I. Definition
Follow-up care after the performance of sterilization by tubal ligation or occlusion; time of follow-up will vary depending upon the procedure performed

II. Etiology
A. Transabdominal surgical procedure: ligation and resection; electrocoagulation
B. Laparoscopy and electrocoagulation, clips or rings
C. Transcervical tubal occlusion

III. History
A. Type of procedure done, when, anesthesia
B. Any sutures to be removed
C. Menstruation: last menstrual period, character
D. Resumption of sexual activity, response; change in sexual habits
E. What patient may present with
  1. Pain, fever, bleeding or discharge from operative site
  2. Abdominal pain; pelvic pain
  3. Vaginal discharge
  4. Urinary symptoms: frequency, dysuria, hematuria
  5. Any new symptoms/concerns with menstrual cycle not experienced prior to tubal ligation such as endocrine manifestations

IV. Physical Examination
A. Vital signs
  1. Blood pressure   2. Pulse   3. Temperature

B. Abdominal examination
   1. Inspection: incision site(s) if any
   2. Auscultation: bowel sounds, hyper-or hypoactive
   3. Palpation: tenderness, guarding, masses
C. Pelvic examination
   1. Uterus: tender, enlarged, masses, fixed or mobile, pain on cervical manipulation
   2. Adnexa: masses, tenderness

V. Laboratory
A. Cervical culture if fever, uterine, adnexal tenderness present (gonorrhea, Chlamydia)
B. Urinalysis and culture if signs of urinary tract infection
C. CBC, differential, sedimentation rate and/or C-reactive protein if fever, tenderness
D. Pregnancy test if uterus enlarged or adnexal mass, signs of ectopic

VI. Differential Diagnosis
A. Urinary tract infection
B. Perforation of bowel
C. Pelvic infection
D. Salpingitis
E. Peritonitis
F. Tubal hemorrhage
G. Problems with sexual expression; lack of libido, responsiveness

VII. Treatment
As indicated by symptoms and diagnosis

VIII. Complications
A. Hemorrhage
B. Pregnancy, increased risk of ectopic
C. Perforation of bowel, bowel burns with electrocoagulation
D. Pelvic inflammatory disease
E. Urinary tract infection
F. Salpingitis
G. Infection of incision site(s)
H. Pelvic abscess
I. Peritonitis
J. Bladder damage
K. Uterine perforation
L. Posttubal ligation syndrome
M. Regrets

IX. Consultation/Referral

A. Consultation/referral to surgeon for differential diagnosis and treatment of any problem
B. Referral for mental health counseling if experiencing sexual maladjustment, regrets

X. Follow-up

A. Return for recheck after resolution of any complications
B. Annual Pap smear, pelvic examination, health examination; mammography per recommendations

See Bibliography.

2

Infertility

I. Definition
Inability to conceive after one full year or more of unprotected intercourse.

II. Etiology
A. Factors in male infertility: faulty sperm production; reproductive tract anomaly; physical and chemical agents (coal tar, radioactive substance, etc.); endocrine disorders; general state of health; blocked vas deferens; testicular infection; injury to reproductive organs/tract; nerve damage; impotence; lifestyle factors (smoking, alcohol, street drugs, etc.); incompatible immunologic factors for sperm—antispermatozoa antibodies
B. Factors in female infertility: blocked fallopian tubes; anovulatory cycles; anatomical anomalies; hormonal imbalance; polycystic ovary syndrome (PCOS); obstruction of vaginal, cervical, and/or uterine cavity; hostile cervical mucus; ovarian cyst or tumor; pituitary tumor; endometriosis; previous STDs, vaginitis, vaginosis, PID, septic abortion, history of and drug treatment for thyroid disease, depression, asthma; lifestyle factors (alcohol, smoking, street drugs, etc.)
C. Factors in couple infertility: improper technique for intercourse; infrequent intercourse; emotional state; male and female factors contributing to infertility

III. History
A. What the patient presents with
   1. History of failure to conceive for period of time with no use of contraception
   2. Desire for pregnancy
B. Additional information to be obtained
   1. Complete medical and surgical history including immunizations; family history
   2. Complete menstrual history including menarche, character of menses, frequency, duration, last menstrual period, postmenarche amenorrhea
   3. Gynecologic history: anomalies, problems, infections, surgery, DES exposure, endometriosis, fibroids, abnormal Paps
   4. Contraceptive history to the present including post method amenorrhea

5. Obstetrical history: any previous conceptions; number of children, abortions, stillbirths; complications
6. Partner's reproductive history; medical, surgical history
7. Employment history: exposure to radiation, viruses, other substances known to cause sterility; teratogens
8. Sexual history: techniques, frequency and timing of intercourse in relation to the menstrual cycle; use of lubricants, douches, sex stimulants or toys; trauma
9. Report of any previous infertility testing, work-ups; diagnoses; interventions; genetic evaluation
10. Lifestyle history: use of recreational (street) drugs, prescription drugs, alcohol, tobacco, caffeine, eating habits, saunas or hot tubs, exercise (including biking and running); stress
11. Age of patient/partner may determine timing of intervention

IV. Physical Examination
A. Vital signs
   1. Temperature
   2. Pulse
   3. Blood pressure
B. Complete physical examination; observation of secondary sex characteristics; signs/symptoms of PCOS
C. External examination (careful observation for signs of infection, lesions, or anomalies)
   1. Clitoris   4. Bartholin's glands
   2. Labia   5. Vulva
   3. Skene's glands   6. Perineum
D. Pelvic examination
   1. Length of vagina
   2. Position and character of cervix
   3. Any anomalies
   4. Sounding of uterus
E. Bimanual examination (examine for palpable masses, tenderness, anomalies, signs of trauma)
   1. Uterus   2. Ovaries   3. Adnexa

V. Laboratory
A. Papanicolaou smear, maturation index; mammogram. as appropriate
B. N. gonorrhea culture; RPR status (syphilis), TB status, HIV, hepatitis status; Rubella titre, varicella titre

C. Chlamydia smear
D. Pregnancy test in amenorrhea
E. Complete blood count; erythrocyte sedimentation rate
F. Mycoplasma and ureaplasma culture
G. Endometrial biopsy during luteal phase
H. Serum progesterone level days 21–23 of cycle
I. Wet mounts, vaginal cultures
J. Prolactin level, FSH, LH, TSH, Rh factor, blood type

VI. Differential Diagnosis
A. Partner infertility, sterility
B. Sterility
C. Anomaly, absence of reproductive organs
D. Cause(s) of infertility

VII. Treatment
A. Infertility work-up for the woman
   1. Basal body temperature charts, may use test for LH surge instead
   2. Commercially available ovulation tests or devices and fertility monitoring devices*
   3. Postcoital test—serial if antispermatozoa antibodies
   4. Cervical mucus test, sperm antibody level; sperm agglutination test; sperm immobilization test; endometrial biopsy 2–3 days before menstruation
   5. Hysterosalpingogram after menses, before ovulation
   6. Hormonal assay (serum) such as FSH, LH, prolactin, estrogen DHEA-S, testosterone, urinary LH 4–5 days at midcycle
   7. Tuboscopy
   8. Ultrasound
   9. Laparoscopy with chromotubation, hydrotubation; hysteroscopy; salpingoscopy
B. Work-up of partner involving tests done by specialist
C. For complete work-up, referral may be in order

VIII. Complications
A. Risks associated with certain tests; costs of testing
B. Persistent infertility, discovery of sterility
C. Effects on couple's relationship

---

*Examples are OvuGen®; Clear Plan Easy®, First Response®, OVu Quick® Self Test for detecting luteinizing hormone (LH) in urine; Clear Plan Easy Fertility Monitor®

IX. Consultation/Referral
To gynecologist or infertility specialist; reproductive technology centers; genetic counseling

X. Follow-up
Long-term process for work-up that is staged, so patient would be asked to return for next phase of testing if conception not achieved

See Bibliography.

3

Vaginal Discharge, Vaginitis, and Sexually Transmitted Diseases

Checklist for Vaginal Discharge Work-up

Subjective Data

A. Social history
  1. Age
  2. Occupation
  3. Partner status
     a Frequency of sexual contact
     b. Last sexual act and type
     c. Age of first intercourse
  4. Pregnancy history
  5. Sexual preference
  6. Number of sexual partners over lifetime; known partner history; history of new partner within past month
  7. Documented STD history including HIV status
  8. Recent weight change
B. Previous gynecologic surgery including abortion, tubal ligation, D&C , Cesarean section
C. Past or current medical illness; chronic diseases
D. Family history of diabetes, personal history of Type 1, 2
E. Diet, alcohol, cigarettes, recent change in habits; use of street drugs including injectables; use of sex toys, stimulants
F. Medications (past and present); recent antibiotics; use of vaginal medications (OTC and prescription)
G. Past history of similar problems
  1. Dates   2. Treatment   3. Follow-up
H. Vaginal discharge
  1. Onset   6. Constant vs. intermittent
  2. Color   7. Related to sexual contact
  3. Odor   8. Relationship to menses
  4. Consistency   9. Relation to other life events
  5. Amount   10. Wear pads, tampons

I. "Sores": anywhere on the body; rashes
J. Genital itching, swelling, or burning; genital sores or tears
K. Abdominal or pelvic pain
L. Fever, chills
M. Achy joints
N. Nausea and vomiting; diarrhea
O. Dyspareunia
P. Known contact with sexually transmitted disease; AIDS risk*
Q. Birth control (including recent changes in method or products used)
    1. Oral contraceptive, vaginal ring, patch: type and length of use
    2. Intrauterine device: type, how long in place
    3. Diaphragm; cervical cap
    4. Depo-Provera®, Lunelle®
    5. Condom (male or female); foam, jelly, cream, vaginal film, tablets, suppositories, gels
R. History of douching; use of soaps, chemicals
S. Personal hygiene
    1. Use of feminine hygiene sprays or deodorant tampons, panty liners, or pads
    2. Poor personal hygiene
T. Clothing: consistent wearing of tight-crotched pants; type of underwear; pantyhose
U. Last menstrual period
V. Urinary problems
    1. Frequency
    2. Dysuria
    3. Urgency
    4. Hematuria: other debris in urine
    5. Odor
    6. Dark or cloudy urine; color
W. Allergies to drugs: reactions
X. Partner problems

Objective Data
A. Vital signs: blood pressure, pulse, respiration, temperature
B. Inguinal lymph nodes
C. Abdominal examination: rebound, bowel sounds, suprapubic tenderness, masses, organomegaly, enlarged bladder, costovertebral angle (CVA) tenderness
D. External genitalia: Bartholin's glands, Skene's glands, "sores," rash, genital warts, swollen reddened urethra, urethral discharge; lesions on labia, between labial folds.

---

*See Appendix F.

E. Vaginal examination (speculum)
   1. Inspection of vaginal walls, vaginal lesions, tears, discharge
   2. Inspection of cervix: friability, ectropion, cervical erosion, discharge from os, cervical tenderness; color
   3. Discharge: if present, characteristically is thick, mucus at cervical os, difficult to remove
F. Bimanual examination: pain on cervical motion, fullness or pain in adnexa, tenderness of uterus, size and shape of uterus

Assessment and Plan
A. Normal discharge: usually clear or white, nonirritating or nonpruritic, pH 3.8–4.2, doesn't pool, has body, can write initials in it
B. Diagnosis
   1. Wet prep will be negative
   2. Gram stain will be negative
   3. pH within normal range
   4. Card test for elevated ph and trimethylamine and for prolineaminopeptidase (Fem Exam, Pip Activity test card).
C. Treatment: none required
D. Patient education
   1. Reassurance
   2. If clinical and/or laboratory findings are not within normal limits, refer to protocol for suspected organism(s) for further work-up

Hints on Preparation of a Wet Smear*
A. Collect a copious amount of vaginal discharge from the
lateral walls with a wooden Pap spatula (some say a cotton swab moistened with saline); repeat so you have two samples to work with
B. Place a drop of the specimen mixture at each end of a clean glass slide, or on 2 separate slides, when you are ready to read the slides; or place a drop of saline on one slide and a drop of KOH on a second before collecting specimens; place in cardboard slide holders if available
C. Add a drop of KOH** (10%) to one specimen or stir one specimen into the KOH on the slide and sniff immediately for the characteristic "fishy" odor of bacterial vaginosis (+ whiff test)
D. Cover both specimens with cover slips once you reach the microscope. Plan to view the plain saline specimen first to allow time for the KOH to

*Adapted from material developed by R. Mini Clarke Secor (1997) *Vaginal microscopy, Clinical Excellence for Nurse Practitioners* 1(1)29–34, and from Fischbach, F. *A Manual of Laboratory and Diagnostic Tests,* 6th ed., Philadelphia: Lippincott, 1999
**Note that KOH should be used with care since it is very damaging to the microscope.

lyse cells prior to looking for Candida.* If you suspect trichomonas, you may want to examine slide without a cover slip, as the slip can sometimes immobilize the trich. Warming the slide will also increase the possibility of seeing trichomonads

E. With the 10X objective in place on the microscope, the light on low power and the condenser in the lowest position, place the slide on the stage and lower the objective until it is as close to the slide as possible

F. Adjust the eyepieces until a single round field is seen. Turn the coarse focus knob until the specimen is focused. Use the fine focus knob to bring the specimen into sharp focus

G. Be sure to use subdued light and a lowered condenser for a wet specimen. Try increasing the light and raising the condenser while viewing the specimen to see how the cells and bacteria disappear from view

H. Move the slide until you have a general impression of the number of squamous cells. Switch to high power (40X); it may be necessary to increase the amount of light slightly

I. Evaluate the slide for bacteria, WBCs, clue cells, trichomonads, hyphae and yeast buds. Even if one organism is identified, continue to scan the slide systematically to fully evaluate the specimen. Vaginitis/vaginosis may have multiple causes

J. Move the KOH slide into position; switch back to low power to scan the slide for Candida. If hyphae are noted, switch to high power to confirm the impression

K. Be sure to wipe spilled fluid from the stage. If the objective becomes contaminated, clean it only with special lens paper

L. To perform gram staining:

1. Spread a *thin* smear of the specimen on a glass slide. Air dry the slide completely, or dry it carefully high above a flame

2. After the specimen is dry, fix it by passing it through a flame several times (with the specimen side away from the flame). Allow it to cool completely; otherwise the reagents used in the staining process may precipitate on the slide

3. Flood the slide with Gram crystal violet. Wait 10 seconds, then rinse with tap water

4. Flood the slide with Gram iodine. Wait 10 seconds, then rinse with tap water

5. Wash the slide with decolorizer just until the fluid dripping from the slide changes from blue to colorless, then immediately rinse the slide with tap water. This step is crucial to ensure correct decolorizing

---

*Candida torulopsis glabrata does not have the same characteristics as Candida albicans so KOH will be negative.

6. Flood the slide with Gram sufranin. Wait 10 seconds, then rinse the slide with tap water
7. Allow the slide to air dry, or blot dry. Place the slide on the microscope stage and put a small drop of oil on the stained specimen. With the oil power objective in place, the condenser tip and the diaphragm open (for bright field illumination), focus and examine several fields on the slide
8. When finished, remove the oil from the lens with lens paper

Appendix A contains information on vaginal discharge to copy or adapt for your patients. See Bibliography.

Work-up for Vaginal Discharge and Odor

I. Definition
Vaginal discharge that may or may not have a distinctive odor may be a vaginitis or vaginosis.

Vaginitis: Inflammation of the vagina, characterized by an increased vaginal discharge containing many white blood cells (WBCs).

Vaginosis: Characterized by increased discharge without inflammatory cells (WBCs).

II. Etiology
A. Foreign body (i.e., forgotten tampon, retained cap, condom, or diaphragm)
B. Allergy to soap or feminine hygiene spray
C. Deodorants
D. Scented toilet tissue
E. Vaginal contamination through oral or rectal intercourse
F. Poor personal hygiene
G. Sensitivity to contraceptive spermicides or lubricants
H. Condom allergy. (Hint: If woman is allergic to latex, then use latex condom with animal skin or polyurethane condom over; if man is allergic to latex, use animal skin condom or polyurethane with a latex condom over)
   1. Presence of a pathogen

III. History
A. What patient may present with
   1. Vaginal discharge, may be chronic
   2. Vaginal odor

   3. Vulvar/vaginal irritation, pruritus, and/or burning made worse by urination, intercourse
   4. Postcoital bleeding
   5. Difficulty urinating or pain with urination
B. Additional information to be considered
   1. Relationship of discharge to birth control method: any ended
   3. Relationship of discharge to sexual contact: recency; partner affected; recent change in partners
   4. Relationship of discharge to personal hygiene: any recent change in hygiene products or toiletries; douching
   5. Any history of vaginal infection associated with sexually transmitted disease or pelvic inflammatory disease
   6. History of
      a. Previous infection or STD
      b. Chronic cervicitis
      c. Cervical surgery
      d. Abnormal Papanicolaou
      e. Diethylstilbestrol (DES) exposure
   7. Description of discharge
      a. Color
      b. Onset
      c. Odor
      d. Consistency
      e. Constant vs. intermittent
      f. Color of discharge on underwear; changes

IV. Physical Examination
A. External examination: external genitalia
   1. Erythema
   2. Excoriations
   3. Lesions
   4. Edema
B. Vaginal examination (speculum)
   1. Presence of foreign body
   2. Erythema and edema of the vaginal vault
   3. Inspection of cervix
      a. Erythema
      b. Erosion
      c. Severe physiological ectropion
      d. Friability
      e. Serous sanguineous discharge
      f. Lesions
C. Bimanual examination if indicated

V. Laboratory Examination
A. As indicated by findings
   1. Wet saline prep; KOH slide

2. Card test for elevated pH and trimethylamine* and prolineaminopeptidase**
3. Gram stain
4. Gonorrhea culture if indicated
5. Chlamydia test if indicated
6. Urinalysis if indicated
7. Herpes culture if indicated
8. Cervical culture
9. pH with nitrazine paper; QuickVue Advance pH & Amines Test; Quick Vue Advance G. VAginalis Test***
10. HIV testing

VI. Differential Diagnosis

A. Normal physiological discharge
B. Diethylstilbestrol (DES) exposure
C. Chlamydia
D. N. gonorrhea
E. Candida albicans or other Candida infection; bacterial vaginosis
F. Urinary tract infection
G. Condylomata
H. Herpes simplex
I. Contact dermatitis
J. Tinea or other fungus

VII. Treatment

A. General measures
   1. Removal of causative factor
   2. Education as to
      a. Personal hygiene
      b. Avoidance through use of alternatives to causative factors
B. Medications
   1. No treatment, depending on evaluation of clinical data
   2. If a pathogen is identified, treat via appropriate protocol
   3. If after one week of no treatment, try Aci-jel®, one application intravaginally at h.s. for 7–14 days or until tube is used up

VIII. Complications

Abnormal Papanicolaou smear resulting from continuing irritation; reparative process

IX. Consultation/Referral

Unresolved symptomatology

---

*Fem Exam (Cooper Surgical, Shelton, CT)
**Pip Activity Test Card (Litmus Concepts, Santa Clara, CA)
***Quidel Corporation, San Diego, CA

X. Follow-up
A. One week if indicated, then prn
B. If no improvement at one week after treatment of Aci-jel®, referral to physician

See Appendix A and Bibliography.

Candidiasis

I. Definition
Candidiasis, or monilia, is a microscopic yeast-like fungal infection of the vagina usually caused by Candida albicans (90%). Candida tropicalis, Torulopsis glabrata, Candida Krusei, Candida parapsilosis and other lesser known Candida species are also clinically implicated.

II. Etiology
A. A fungus of the genus Candida, species albicans, tropicalis, or Torulopsis glabrata, part of the normal flora of the mouth, gastrointestinal tract, and vagina; may become pathogenic under variable conditions, such as change in the vaginal pH, which encourage an overgrowth of the organism
B. Incubation period: about 96 hours

III. History
A. What patient may present with
  1. Pruritus
  2. Vulvar and vaginal swelling
  3. Vulvar excoriation
  4. Vulvar burning with urination
  5. Dyspareunia or burning during and/or after intercourse
B. Additional information to be considered
  1. Previous vaginal infections or vaginosis; diagnosis, treatment and compliance with treatment
  2. Chronic illness (diabetes); immunocompromised
  3. Sexual activity including oral and anal sex
  4. History of sexually transmitted disease or pelvic inflammatory disease
  5. Last intercourse; changes in frequency; new partner
  6. Last menstrual period
  7. Method(s) of birth control
  8. Other medications
     a. Antibiotics   b. Steroids   c. Estrogens

9. Description of discharge
   a. Color
   b. Onset
   c. Odor
   d. Consistency
   e. Constant vs. intermittent
   f. Relationship to sexual contact
   g. Relationship to menses
   h. Use of vaginal deodorant sprays, deodorant or scented tampons, panty liners, or pads, douches, perfumed toilet tissue
   i. Change in laundry soaps, fabric softener, body soap (amount of soap used and application inside labia)
   j. Clothing: consistent wearing of tight-crotched pants; wearing nylon underwear, panty hose under slacks; wearing underwear to bed
10. "Jock" itch (partner), athlete's foot (self or partner), itchy rash on thighs, buttocks, under breasts; oral candidiasis (thrush)
11. Diet high in refined sugar

IV. Physical Examination
A. External examination
Observe perineum for excoriation, erythema, edema, ulcerations, lesions
B. Vaginal examination (speculum)
   1. Inspection of vaginal mucosa: may be erythematous, irritated, with white patches along side walls
   2. Cervix
   3. Discharge: characteristically thick, odorless, white, curd-like, resembling cottage cheese, with pH remaining in the normal range of 3.8–4.2 (nitrazine paper)
C. Bimanual examination

V. Laboratory Examination*
A. Wet prep microscopic examination to visualize hyphae, pseudohyphae, spores or buds
B. Consider vaginal or cervical culture.
C. Consider fasting blood sugar and 2° postprandial on women with chronic yeast infections
D. Further laboratory work as indicated by history including HIV testing

---

*Biomed Diagnostic has introduced In Tray Colorex Yeast Test to differentiate the 4 species. 1–800–964–6466.

VI. Differential Diagnosis
A. Herpes genitalis
B. Chemical vaginitis
C. Contact dermatitis
D. Normal physiologic discharge
E. Candidiasis 2° to diabetes, pregnancy, + HIV status
F. Candida Torulopsis glabrata or Candida tropicalis or lesser known species (C. Krusei, C. parapsilosis, other C. species)
G. Trichomonas, bacterial vaginosis, Chlamydia, or gonococcal infection

VII. Treatment
A. Medications (some of these are now over the counter)*†
1. Butoconazole 2% cream 5 grams intravaginally x 3 days (Femstat3®) OR Gynazole1®
2. Butoconazole1 2% cream, 5 grams (sustained release) 1 applicator full OR
3. Clotrimazole (Gyne-Lotrimin®, Lotrimin®, Mycelex®, Mycelex-GS) 1% cream 5 grams (1 applicator full) intravaginally qhs x 7–14 days OR
4. Clotrimazole 100 mg vaginal tablet qhs x 7 days OR
5. Clotrimazole 100 mg vaginal tablet, 2 tablets for 3 days OR
6. Clotrimazole 500 mg vaginal tablet 1 single dose OR
7. Coltrimazole (Gyne-Lotrimin) suppositories 100 mg qhs x 7 nights OR
8. Miconazole (Monistat®) 2% cream 5 grams (1 applicator full) intravaginally x 7 days OR
9. Miconazole 200 mg vaginal suppository 1 each for 3 days OR
10. Miconazole (Monistat®) ovule 1200 mg single dose OR
11. Miconazole 100 mg vaginal suppository 1 each for 7 days OR
12. Nystatin® 100,000 unit vaginal tablet 1 tablet qd for 14 days OR
13. Tioconazole (Vagistat-1®) 6.5% ointment 5 grams intravaginally single dose hs (pregnancy category C) OR
14. Terconazole (Terazol®) 0.4% cream 5 grams (1 applicator full) intravaginally x 7 days OR
15. Terconazole 0.8% cream 5 grams (1 applicator full) intravaginally x 3 days OR
16. Terconazole 80 mg suppository 1 each x 3 days

---

*Imidazole drugs (Miconazole, Clotrimazole, Econazole, Butaconazone) are not as effective for non-Candida albicans infections as are triazole compounds including terconazole and tioconazole.

†Note serious adverse effects can occur; use with caution when patient is taking other drugs, so check carefully for drug interactions before recommending or prescribing.

17. Oral therapy: Fluconazole (Diflucan®) 150 mg oral tablet, one tablet in a single dose (pregnancy category C)
18. In pregnancy: use only topical azole therapies; most effective in pregnancy are butoconazole, clotrimazole, miconazole, and terconazole; most experts recommend 7–day therapy
19. Miconazole cream (Monistat-Derm®) or clotrimazole cream (Mycelex®) can be used for external irritation
20. If treatment is unsuccessful, may refill script x 1; if still unsuccessful, consider treating partner and/or fasting blood sugar and 20 postprandial. Review history carefully with woman
21. If fasting blood sugar and 2° postprandial are within normal limits several options may be considered
    a. Clotrimazole® 1 applicator full intravaginally every other week x 2 months. If patient remains symptom free, reduce treatment to q month, the week prior to menses
    b. If 12 is not successful, Candida torulopsis glabrata or Candida Tropicalis should be considered. If lab confirms diagnosis, treat with gentian violet one tampon q hs x 12 days; triazole compounds have also been found to be effective (Terazol®—terconazole)
    c. Boric acid capsules. 600 mg 1 capsule 2 x/week intravaginally for recurrent candida vaginitis (4 or > episodes year) as organism may be Torulopsis glabrata (less sensitive to fluconazole or imidazoles)
    d. Clove of garlic in gauze placed in vagina for 10–12 hours; other complementary therapies (see guideline and Bibliography)
B. General measures
  1. No intercourse until symptoms subside; then use condoms until end of treatment
  2. No douching
  3. Stress importance of continuing medication even if menses begin
  4. Do not use tampons during treatment
  5. Stress hygiene, cotton underwear, loose clothing, no underpants while sleeping, wipe front first and then back
  6. Do not use feminine hygiene sprays, deodorants, etc.
  7. Treat athlete's foot, "jock" itch, or rash with OTC antifungals (such as Lotrimin®, Tinactin®) or prescription Dual-action Lotrisone®
  8. Consider the use of vitamin C 500 mg BID-QID to ↑ acidity of vaginal secretions or oral acidophilous tablets 40 million to 1 billion units QD (1 tablet); eat live culture yogurt several times a week

VIII. Complications
Drug interactions; adverse reactions to treatment

IX. Consultation/Referral
A. No response to treatment as outlined above
B. Elevated fasting blood sugar or 2° postprandial
C. Presence of concurrent systemic disease

X. Follow-up
None necessary unless
A. Symptoms persist after treatment
B. Symptoms recur or exacerbate

Appendix A has information on candidiasis which you may wish to photocopy or adapt for your patients.

See Bibliography.

Trichomoniasis

I. Definition
Infection with the organism Trichomonas, usually sexually transmitted; found in the vagina and urethra of women and the urethra of males.

II. Etiology
The parasitic protozoan flagellate, Trichomonas vaginalis

III. History
A. What the patient may present with
   1. Foul-smelling vaginal discharge, often fishy
   2. Burning and soreness of vulva, perineum, thighs
   3. Vaginal and perineal itching
   4. Dyspareunia, dysuria
   5. Postcoital bleeding
   6. Possibly no objective symptoms
B. Additional information to be considered
   1. Previous vaginal infection, vaginosis; diagnosis, treatment; compliance with treatment
   2. Sexual activity; partner preference (do not disregard possibility of women having sex with women)
   3. History of sexually transmitted disease or pelvic inflammatory disease
   4. Last menstrual period
   5. Last intercourse, sexual contact
   6. Method of birth control; other medications

7. History of chronic illness (especially seizure disorders)
8. Description of discharge
   a. Color
   b. Onset
   c. Odor
   d. Consistency
   e. Amount

   f. Constant vs intermittent
   g. Relationship to menses
   h. Relationship to sexual contact
9. Partner has symptoms

IV. Physical Examination
A. External examination
Observe perineum for excoriation, erythema, edema, ulceration, lesions
B. Vaginal examination (speculum)
   1. Inspection of vaginal walls; red papules may appear
   2. Inspection of cervix: strawberry appearance of cervix and upper vagina due to petechiae
   3. Discharge: greenish, yellow, malodorous, frothy with >4.5 pH (5.0–7.0)
C. Bimanual examination

V. Laboratory Examination
A. Wet prep microscopic examination; should see highly motile cells, slightly larger than leukocytes, smaller than epithelial cells; > 10 WBCs/high power field
B. Gonococcus culture, Chlamydia test, serology testing for syphilis if history indicates; culture for T. vaginalis; DNA probe for T. vaginalis
C. CBC should be done if more than two courses of Metronidazole® taken within 2-month period
D. KOH "whiff" test: sometimes fishy but not always

VI. Differential Diagnosis
A. Candidiasis
B. Bacterial vaginosis
C. Urinary tract infection

D. Gonorrhea
E. Chlamydia infection

VII. Treatment*
A. Medications
   1. Metronidazole (Flagyl®, Metryl®, Protostat®, Satric®) 2 grams orally in single dose (review history for seizure disorder)

*Vaginal gel Metronidazole® is not recommended for trichomoniasis as the protozoa are multifocal including the urethra, Skene's glands, and so on.

2. Metronidazole 500 mg BID x 7 days (recommended for treatment failures)
3. Metronidazole capsules 375 mg BID x 7 days*
4. In pregnancy, Metronidazole 2 grains orally in single dose

B. General Measures
   1. Stress importance of not drinking alcohol during treatment or for 48 hours after treatment
   2. Metronidazole® can cause gastrointestinal upset; also causes urine to darken
   3. Stress avoidance of intercourse during treatment; if intercourse does occur, condoms should be used
   4. Stress importance of completing medication
   5. Stress personal hygiene; cotton underpants, no underpants while sleeping, wipe front first, and then back
   6. Patient should be given informational handout to deliver to sexual partner advising need for partner's treatment
   7. Comfort measures for severe symptoms: sitz baths
   8. Stress that if partner is not treated before next act of unprotected intercourse, reinfection can occur

VIII. Complications**

A. Of the disease
   Spread of the infection to urethra, or prostate in the male
B. Untreated Trichomonas vaginalis may result in atypia on Papanicolaou smear; may also be associated with adverse pregnancy outcomes (premature rupture of membranes and preterm delivery); ↑ susceptibility to HIV acquisition
C. Of the treatment
   1. Nausea
   2. Neurological symptoms: seizures
   3. Vomiting (may be severe) if alcohol is consumed while on treatment or within 48 hours after treatment
   4. Possibility of blood dyscrasia posttreatment

IX. Consultation/Referral

A. Refer to physician if woman has seizure disorder prior to initiating therapy
B. Consult if treatment (VII A. 1. and 2.) fails

---

*Not yet approved by CDC—not in guidelines but approved by the FDA with pharmacological equivalency of metronidazole 250 mg tid for 7 days; no clinical data available to demonstrate clinical equivalency.

**Tinidazole available from Presutti Labs (Arlington Heights, IL) on compassionate use protocol for metronidazole-resistant trichomonas in women.

X. Follow-up
None necessary unless symptoms persist or recur after treatment
    See Appendix A and Bibliography.

Bacterial Vaginosis

I. Definition
A clinical syndrome characterized by an overgrowth of anaerobic bacteria (bacteroides, peptostreptococcus, mobiluncus curtesii, eubacterium, and pre-voltella) and facultative bacteria (gardnerella vaginalis, mycoplasma hominis, enterococcus, group B Streptococcus and decrease in H_2O_2–producing lactobacilli).

II. Etiology
A. Bacterial vaginosis (BV) is a vaginosis rather than vaginitis. As such, there is usually little or no inflammation of epithelium associated with the syndrome (relative absence of polymorphonuclear leukocytes). It is not caused by a single pathogen, but is probably a disturbance of the vaginal microbial ecology, with a displacement of normal lactobacillary flora by anerobic microorganisms
B. It is a sexually associated rather than a sexually transmitted syndrome. (Bacterial vaginosis is found more often in sexually active women.) A male version of BV has not been identified

III. History
A. What the patient may present with
    1. Vaginal odor (fishy)
    2. Increased vaginal discharge—milky white, thin adherent discharge or dark or dull gray discharge
    3. Vaginal burning after intercourse; vulvar pruritis (15% of women)
    4. No symptoms in many patients
B. Additional information to be considered
    1. Previous vaginal infections; diagnosis, treatment; compliance with treatment
    2. Chronic illness; careful history of seizure disorders
    3. Sexual activity; partner preference
    4. History of sexually transmitted disease or pelvic inflammatory disease
    5. Last intercourse
    6. Last menstrual period; pregnancy
    7. Method of birth control; other medications

8. Description of discharge
   a. Onset
   b. Color
   c. Odor stronger during intercourse
   d. Consistency
   e. Constant vs. intermittent
   f. Relationship of symptoms to sexual contact
   g. Relationship of symptoms to menses
   h. Amount
9. Use of vaginal deodorant sprays, deodorant tampons, pantyliners, or pads, douches, perfumed toilet tissue
10. Change in laundry soaps, fabric softener, body soap
11. Clothing: consistent wearing of tight-crotched pants; nylon underwear, underwear to bed
12. Personal hygiene
13. Recent change in lifestyle (stress, personal crisis)
14. Partner symptoms

IV. Physical Examination
A. External examination
Perineum usually has a normal appearance; occasional irritation
B. Vaginal examination (speculum)
   1. Inspection of vaginal walls
   2. Inspection of cervix
   3. Discharge: characteristically adherent homogenous, whitish in color, and of a fishy, musty odor with pH >4.5. Take smear from lateral walls of vagina, not cervix, for accurate pH (use nitrazine paper for test)
C. Bimanual examination if indicated

V. Laboratory Examination May Include
A. Diagnosis (3 of 4Amsel criteria)
   1. White, thin adherent discharge
   2. ph ≥ 4.5
   3. + whiff test (fishy amine odor from vaginal fluid mixed with 10% KOH)
   4. Clue cells on wet mount: epithelial cells dotted with large numbers of bacteria that obscure cell borders, should see ≥ 20% clue cells
B. Card Test (FemExam, Pip Activity Test Card)
C. Few WBCs seen on wet mount; decreased Lactobacilli
D. Further laboratory work as indicated by history or wet prep/card test results

VI. Differential Diagnosis

A. Trichomoniasis   B. Presence of foreign body

VII. Treatment

A. Medications

1. Vaginal preparation
   a. Metronidazole gel (MetroGel®) 0.75% one applicatorful (5 grams) intravaginally BID x 5 days or one applicatorful HS x 5 days (if additional treatment is necessary within 2 months, a CBC will be necessary)
   b. Clindamycin phosphate cream (Cleocin® vaginal cream 2% one applicatorful, 5 grams) intravaginally HS x 7 nights. Clindamycin is contraindicated with colitis, other chronic bowel disease. Use cautiously in patients with asthma, impaired renal or hepatic function. *Note:* the mineral oil in Cleocin® vaginal cream may weaken latex or rubber products such as condoms or vaginal diaphragms. Use of these products within 72 hours following treatment is not recommended
   c. Clindamycin (Cleocin®) vaginal ovules 100 mg hs x 3 nights
2. Oral preparation:
   a. Metronidazole (Flagyl® ER) 750 mg orally 1 qd x 7 days*
   b. Metronidazole (Flagyl®) 500 mg orally BID x 7 days
3. Alternative treatment:
   a. Metronidazole 2 grams orally single dose OR
   b. Clindamycin 300 mg orally BID x 7 days OR
   c. Clindamycin vaginal ovules 100 mg x 3 days
4. In pregnancy:**
   For women at high risk (previous preterm delivery)
   a. Metronidazole 250 mg orally TID for 7 days
   b. Clindamycin 300 mg orally BID for 7 days
   For asymptomatic women at low risk (no history of preterm delivery) *data are conflicting; some data suggest ↓ in preterm birth, postpartum infection with screening and treatment*
5. Treatment for partner not recommended by CDC (no decrease in recurrences with partner treatment and no effect on cure rates)
6. Note: If bacterial vaginosis coexists with candidiasis:
   a. Treat a predominant organism first. If symptoms persist, recheck and treat as indicated

---

*FDA approved but data on equivalency with other clinical regimens not published.
**Clindamycin not recommended with breast feeding

  b. Consider local treatment for candidiasis concurrently with oral treatment for bacteria vaginosis as above
  c. Cleocin® also kills lactobacilli, so candidiasis is common after treatment. Consider sequential treatment
  d. If bacterial vaginosis coexists with Strep B treat concurrently
B. General measures
  1. Stress avoidance of intercourse until symptoms subside, then use condoms until end of treatment; condom therapy for 4–6 weeks (without antibiotic treatment) often results in resolution of BV
  2. Stress no douching during treatment or after
  3. Stress necessity of completing course of medication
  4. Nausea, vomiting, and cramps can occur (if patient is on Metronidazole®). Stress no alcohol intake during treatment and for 48 hours after completing medications
  5. Stress appropriate choice of medications if pregnant/ possibly pregnant, nursing
  6. Stress hygiene: cotton underwear, loose clothing, no underpants while sleeping, wipe front first and then back, no feminine deodorants or hygiene sprays
  7. Careful history of seizure disorders
  8. Metronidazole® can cause GI upset even with no alcohol
  9. For recurring BV, consider maintenance therapy with oral metronidazole, or hydrogen peroxide douche, or acid lactate gel vaginally*

XIII. Complications
Bacterial vaginosis has been associated with PID, endometritis, cervicitis, inflammation or ASC on Pap smears, possible link to LGSIL on Pap smears, preterm rupture of membranes, preterm labor, low birth weight, chorioamnitis; ↑ risk of HIV acquisition

IX. Consultation/Referral
If no response to treatment as discussed above

X. Follow-up
None necessary unless:
A. Symptoms persist after treatment
B. Symptoms recur

*Nyirjesy, P. (2000, November). Emerging challenges in bacterial vaginosis. *Contemporary Ob/Gyn*, 15–24, 28.
Berkhoudt, K. (2001). *Clinical management of bacterial vaginosis.* Educational session, October 23, Chestnut Hill, MA.

C. Pregnancy—asymptomatic women @ high risk consider 1 month after completion of treatment

See Appendix A and Bibliography.

Chlamydia Trachomatis Infection

I. Definition
Chlamydia trachomatis infection is a parasitic sexually transmitted disease of the reproductive tract mucous membrane of either sex.

II. Etiology
A. The causative organism is a small, obligate, intracellular, bacterium-like parasite (Chlamydia trachomatis or C. trachomatis) that develops within inclusion bodies in the cytoplasm of the host cells.
B. The incubation period is unknown

III. History
A. What the patient may present with
  1. Female
    a. Vaginal discharge
    b. Dysuria
    c. Pelvic pain
    d. Changes in menses
    e. Intermenstrual spotting
    f. Postcoital bleeding
    g. Frequently asymptomatic
    h. Mucopurulent discharge in cervical os
  2. Male
    a. Dysuria
    b. Thick, cloudy penile discharge
    c. Rarely asymptomatic
B. Additional information to be considered
  1. Previous vaginal infections; diagnosis, treatment; compliance with treatment
  2. Chronic illness
  3. Sexual activity; new partner(s)
  4. History of sexually transmitted disease or pelvic inflammatory disease
  5. Known contact
  6. Last intercourse, sexual contact, sex toys
  7. Method(s) of birth control, other medications

Description of discharge

a. Onset	e. Amount
b. Color	f. Constant vs intermittent
c. Odor	g. Relationship to sexual contact
d. Consistency	h. Relationship to menses

9. Use of vaginal deodorant sprays, deodorant tampons, panty liners, pads, perfumed toilet tissue, douches
10. Change in laundry soaps, fabric softener, body soap
11. Clothing: consistent wearing of tight-crotched pants
12. Personal hygiene
13. Any drug allergies
14. Travel to Asia, Africa

IV. Physical Examination
A. Vital signs
　1. Blood pressure　　　　　2. Temperature
B. Abdominal examination: check for guarded referred pain, rebound pain
C. External examination
　Observe perineum for edema, ulcerations, lesions, excoriations, erythema, enlarged, tender Bartholin's glands
D. Vaginal examination (speculum)
　1. Inspection of vaginal walls
　2. Cervix (cervicitis), friability
　3. Discharge: if present, is characteristically mucopurulent
E. Bimanual examination
　Pain on cervical motion (positive Chandelier sign), fullness in adnexa, tender uterus

V. Laboratory Examination
A. DFA: secretions fixed on slide and stained with fluorescein labelled monoclonal antibody specific for chlamydial antigens
B. Laboratory test for chlamydia (sensitivities and specificities vary):
　1. Enzyme-linked immunoassays (EIA) detection of chlamydial antigens
　2. DNA probe (Genprobe®) (PRC + LCR = amplified tests done on Genprobe®)
　3. Polymerase chain reaction (PCR)
　4. Ligase chain reaction (LCR)
C. Endocervical culture (only 100% specific test in transport media—do in medicolegal cases—rape, child sexual abuse)
D. Serology test for syphilis if history indicates

E. Consider HIV testing
F. Consider hepatitis B & C testing
G. GC culture

VI. Differential Diagnosis
A. Gonorrhea   B. Appendicitis   C. Cystitis

VII. Treatment
A. Medication
  1. Azithromycin 1 gram orally in a single dose OR Doxycycline 100 mg orally BID x 7 days
  2. Alternative regimens
    a. Erythromycin base 500 mg orally QID x 7 days OR
    b. Erythromycin ethylsuccinate 800 mg orally QID x 7 days OR
    c. Ofloxacin 300 mg orally BID x 7 days OR
    d. Levofloxacin 500 mg orally qd for 7 days
  3. In pregnancy
    a. Erythromycin base 500 mg orally QID x 7 days
    b. Amoxicillin 500 mg orally TID x 7–10 days (for erythromycin intolerance)
  4. Alternative regimens in pregnancy
    a. Erythromycin base 250 mg orally QID x 7 days
    b. Erythromycin ethylsuccinate 800 mg QID, x 7 days
    c. Erythromycin ethylsuccinate 400 mg orally QID x 14 days
    d. Azithromycin 1 gram orally in single dose
B. For sexual contacts during 60 days preceding onset of symptoms or diagnosis of chlamydia
  1. Offer chlamydia test prior to treatment
  2. Start treatment prior to results of testing
  3. Treat same as for woman; do follow-up if symptoms persist and re-screening per CDC Guidelines
    General measures
  1. Stress partner should be treated
  2. No intercourse until both partners are treated, or use condoms, but abstinence is preferred
  3. Condom for back-up birth control method for remainder of cycle if on oral contraceptives
  4. Stress importance of completing medication for woman and partner
  5. Stress no use of feminine hygiene sprays, deodorants, douches
  6. Stress possibility of increased photosensitivity with Doxycycline®
  7. Inform patient taking tetracycline that medication should be taken 1

hour before or 2 hours after meals and/or consumption of dairy products, antacids, mineral-containing products
8. Return for reevaluation if symptoms persist or return after treatment

VIII. Complications
A. Women
  1. Pelvic inflammatory disease
     a. Pelvic abscess (ovarian)
     b. Infertility; chronic pelvic pain
  2. Abnormal Papanicolaou smear with cervicitis (30–50%)
  3. Postpartum endometritis
B. Men
  1. Epididymitis, prostatitis
  2. Reiter's syndrome (primarily men)
C. ↑ Risk of acquiring HIV
D. Newborn
  1. Conjunctivitis
  2. Pneumonia
  3. Urogenital tract, rectal infection
E. Urethritis

IX. Consultation/Referral
A. If no response to treatment as discussed above
B. If complications develop

X. Follow-up
A. If no response to treatment or possibility of reinfection
B. Test of cure not routinely required per CDC Guidelines. If symptoms persist or reinfection is suspected, consider retesting women after treatment. (↑ rate of reinfection). Consider rescreening all women with chlamydia infection 3–4 months after treatment. Rescreen all women treated when they next present for care within 12 months.
C. Consider retesting 3 weeks after completion of treatment with erythromycin
D. Repeat Pap if abnormal prior to treatment
E. Gonorrhea cultures if not done
F. Serology test for syphilis
G. In some states, chlamydia is a reportable disease

Appendix A has information on chlamydia trachomatis infection to photocopy or adapt for your patients. See Bibliography.

Genital Herpes Simplex

I. Definition
Genital herpes simplex is a recurrent viral infection of the skin and mucous membranes of the genitalia, characterized by eruptions on a lightly raised erythematous base.

II. Etiology
A. Herpes simplex virus (HSV). There are two HSV strains:
    1. HSV Type 1 (HSV-1): commonly causes herpes labialis ("cold sores") and herpes keratitis
        a. Usually seen in childhood (as acute gingivostomatitis)
        b. May be seen in adults who engage in oral sex, kissing
        c. Incubation period 3–7 days, course 1–3 weeks
        d. May be recurrent and has no cure
        e. Offers no protection against getting HSV-2 but makes HSV-2 more likely to be subclinical
    2. HSV Type 2 (HSV-2)
        a. Genital counterpart of acute gingivostomatitis; primarily sexually transmitted
        b. Incubation period 4–7 days up to 4 weeks, course may last 2–3 weeks
        c. HSV-2 remains dormant in dorsal nerve ganglia; may be recurrent and has no cure
        d. May be present for many years with no symptoms or no recognizable symptoms
        e. HSV-2 does provide immunity against HSV-1
        f. 25% of population has HSV-2
    3. Both HSV-1 (10%) and 2 (90%) have been implicated in genital infections but rarely is type 2 found orally

III. History
A. Genital herpes
    1. Primary infection (may actually be caused by HSV-1 or 2); mean duration 12 days
        a. Multiple lesions
            1) Male: penis, buttocks, thigh
            2) Female: labia, fourchette, cervix, buttocks, thigh, nipples
        b. Myalgia
        c. Arthralgia
        d. Malaise

      e. Fever, lymphadenopathy

      f. Dysuria, male and female (urinary retention may occur, especially in women with lesions close to meatus)

      g. Dyspareunia

      h. Headache (can be sign of herpes meningitis)

   2. Recurrent genital lesions

      a. Lesions less painful

      b. Less or no systemic symptoms

      c. Unilateral

      d. Prodromal symptoms (itching, burning, and/or tingling at site where lesions then appear)

B. Additional information to be considered

   1. Genital herpes: primary infection

      a. Known exposure

      b. Sexual preference

      c. Recent participation in oral sex with partner having herpes labialis

   2. Genital herpes: recurrent infection

      a. History of recent exposure to reactivating factors: physical trauma, exposure to sunlight, stress, menses

      b. Prodrome

         1) Pruritus

         2) Burning at site of previous lesion(s)

         3) Tingling at site of previous lesion(s)

         4) Symptoms as in 1, 2, and/or 3 across nerve tract serving site of previous lesion(s); i.e., sciatic pain with lesion on labia

IV. Physical Examination

A. Genital herpes

   1. Primary infection

      a. Temperature, blood pressure

      b. Examination of genitalia: vesicular lesions containing cloudy liquid on erythematous base. Vesicles break, lesions coalesce forming ulcerative lesions with irregular borders, macerated if in moist areas

         1) Female: lesions (painful), examination will be difficult; use of speculum may be impossible. Lesions present as described in III.A. cervicitis may be present

         2) Male: lesions (painful) present in areas previously described in III.A. Urethral discharge may be present

      c. Groin: inguinal adenopathy may be present

      d. Abdomen: bladder distension, secondary to urinary retention may be present; more common in women

   e. Check for atypical presentation as cystitis, meningitis, encephalitis, urethritis, ocular lesions
 2. Recurrent infection genital herpes
As above (III.B.2.) but clinical picture is less severe

V. Laboratory Examination May Include HSV Types I and II
A. Scrape lesion for samples for
 1. Virology culture (within 7 days of 1st episode, 2 days of recurrence)
 2. Genital lesions: consider gonococcus culture, serology test for syphilis, chlamydia test (may need to wait until follow-up visit if infection is severe)
 3. Antibody E detection (such as HerpeSelect-1 & HerpeSelect-2 ELISA IgG; Herpe-Select-1 & 2 Immunoblot IgG; POCKit-HSV-2 assay*)
B. Consider HIV testing

VI. Differential Diagnosis
A. Syphilis   C. Lymphogranuloma inguinale
B. Chancroid   D. Granuloma inguinale

VII. Treatment of Genital Herpes
A. General therapy
 1. Consider immune status of patient with frequent outbreaks and/or long duration outbreaks, plus the degree of systemic involvement
 2. Consider also the potential for asymptomatic shedding
 3. Comfort measures
    a. Tepid water sitz baths, plain or with Betadine solution; dry carefully with cool air hair dryer making sure to hold it away from body
    b. If voiding over lesions is painful, instruct patient to void while sitting in water in bathtub
    c. Stress avoidance of tight, restricting clothing. The vulva should be exposed to air flow as much as possible (patient may wear a skirt or robe without underpants when at home)
    d. Peri-irrigation for comfort
 4. Patient education
    a. Explain the disease process and route of transmission to the patient (i.e., oral/genital sex during outbreaks)
       1) 90% of those infected don't know
       2) Majority of transmission occurs without symptoms in the infected person

*Many new blood tests for HSV are available depending on geographic locastion. Check with your local laboratories.

3) Viral shedding occurs 5–70% of day
4) Condom use protects women not men

b. Patients should be advised to abstain from sexual activity while lesions are present
c. Explain the dangers associated with herpes during pregnancy
d. Discuss possible factors involved with recurrences
e. Discuss need for yearly Papanicolaou smear
f. Support group: alt.support.herpes (usenet news group)

B. Medication
1. Initial genital outbreak
   a. Acyclovir 400 mg orally TID x 7–10 days OR
   b. Acyclovir 200 mg orally 5x day for 7–10 days OR
   c. Famciclovir (Famvir®) 250 mg orally TID for 7–10 days OR
   d. Valacyclovir (Valtrex®) 1 gm orally BID x 7–10 days OR
   e. Zylocaine 2% gel or cream; apply 3–4 times daily (do not use around urethra) for comfort measure
   f. Bacitracin ointment, apply locally, for secondary infection only 2–5 x daily
2. Episodic recurrent infection
   a. Episodic—infrequent outbreaks 6 times or fewer a year. Therapy should be initiated within 1 day of lesion onset or during prodrome for best effect
   b. Acyclovir 400 mg orally TID for 5 days OR
   c. Acyclovir 200 mg orally 5 times a day for 5 days OR
   d. Acyclovir 800 mg orally BID for 5 days OR
   e. Famciclovir 125 mg orally BID for 5 days OR
   f. Valacyclovir 500 mg orally BID for 3–5 days OR
   g. Valacyclovir 1.0 g orally qd x 5 days (3–day course may be as effective per CDC)
3. Suppressive therapy* Evidence is growing showing benefits of beginning suppressive therapy with first episode, not waiting for chronic outbreaks to be established. Early intervention will decrease recurrences during the first year when outbreaks are the most frequent as well as decrease the likelihood of viral shedding. Safety has been established for up to 15 years of continuous use
   a. Acyclovir 400 mg orally BID OR
   b. Famciclovir 250 mg orally BID OR
   c. Valacyclovir 500 mg orally QD for persons with 9 or < outbreaks per year OR

---

*A topical gel resiquimod applied to active lesions during a recurrence to delay recurrence time and is in clinical trials.

      d. Valacyclovir 1g orally QD for persons with 10 > per year
  4. In pregnancy (report treatment—see CDC 2002 Guidelines)
      a. First clinical episode or severe recurrent—treat with oral acyclovir
      b. In life-threatening, severe maternal HSV infection, treat with IV acyclovir
  5. Unresolved herpes—herpes outbreaks lasting several weeks or more
      a. Immunological status should be evaluated with physician consultation
  6. Oral lesions—treat with Idoxuridine (Stoxil, Herplex), Peridin-C (ascorbic acid, Hesperidin methyl Chalcone, and Hesperidin Complex); penciclovir cream 1% (Denavir); Valacyclovir 1 gm q 12° × 1 day.

VIII. Complications
A. Secondary infection of lesion
B. Keratitis (keep fingers away from eyes)
C. Generalized herpetic skin eruptions
D. Meningitis
E. Encephalitis
F. Pneumonitis
G. Hepatitis
H. Fetal-neonatal infection
I. Spread to other persons at risk of developing disseminated herpes
  1. Immunosuppressed or deficient individuals including persons with HIV
  2. Patients with open skin lesions, e.g., burns, atopic dermatitis
  3. Infants, small children

IX. Consultation/Referral
A. Secondary infections
B. Urinary retention if unable to void in bathtub
C. Suspected ocular lesion
D. Severe primary episode
E. Poor fluid intake associated with severe primary episode
F. Persistent headache, nausea, vomiting, photophobia, convulsions, pain in upper right quadrant, chest pain, SOB
G. Unresolved outbreaks lasting several weeks or more
H. Life-threatening episode in pregnant woman

X. Follow-up
As needed
    See Appendix A for information you may want to photocopy or adapt for your patients. See Bibliography.

Herpes Resources online:
www.herpes.com
www.ashastd.org/herpes/hrc.html
www.webmd.com
America on-line keyword Better Health
www.thrive.com
www.viridas.com
www.diagnology

American Social Health Assoc. (ASHA) booklets, books, handouts
The Helper 800–230–6039
ASHA patient herpes hotline
919–361–8488

Condylomata Acuminata (Genital Warts)

I. Definition
Condylomata acuminata is a sexually transmitted condition (but it may also be a fomite) caused by a virus, Human Papilloma Virus (HPV), and characterized by the formation of warty excrescences on the external genitalia, and on the cervix, vagina, anal area, nipples, umbilicus, pharynx. Virus does not always cause a lesion; subclinical infection occurs on cervix and externally.

II. Etiology
A. The cause of the condition is a DNA virus of the Papilloma group (HPV) more than 30 types of HPV can affect the genital tract
B. Incubation period: 1 to 6 months; may be much longer (up to 30 years); up to 70% may regress spontaneously
C. Period of communicability is unknown

III. History
A. What the patient may present with
  1. "Feeling a lump" in vulvar area
  2. Increased vaginal discharge
  3. Vulvar itch, burning, pain, bleeding
B. Additional information to be considered
  1. Previous vaginitis/vaginosis; diagnosis, treatment
  2. Sexual activity, last intercourse, sexual contact
  3. Last menstrual period: any chance of pregnancy
  4. Method of birth control

     5. Previous history of condylomata, herpes simplex
     6. Known contact; consider any contact with person with condylomata on any body part
     7. History of sexually transmitted disease or pelvic inflammatory disease
     8. Description of discharge (odor, consistency, amount, color)
     9. Any drug allergies
    10. History of abnormal Papanicolaou smear, colposcopy, treatment
    11. Reactivation of subclinical infection with sexual activity
    12. Self-infection from condyloma on any body part
    13. Lifestyle: smoking, sexual practices such as anal intercourse, sex toys, exposure to utraviolet light, nutrition

IV. Physical Examination
A. External Examination
     1. Small, pink, or flesh colored, soft papillomatous or raised "warty" lesion visualized in
       a. Periclitoral area
       b. Vestibule
       c. Posterior perineal and perianal areas
       d. Extragenital areas
     2. Confluence of many individual warts may give impression of a single, fleshy, proliferative lesion
     3. Secondary infection of lesions (from scratching)
     4. On hair-bearing skin keratotic appearance
B. Vaginal examination (speculum); observe for same lesions as above
     1. Vaginal walls
     2. Cervix (more often subclinical and no visible lesions on inspection)

V. Laboratory Examination May Include
A. Visual examination (classic appearance, as above); often visible after application of 5% acetic acid (white vinegar)
B. Gonococcal culture
C. Chlamydia smear
D. Serology test for syphilis
E. Other laboratory work as indicated by history and examination
F. Colposcopy
G. Papanicolaou test
H. DNA testing—such as the Hybrid Capture Tube Test®
I. Biopsy of cervix or unresponsive or unusual lesion on vulva for histologic examination
J. HIV testing

VI. Differential Diagnosis
Condylomata lata (associated with syphilis), molluscum contagiosum, lipomas, fibroma, adenomas, squamous cell carcinoma, nevi, seborrheic keratoses, psoriatic plaques, carcinoma in situ, micropapillometosis labialis, giant condyloma (Buschke-Löwenstein tumor), Bowenoid papulosis, malignant melanoma, skin tags, lichen nitidus, lichen planus, sebaceous Tyson's glands, herpes simplex, angiokeratoma

VII. Treatment
A. Medical treatment
  1. Patient applied
    a. Podofilox (Condylox®) 0.5% solution or gel BID for 3 days; no therapy 4 days; repeat prn up to 4 cycles
    b. Imiquinod (Aldara®) (an immune response modifier inducing cytokines), 5% cream 3 times a week h.s. for up to 16 weeks (may weaken rubber in diaphragms, condoms); needs to be washed off after 6–10 hours
  2. Provider applied for visible genital warts
Apply trichloracetic acid (TCA) or bichloracetic (BCA) acid (80–90%)* (topical) or podophyllin resin (podophyllin), 10–25% in tincture of benzoin (10%) and isopropyl alcohol: allow to dry (apply vaseline collar with podophyllin**)
    a. No need to wash trichloracetic acid off, wash podophyllin off in 1–4 hours
    b. May burn on application; if excess amount of TCA or BCA is applied, powder treatment area with talc, Na bicarb or liquid soap to remove unreacted acid
    c. Only use once a week x 8–12 weeks
    d. Intralesional interferon
  3. Cervical warts—colpo/consultation; Vaginal warts—cryotherapy, TCA or BCA repeat weekly; Urethral meatus—cryotherapy OR podophyllin; Oral & Anal—cryotherapy, BCA or TCA or surgical removal
  4. Pregnancy: Podofilox, imiquimod, and podophyllin should NOT be used in pregnancy.
B. Surgical treatment
  1. Cryotherapy with liquid nitrogen or cryoprobe; dimethylether (Histofrezer®) repeat q 1–2 weeks

---

*No data on BCA efficacy are available.
**Podophyllin is now considered ineffective; its use has been discontinued in many settings. Use should be limited to >0.5 ML or <10CW^2/session to ↓ potential systemic effects

    2. CO_2 laser vaporization

    3. Surgical excision

    4. LEEP (Loop electrosurgical excision procedure)

C. General measures

    1. Sexual partner(s) should be checked if lesions are present; CDC recommends that the role of reinfection is probably minimal

    2. Stress importance of personal hygiene

D. Use of condoms to help prevent further infection with partners likely to be uninfected (note precaution with imiquimod)

E. Education that even after treatment and elimination of visible warts, the potential for transmission exists

VIII. Complications

A. Lesions can become numerous and large requiring more extensive treatment

B. Visible genital warts are usually caused by HPV types 6 or 11. Other HPV types in the anogenital region (types 16, 18, 26, 31, 33, 35, 39, 45, 51, 52, 53, 56, 58, 59, 66, 68, 73, 82) have been strongly associated with cervical neoplasia

C. Laryngeal papillomatosis in infant

D. Men with HPV are at increased risk for dysplastic changes and cancers in the penile and anorectal areas

IX. Consultation/Referral

Refer to or consult with physician

A. After 8–12 treatments for evaluation

B. If warts are present on vaginal walls or cervix or rectal mucosa (see VII.C.)

C. Extensive or deep anorectal warts for proctologic examination; urethroscopy as indicated

D. If any wart is over 2 cm in size or for large cluster of warts, consider referral

E. Abnormal Pap smear (per protocol)

F. For possible biopsy in older age groups; atypical appearance of lesions, poor response to treatment in younger patients

G. Pregnant women

X. Follow-up

A. Weekly x 8–12 weeks

B. Patient advised to check self periodically and return if warts recur

C. Stress importance of q 6 month Papanicolaou smear in woman treated for condylomata (some settings repeat q 3 months x 1 year, then q 6 months x 1 year; if normal, then yearly, and some now say yearly if none over 1 year are abnormal) See Papanicolaou guidelines

See Appendix A on condylomata acuminata, and information you may want to photocopy or adapt for your patients. See Bibliography. National Cancer Institute: www.nci.nih.gov; www.ashastd.org

Gonorrhea

I. Definition
Gonorrhea is a sexually transmitted bacterial infection of the urethra, rectum, and/or cervix; the causative organism can also be cultured in the nasopharynx. As many as 80% of infected women may be asymptomatic.

II. Etiology
A. The causative organism is Neisseria gonorrhoea, a gram negative, intracellular, nonmotile diplococcus. Increasingly, plasmid-mediated penicillinase-producing N. gonorrhoea (PPNG), plasmid-mediated tetracycline resistant (TRNG), chromosomally mediated resistant (CMRNG), Spectinomycin-resistant, and quinolone resistant strains exist. Incubation: 1–13 days.

III. History
A. What patient may present with
  1. Females: a large percentage (perhaps 80%) of infected women are asymptomatic in the early disease stage
    a. Early symptoms
      1) Dysuria, dyspareunia
      2) Leukorrhea; change in vaginal discharge
      3) Unilateral labial pain and swelling
      4) Lower abdominal discomfort
      5) Pharyngitis
    b. Later symptoms
      1) Purulent, irritating vaginal discharge
      2) Fever (possibly high)
      3) Rectal pain and discharge
      4) Abnormal menstrual bleeding
      5) Increased dysmenorrhea
      6) Nausea, vomiting
      7) Lesions in genital area; labia pain

        8) Joint pain and swelling
        9) Upper abdominal pain (perihepatitis)
       10) Pain, tenderness in pelvic organs; urethral pain
  2. Males: usually symptomatic (up to 10% asymptomatic)
    a. Early symptoms
      1) Dysuria with frequency
      2) Whitish discharge from penis
      3) Pharyngitis
    b. Later symptoms
      1) Yellow or greenish discharge from penis
      2) Epididymitis
      3) Proctitis
B. Additional information to be considered
  1. Previous vaginal infections, diagnosis and treatment
  2. Chronic illness
  3. Sexual activity; number, new sexual partner(s)
  4. History of sexually transmitted disease or pelvic inflammatory disease
  5. Known contact
  6. Last intercourse, sexual contact
  7. Method of birth control, other medications
  8. History of cervical ectopy, friability in known patient
  9. Post-coital bleeding
  10. Description of discharge

a. Onset	d. Consistency
b. Color	e. Amount
c. Odor	f. Relationship to sexual contact

  11. Any change in menses (increased flow or dysmenorrhea)
  12. Any drug allergies
  13. HIV risk or exposure
  14. Travel to Asia, Africa, the Pacific, US West Coast

IV. Physical Examination
A. Vital signs
  1. Blood Pressure   2. Temperature 3. Pulse
B. Abdominal examination
  1. Guarding   2. Referred pain
  3. Rebound pain   4. Upper bilateral quadrant pain
  5. Bowel sounds indicating intestinal hyperactivity
C. External examination
  1. Inspection of Skene's glands
  2. Inspection of urethra

3. Inspection of Bartholin's glands
D. Vaginal examination (speculum)
1. Vaginal walls: discharge, redness
2. Cervix: mucopurulent discharge, ectopy, friability
3. Vaginal discharge
E. Bimanual examination
1. Pain when cervix is moved by examiner
2. Uterine tenderness
3. Adnexal tenderness
4. Adnexal mass
F. Throat examination
1. Erythema including tonsils
2. Edema of posterior pharynx
3. Erythema

V. Laboratory Examination
A. Gonococcus culture/Chlamydia test (Thayer-Martin still the gold standard for GC; polymerase chain reaction (PCR) and ligase chain reaction (LCR) tests useful; for rectal and throat need to culture (Thayer-Martin); gram stain >20 polys (in males sufficient for diagnosis)
B. Serology test for syphilis

VI. Differential Diagnosis
A. Chlamydia   B. Appendicitis   C. Ectopic pregnancy

VII. Treatment: Cervix, Urethra, Rectum
A. Medication
1. Ceftriaxone 125 mg IM single dose, OR Ciprofloxacin 500 mg orally single dose (not in women < 18) OR Ofloxacin* 400 mg orally single dose OR Levofloxacin 250 mg orally single dose (for Chlamydia coverage if not ruled out) PLUS (250 mg orally single dose)
   a. Azithromycin 1 gram orally in a single dose OR
   b. Doxycycline 100 mg orally BID x 7 days
2. Alternative regimens
   a. Spectinomycin 2 grams IM in a single dose OR
   b. Ceftizoxime 500 mg IM single dose OR
   c. Cefoxitin 2 grams IM single dose with probenecid 1 gram orally OR
   d. Cefotaxime 500 mg IM single dose OR

*Not in Hawaii as noted in 2002 CDC guidelines

       e. Gatifloxacin 400 mg orally single dose OR

       f. Norfloxacin 800 mg orally single dose

       g. Lomefloxacin 400 mg orally single dose

       h. PLUS Chlamydia regimen

   3. Pregnancy: Cephalosporins such as Ceftriaxone 125 mg IM single dose; if not tolerated use Spectinomycin 2 grams IM single dose

      PLUS Chlamydia regimen for pregnancy

      Do not use quininolones (Ciprofloxacin, Ofloxacin, Enoxacin, Lomefloxacin, Norfloxacin) or tetracyclines in pregnancy

   4. Pharynx

      Ceftriaxone 125 mg IM single dose OR

      Ciprofloxacin 500 mg PO single dose

      PLUS Chlamydia regimen

   5. Conjunctiva 1 gram IM Ceftriaxone plus lavage infected eye with saline solution x 1

   6. For contacts: verify if partner had diagnosed infection; also try to ascertain if culture was betalactinase positive or negative, then after appropriate culture treat with same regimen as patient depending on history of sensitivities

B. General measures

   1. All sexual partners should be treated if last sexual contact was within 60 days of onset of symptoms in patient or diagnosis of infection. If > 60 days, treat patient's most recent sexual partner

   2. No intercourse until both partners are treated, or use condoms, but abstinence is preferred

   3. Stress importance of completing medication

   4. Stress personal hygiene

   5. Stress need for follow-up culture if symptoms persist, recur, or exacerbate

VIII. Complications

A. Females

   1. Pelvic inflammatory disease

      a. Pelvic abscess or Bartholin's abscess

      b. Infertility

   2. Disseminated gonococcal infection—gonococcal bacteremia

   3. In pregnancy: spontaneous abortion, premature rupture of membranes, premature delivery, chorioamnionitis

B. Males

   1. Proctitis

   2. Infertility due to epididymitis, prostatitis and/or seminal vesiculitis

   3. Urethral stricture

4. Disseminated gonococcal infection—gonococcal bacteremia
C. Newborns: ophthalmia neonatorum, sepsis, arthritis, meningitis, rhinitis, urethritis, vaginitis, inflammation at sites of fetal monitoring
D. Males and females
   1. Meningitis
   2. Endocarditis
   3. Gonococcal conjunctivitis

IX. Consultation/Referral
A. If no response to treatment as discussed above
B. If complications develop

X. Follow-up
A. Test of cure not recommended by CDC unless symptoms recur, exacerbate, or do not resolve
B. Serology test for syphilis in 30 days
C. Chlamydia test if not done at initial visit prior to treatment
D. Consider HIV and hepatitis B and C screening

Appendix A has information about gonorrhea that you can photocopy or adapt for your patients. See Bibliography.

Syphilis

I. Definition
Syphilis is a sexually transmitted systemic disease characterized by periods of active florid manifestations and periods of symptomless latency. It can affect any tissue or vascular organ of the body and can be passed on from mother to fetus.

II. Etiology
A. The causative organism is a motile spirochete, Treponema pallidum (T. pallidum)
B. Incubation period, 10–90 days; average 21 days

III. History
A. What the patient may present with
   1. Primary symptoms
      a. Painless lesion (chancre) at site of entry of T. pallidum. Chancre appears on average about 3 wks after sexual contact and heals in 3–6 wk with a small inculun—this incubation period may be as long

as 90 days. Sites include vulva, labia, fourchette, clitoris, cervix, nipple, lip, roof of mouth, tonsils, bite area, finger, urethra, rectum, and smooth, firm borders of ulcer

   b. Enlarged inguinal or regional nodes; trochlear

  2. Secondary symptoms that may or may not occur in untreated patients within 4–10 weeks of resolution of primary symptoms

   a. Generalized symmetrical papillo-squamous eruption of palms, soles or mucous membrane (condylomata lata)

   b. Alopecia; may have "moth-eaten look"

   c. Loss of lateral 1/3 of eyebrow

   d. Generalized nontender lymphadenopathy with firm, rubbery feel

   e. Symptoms of upper respiratory tract infection

   f. Low grade fever

   g. Malaise, anorexia, and arthralgia

   h. Mild hepatitis, splenomegaly or nephrotic syndrome in about 10% of cases

   i. Mucus patches on tongue, under foreskin and in intertriginous areas

  3. Latent stage

No clinical symptoms although 25% may have recurrence of cutaneous lesion; however demonstrate seriologic evidence

   a. Early latency: infection within the preceding year

   b. Late latency: over a year from date of initial infection. Patient may remain in latent stage for remainder of his/her life; however, 1/3 will develop the tertiary form of disease

   c. Tertiary stage

Osseous or cutaneous structures, cardiovascular system or nervous system become involved; most common developments are cardio-vascular syphilis and neurosyphilis

   d. Neurosyphilis (exceedingly uncommon today) can occur at any stage from 1–30 or more years after original infection

B. Additional information to be considered

  1. Sexual preference

  2. Current sexual activity

  3. Last sexual contact

  4. Birth control method(s)

  5. History of known contacts

  6. History of previous sexually transmitted disease

  7. History of recurrent infectious illness (e.g. mononucleosis)

  8. History of fever, malaise, arthralgia, or rash of unknown etiology

    9. History of cognitive dysfunction, sensory deficits, other neurological symptoms

  10. Current medical therapy

  11. Risk for HIV exposure

IV. Physical Examination

A. Vital signs

    1. Temperature   2. Blood pressure   3. Pulse

B. General examination of skin

    1. Alopecia

    2. Rash including soles of feet, palms, condyloma lata

C. Pharyngeal examination

D. Examine for enlarged inguinal nodes

E. External examination of genitalia

    Vulvar lesions; chancre at point of inoculation

F. Internal examination (speculum)

    1. Inspection of vaginal walls for lesions

    2. Inspection of cervix for lesions

    3. Inspection of discharge

G. Bimanual examination

H. Neurological examination per history and clinical findings

V. Laboratory Examination

A. Nontreponemal: venereal disease research laboratory (VDRL) and rapid plasma reagin (RPR) (these are nonspecific serum tests) detect cross-reaction of antibody to syphilis with cardiolipin. Reported as reactive or nonreactive. Reactive test is reported by a quantitative titre and reactive tests should be confirmed with treponemal testing

    1. Biological false positives occur with cardiolipin antigens sometimes present in drug abuse and in such diseases and conditions as

        a. Lupus erythematosus

        b. Mononucleosis

        c. Malaria

        d. Leprosy

        e. Viral pneumonia

        f. After smallpox vaccinations or other recent vaccinations

        g. Persons with HIV

        h. Narcotic addiction

        i. Arthritis

        j. Scleroderma

    k. Tuberculosis

    l. Chronic fatigue syndrome

    m. Pregnancy

B. Specific serum treponemal antibody tests (correlate poorly with disease activity; persons who have a reactive test will have it for life unless diagnosis and treatment are very early)

    1. Fluorescent Treponemal Antibody-Absorption Test (FTA-ABS)

    2. Microhemagglutination Assay for T. Pallidum (MHA-TP)

    3. TPHA (Treponema pallidum hemagglutination)

C. Gonococcus culture

D. Chlamydia test

E. Biopsy of the lesion

F. Darkfield microscopy exam (rarely available in free-standing clinics or offices)—most useful for males

G. Consider HIV testing; testing for Hepatitis B, C

VI. Differential Diagnosis

A. Herpes simplex

B. Condylomata acuminata

C. Granuloma inguinale

G. Pyoderma

C. Chancroid

E. Lymphogranuloma venereum

F. Carcinoma

VII. Treatment (with physician consult in some settings)

A. Medication (for primary and secondary syphilis

    1. Benzathine penicillin G (BiCillin®) 2.4 million units IM stat.* Caution re: Jarisch-Herxheimer Reaction: in 50% of cases, 6–12 hours after injection, patient develops high fever, malaise, and exacerbation of symptoms lasting 24 hours. (This is a sign that the spirochete is breaking down)

    2. For penicillin allergy: Doxycycline 100 mg orally BID x 14 days OR Tetracycline 500 mg orally QID x 14 days

B. For early latent syphilis (<1 year)

    1. Benzathine penicillin G, 2.4 million units IM single dose

C. For late latent syphilis or unknown duration

    1. Benzathine penicillin G, 7.2 million units total, in 3 doses of 2.4 million units IM each at 7–day intervals

D. For later syphilis or unknown duration

---

*In some states the guideline is two doses of benzathin-penicillin 2.4 million units 1 week apart.

1. Benzathine penicillin G, 7.2 million units total, in 3 doses of 2.4 million units IM each at 7–day intervals
E. In pregnancy
    1. Treat with penicillin regimen appropriate for stage of syphilis
    2. Hospitalize pregnant patients with history of penicillin allergies to undergo skin testing. If positive, should be desensitized and treated with penicillin. See current CDC guidelines
F. General measures
    1. Support, especially in regard to possible Jarisch-Herxheimer Reaction
    2. Stress importance of completing all medication
    3. Partner should be treated concurrently; all contacts exposed within 90 days of diagnosis of primary, secondary, or early latent syphilis

VIII. Complications
A. Progression of disease to tertiary stage
B. 100% transmission to fetus with primary and secondary in pregnancy; 50% fetal mortality and 50% congenital syphilis. Early latent: 80% fetal infection (20% premature, 20% fetal death, 40% congenital syphilis). Late latent: 30% fetal transmission, 11% fetal death.

IX. Consultation/Referral
Positive diagnosis of disease

X. Follow-up
Serology tests for primary and secondary syphilis (nontreponemal serologic) should be obtained at 6 and 12 months (falling titer should be demonstrated if treatment is adequate—at least a 4–fold drop by 6 months using same test). If repeat titre does not decrease, patient should be followed with titres, or re-treated. For latent syphilis, repeat testing at 6, 12, and 24 months.

See Appendix A and Bibliography.

Chancroid

I. Definition
Chancroid is a bacterial infection of the genitourinary tract in which a rapidly growing ulcerated lesion forms on external genitalia. Definitive diagnosis requires the identification of H. ducreyi using special culture media. Even with the use of these media, sensitivity is ≤ 80%. Diagnosis is usually based on clinical findings.

II. Etiology
A. Causative agent is Haemophilus ducreyi, a short gram negative bacillus with rounded ends, usually found in chains and groups
B. Incubation period, 4–7 days after exposure (rare <3 or >10 days); lesion appears 3–14 days after exposure

III. History
A. What patient may present with
   1. History of (1–3) painful macules on the external genitalia which rapidly changed to a pustule and then to an ulcerated lesion; may have "kissing ulcers" from autoinoculation; can also be painless
   2. Enlarged inguinal nodes
   3. Abscess in inguinal region
   4. A sinus formed over the healed lesion
   5. New lesions forming when exposed to lesions already present
   6. Pain on voiding or defecating
   7. Rectal bleeding
   8. Dyspareunia
B. Additional information to be obtained
   1. History of sexually transmitted disease or pelvic inflammatory disease
   2. Previous vaginal infections; diagnosis, treatment
   3. Previous urinary tract infections
   4. Sexually active
   5. Last sexual contact; new partner
   6. Did partner complain of "sores"
   7. Last menstrual period
   8. Method of birth control; other medications (antibiotics may mask symptoms)
   9. Any associated vaginal discharge; duration of ulcers
   10. Any associated pain
   11. Travel to Asia (Thailand especially), Africa, South America, Philippines in past month

IV. Physical Examination
A. Vital signs
   1. Temperature   2. Blood pressure   3. Pulse
B. Inguinal nodes
   1. Size
   2. Tenderness
   3. Nodes matted together forming a fluctuant abscess (buboes) in groin; usually unilateral inguinal lymphadenopathy

C. External examination
  1. Observe labia, fourchette, clitoris, vagina, anal area for macules, papules
  2. Observe for shallow, nonindurated, painful ulcers with ragged, unde-termined edges, varying in size and often coalesced; base of ulcers may be gray/bluish gray; surrounding red halo
  3. Observe for sinuses which may have formed when skin over abscesses has broken down
  4. Look for new lesions which may be forming as a result of autoinoculation
D. Vaginal examination (speculum); observe for lesions in vagina, on cervix
E. Bimanual examination

V. Laboratory Examination
A. Usually based on clinical findings and history
B. Cultures to laboratory; use media containing fresh defibrinated rabbit's blood or patient's own serum
C. Darkfield exam for T. pallidum or serologic test for syphilis performed at least 7 days after onset of lesions and repeated in 3 months
D. Gonococcus culture, Chlamydia test
E. Herpes antibodies
F. HIV testing should be done at the time of this diagnosis and again in 3 months if initial results are negative
G. Further laboratory work as indicated
H. PCR testing for H. ducreyi when it becomes available

VI. Differential Diagnosis
A. Herpes simplex
B. Syphilis

VII. Treatment
A. Medications
  1. Azithromycin 1 gram orally single dose OR
  2. Ceftriaxone 250 mg IM single dose OR
  3. Ciprofloxacin 500 mg orally BID for 3 days (safety in children <15 years of age or in pregnancy or lactation has not been established) OR
  4. Erythromycin base 500 mg orally TID x 7 days
B. Medications in Pregnancy
  1. Ceftriaxone 250 mg IM single dose OR
  2. Erythromycin base 500 mg orally TID for 7 days
C. General measures
  1. Buboes should be aspirated through adjacent intact skin, not incised
  2. No sexual contact until course of medication is finished
  3. Stress importance of completing course of medication

4. Comfort measures
   a. Tepid water sitz baths; dry carefully with cool air hair dryer making sure to hold it away from body
   b. Avoid tight, restricting clothing
   c. Expose perineum to air flow as much as possible (wear a skirt without underpants when at home)
   d. Recommend peri-irrigation set for comfort
5. Patient education
   a. Explain disease process and route of transmission
   b. Stress that sexual partner(s) need to be checked regularly (see X.C.)

VIII. Complications
A. Phimosis in the male
B. Urethral stricture
C. Urethral fistula
D. Severe tissue destruction
E. Ulcers may take years to heal
F. Perineal fistulas

IX. Consultation/Referral
A. Physician if infection is suspected
B. If no response after 7 days of treatment, treatment as outlined above
C. Secondary infections
D. All HIV positive persons diagnosed with chancroid

X. Follow-up
A. Patient should be reexamined 3–7 days after initiation of therapy. If treatment is successful, there should be symptomatic improvement within 3 days of starting therapy. Clinical improvement should be evident within 7 days. If no improvement, consultation as above
B. It should be noted that it may take ≥ 2 weeks for complete healing of ulcers. The amount of time is related to the size of the ulcer
C. All sexual partners who have had sexual contact within 10 days preceding symptoms with a person diagnosed with chancroid should be evaluated and treated even in the absence of symptoms

See Bibliography.

Lymphogranuloma Venereum

I. Definition
Lymphogranuloma venereum is a sexually transmitted disease characterized by a transitory primary lesion followed by suppurative lymphangitis and serious local complications.

II. Etiology
A. Causative agent: Chlamydia trachomatis, serotypes, L1, L2, L3
B. Incubation period 3–12 days up to 3 weeks
C. Found mainly in tropical or subtropical climates (Asia, Africa, South America); rare in USA

III. History
A. What the patient may present with
   1. "Sore" in genital area, mouth, anus, penis (of short duration, may go unnoticed); usually single and painless vesicle or nonindurated
   2. Fever
   3. Malaise
   4. Headaches
   5. Joint pain
   6. Anorexia
   7. Vomiting
   8. Unilateral tender enlargement of inguinal lymph node; stiffness, aching of groin
   9. Abscess in groin after 2–3 weeks
  10. Sinuses, scars in lower vagina or around introitus or (in males) on penis
  11. Rectal discharge; perirectal/perianal fistulas and strictures
  12. Vaginal discharge
B. Additional information to be considered
   1. Sexual preference; sexual practices
   2. Last sexual contact; new partner
   3. Known contact
   4. History of sexually transmitted disease or pelvic inflammatory disease
   5. Last menstrual period
   6. Method of birth control; other medications (antibiotics may mask symptoms)
   7. History of chronic infections
   8. Recent trip out of country or new immigrant from a country where LGV is common
   9. Duration of lesion

IV. Physical Examination
A. Vital signs
   1. Blood pressure   3. Respiration
   2. Pulse   4. Temperature
B. Inguinal nodes
   1. First symptoms unilateral tender enlargement of nodes

   2. Disease progresses for 2–3 weeks to form a large, tender, fluctuant mass that adheres to deep tissues and has overlying reddened skin (bubo)
   3. Multiple sinuses develop with purulent or serosanguineous discharge
   4. Healing occurs with scar formation, but sinuses persist or recur
   5. Chronic inflammation causes blockage of the lymphatic vessels leading to edema, ulceration and fistula formation
C. Vaginal examination (speculum)
   1. Vaginal walls: initial lesion may be on upper vaginal wall, resulting in enlargement and suppuration of perirectal and pelvic lymphatic vessels
   2. Cervix: initial lesion could be on the cervix
D. Bimanual examination
Tenderness in groin, vulva
E. Rectovaginal examination
Rectal wall may be involved, resulting in ulcerative proctitis with serosanguineous rectal discharge

V. Laboratory Examination and Diagnosis
A. LGV complement fixation test: fourfold rise or single titer of $\geq$ 1:64; (80% of patients have titer 1:16 or higher)
B. Serology test for syphilis, gonorrhea culture, Chlamydia test
C. Biopsy of chronic anorectal lesions to rule out carcinoma
D. Microimmunofluorescence test (microl F) measures specific antibody and distinguishes various serotypes of antibody (use if titer $\geq$ 1:512
E. In absence of microimmunofluorescence test, diagnosis may be made by careful history, clinical examination, and presence of high or rising titers of LGV complement fixation antibodies

VI. Differential Diagnosis
A. Syphilis
B. Herpes simplex
C. Carcinoma
D. Chancroid
E. Granuloma inguinale
F. Chlamydia
G. Hodgkin's disease

VII. Treatment
A. Medications
   1. Doxycycline 100 mg orally BID x 21 days

2. Alternative regimen Erythromycin base 500 mg orally QID for 21 days
B. Medications in pregnancy and lactation
   1. Erythromycin base 500 mg orally QID for 21 days
C. General measures
   1. Sitz bath
   2. Stress importance of completing the course of medication
   3. All sexual partners should be treated if contact within 30 days before onset of symptoms; examine and test for Chlamydia/gonorrhea in urethra, cervix
   4. Comfort measures
      a. Tepid water sitz baths; dry carefully with cool air hair dryer making sure to hold it sufficiently away from body
      b. Avoid tight, restricting clothing
      c. Expose perineum to air flow as much as possible (wear a skirt or robe without underpants at home)
      d. Recommend peri-irrigation set
   5. Patient education
      a. Explain disease process and route of transmission
      b. Stress importance of sexual partner(s) within 30 days of onset of symptoms being checked for urethral or cervical chlamydia

VIII. Complications
A. Scar formation
B. Sinuses causing blockage of the lymphatic vessels which leads to edema
C. Fistula formation: rectovaginal, vulvar, other
D. Suppuration of perirectal and lymphatic vessels
E. Rectal stricture
F. Systemic: phlebitis, hepatomegaly, nephropathy

IX. Consultation/Referral
A. With physician prior to treatment if infection is suspected
B. If no response to treatment as outlined above
C. If any of the above complications occur

X. Follow-up
A. Reevaluate 3–5 days after treatment
B. Then evaluate every 1–2 weeks until healing is complete

See Bibliography.

Granuloma Inguinale

I. Definition
Granuloma inguinale (Donovanosis) is a chronic granulomatous bacterial infection usually involving the genitalia and surrounding tissues, and probably spread by sexual contact.

II. Etiology
A. Usually found in tropical and subtropical areas
B. Calymmato bacterium granulomatis (a difficult-to-grow encapsulated bacillus organism)
C. Incubation period, 5–6 weeks (some sources say anywhere from 1–12 weeks)

III. History
A. What the patient presents with
   1. Female
      a. Painless papular or nodular ulcerative lesions arising on the vulva, in the vagina, urethra, anal area, inguinal region or on the perineum with proliferation of granulation tissue and local destruction with scar tissue formation; single or mutiple
      b. Beefy red proliferative lesion of fourchette with elevated rolled borders; bleeds easily
      c. Inguinal adenopathy (due to secondary infection)—bilateral
      d. Malodorous vaginal discharge
   2. Male
      a. Lesion same as in the female and appearing on penis, scrotum, groin or thighs
      b. In homosexual males, lesions on anus and buttocks
B. Additional information to be obtained
   1. History of sexually transmitted disease or pelvic inflammatory disease
   2. History of chronic illness
   3. Has patient recently been out of country? Where? (Especially India, Papua New Guinea, central Australia, southern Africa.) Is patient or patient's partner from, or has either visited, southeastern U.S.?
   4. Sexual preference; sexual practices (anal intercourse; sex toys)
   5. Last sexual contact
   6. Birth control method, current medications
   7. Last menstrual period

IV. Physical Examination
A. Vital signs

1. Temperature   3. Pulse
2. Blood pressure   4. Respirations
B. External examination
   Observe vulva for lesions (papular, nodular, or vesicular), beefy red nod-
   ules which develop into a rounded, elevated, velvety granulomatous mass;
   sharply defined rolled borders; signs of secondary infection
C. Vaginal examination (speculum)
   1. Inspect vaginal walls for lesions
   2. Inspect cervix for lesions
D. Bimanual examination

V. Laboratory Diagnosis
A. Giemsa-stained smears of ulcer (diagnosis is confirmed by identifying Donovan bodies, large mononuclear cells with intracytoplasmic
   vacuoles containing the organism)—scrape at base of ulcer to get
   some fluid
B. Syphilis serology
C. HSV culture

VI. Differential Diagnosis
A. Syphilis   E. Carcinoma
B. Herpes simplex   F. Fungal infection
C. Lymphogranuloma venereum   G. Genital Amoebiasis
D. Chancroid

VII. Treatment
A. Medication
   1. Doxycycline 100 mg orally BID for at least 3 weeks OR
   2. Trimethoprim-sulfamethoxazole one double-strength tablet (800 mg/
      160 mg) orally BID for at least 3 weeks
B. Alternative regimens
   1. Ciprofloxacin 750 mg BID for at least 3 weeks OR
   2. Erythromycin base 500 mg orally QID for at least 3 weeks OR
   3. Azithromycin 1 g. orally once a week for at least 3 weeks
C. In pregnancy and lactation
   1. Erythromycin base 500 mg orally BID for minimum of 3 weeks plus
      strongly consider gentamicin parenterally (or other parenteral aminogly-
      coside)
D. Additional therapy for all adults
   1. Gentamicin 1 mg/kg IV every 8 hours if lesions do not respond within
      first few days of therapy (or other parenteral aminoglycoside)

E. General measures
   1. No sexual contact until treatment is completed
   2. Stress importance of completing course of medication
   3. Stress importance of examination of sexual contacts (within 60 days preceding onset of symptoms)

VIII. Complications
A. Scar tissue secondary to slow healing formation
B. Secondary infection, a common occurrence that results in gross tissue necrosis of genitalia
C. Deformity of genitalia
D. Dyspareunia
E. Systemic infection
F. Massive edema of vulva; penis (may be chronic)

IX. Consultation/Referral
A. With physician prior to treatment if disease is suspected
B. No response to treatment as discussed above in 7 days—contact CDC or state health department

X. Follow-up
A. After completion of 2 to 5 days of medication
B. Follow clinically until signs and symptoms have resolved
C. Annual follow-up visits as disease can reappear and there is a possibility of scar carcinoma

   See Bibliography.

Molluscum Contagiosum

I. Definition
Molluscum contagiosum is an infectious disease of the skin affecting the face, arms, genitals, abdomen, and thighs. It is caused by a virus (molluscipox virus) and is seen in all age groups and in both sexes.

II. Etiology
A. Unknown
B. Probably transmitted through direct skin contact
C. Incubation 1 week–6 months (usual 2–7 weeks)

III. History
A. What the patient may present with
  1. Fleshy growths (1–20), dome-shaped, waxy or pearly white papules with central caseous white core, primarily in genital area, but may be found on other body surfaces; may be 1–5 mm in diameter (but up to 15 mm), may be pedunculated; can be single or grouped
  2. No other symptoms or complaints but occasional pruritus, tenderness and/or pain
B. Additional information to be considered
  1. Previous episode of similar lesions
  2. History of sexually transmitted disease
  3. Sexual activity, last intercourse
  4. Known contact
  5. Method of birth control; other medications
  6. Any drug allergies
  7. HIV risk/exposure, especially with widespread lesions ≥ 100

IV. Physical Examination
A. External examination
  1. Observe perineum for fleshy, usually papular, skin-colored lesions with indented centers that contain white, curd-like material
  2. Observe any other involved body area

V. Laboratory Examination
A. Visual examination
B. Pathology report on crushed excised lesion using Papanicolaou smear, Wright's, Giemsa's, or Gram stain
C. Serology test for syphilis
D. Gonococcus culture/Chlamydia test
E. Further laboratory work as indicated by history
F. Consider HIV screen especially with 100 or more lesions

VI. Differential Diagnosis
A. Genital warts (condylomata acuminata)
B. Herpes simplex
C. Pyogenic granuloma
D. Folliculitis
E. Small epidermal cysts
F. Closed comedones
G. Basal cell carcinoma

H. Furunculosis

VII. Treatment
A. Removal of lesion
   1. Cytotoxic agents—TCA (trichloracetic acid), BCA (bichloracetic acid), podophyllin
   2. Excision of lesions by curettage with topical anesthetic followed by application of silver nitrate
   3. Destruction of lesions by cryotherapy; consider MD consult
   4. Topical 5% imiquimod qd x 5 days/week hs
B. General measures
   1. Return for weekly or biweekly evaluation and treatment until lesions have healed
   2. Refer sexual partner(s) for evaluation

VIII. Complications
A. Secondary staphylococcus infection

IX. Consultation/Referral
A. For treatment stated above
B. Patients with extensive molluscum, lesions on face, or repeated recurrence after treatment should be reevaluated for HIV infection

X. Follow-up
A. Return for reevaluation if lesions persist/recur after treatment

   See Bibliography.

Hepatitis

I. Definition
Hepatitis is an acute or chronic inflammation of the liver with or without permanent tissue damage and can be caused by many viruses including influenza viruses, mononucleosis and CMV; there are also hepatitis viruses whose only target is the liver. At least 6 are known at present and are designated by the letters A, B, C, D, E and G.

II. Etiology
Causative organisms include hepatitis viruses A to E and G, mononucleosis virus, CMV, and various influenza viruses

A. Hepatitis A (HAV) is transmitted enterically (rarely parenterally) with an incubation of 15–50 days, 28 day average
B. Hepatitis B (HBV) is transmitted parenterally, sexually via body fluids, perinatally, or from saliva from human bites; incubation 45–180 days, 60–90 days average
C. Hepatitis C (HCV) is transmitted parenterally and permucosally, with an incubation of 2–26 weeks, average 8–9 weeks; major cause of posttransfusion hepatitis. It is thought that sexual and perinatal transmission may be possible, but is rare unless mother is co-infected with HIV
D. Hepatitis D (HDV), known as Delta virus, only affects persons who have active hepatitis B; transmitted parenterally, sexually and perinatally. Incubation 3–13 weeks.
E. Hepatitis E (HEV) is transmitted enterically (rarely parenterally) with 15–60 days, mean 40 days incubation
F. Hepatitis G: Percutaneous route

III. History
A. What the patient may present with
   1. Right upper quadrant pain (may be intermittent)
   2. Loss of appetite
   3. Malaise, fatigue (increased sleep, ↓ activity level, ↓ libido)
   4. Fever, often low grade
   5. Flulike symptoms, including headache
   6. Adenopathy
   7. Jaundice
   8. Nausea and vomiting
   9. Rash, hives
   10. Joint and muscle pain
   11. Darkened urine
   12. Light-colored stools
   13. Taste and smell peculiarities
   14. Intolerance of fatty foods, cigarettes
B. Additional information to consider
   1. Use of recreational drugs
   2. Alcohol use, quantity and frequency
   3. Medication use (including nontraditional remedies, herbal preparations)
   4. Partner an injectable drug user
   5. Recent transfusion of blood or blood products
   6. Recent surgery
   7. Eating raw or undercooked shellfish

8. Daycare worker or has child/children in day care
9. Occupational risks including exposure to body fluids, excrement; blood, blood products
10. Sexual history and habits, especially anal intercourse; number of partners; use of sex toys; human bites
11. History of sexually transmitted diseases
12. Sexual partner and/or household member with symptoms
13. Known exposure to someone with hepatitis
14. Military or civilian service in the Middle East; travel to Africa, Asia, Central & South America, Eastern Europe, Alaska
15. History of hepatitis B
16. Visited or from disease-endemic areas of world
17. Hemodialysis patient; transplant recipient; hemophiliac
18. Inmate of correctional institution
19. Contraceptive history
20. History of needlestick injury, tattoos, body piercing; acupuncture, sharing toothbrushes, razors, nail files, clippers
21. Infants of HBV & HCV mothers

IV. Physical Examination
A. Vital signs
  1. Temperature
  2. Pulse
  2. Respirations
  4. Blood pressure
B. Abdomen
  1. Liver percussion, palpation
  2. Observation of skin color, turgor
  3. Organomegaly, tenderness
  4. Masses
  5. Adenopathy
C. Complete physical examination with careful attention to
  1. Skin: rash, hives, color, turgor
  2. Joints: joint pain on range of motion; muscle pain
  3. Adenopathy

V. Laboratory Examination
A. Feces for virus
B. Liver function tests
C. Mononucleosis screen
D. Serology to determine type of hepatitis
  HAV: IgM anti-HAV in serum with acute or convalescent phase (5–10 days into incubation up to 6 months)

HBV: several including HBsAg (HBV surface antigen); IgM Anti-HBc
HCV: test for antibody with ELISA followed by the RIBA (recombinant immunoblot assay); for ambiguous results PCR assay is used
HDV: HBsAg, Anti-HDV
HEV: Ig Manti-HEV; IgG anti-HEV
HGV: PCR testing, test for HAV, HBV, HCV, HDV, HEV
E. CMV
F. HIV testing
G. In severe hepatitis, serum albumin, prothrombin, and partial thromboplastin times, electrolytes, glucose, CBC, platelets
H. Pregnancy test

VI. Differential Diagnosis
Infectious mononucleosis, primary or secondary hepatic malignancy, ischemic hepatitis, drug-induced hepatitis, alcoholic hepatitis, acute fatty liver (acute fatty metamorphosis) of pregnancy

VII. Treatment
A. As needed according to laboratory report and etiology; generally referral for medical management and follow-up
B. Supportive for symptoms
   1. No alcohol during acute phase of hepatitis and for 6–12 months thereafter
   2. Adequate calories; balanced diet
C. Interferon is being used for HBV, HCV*
D. Gamma globulin to household and daycare center contacts for hepatitis A within 2 weeks of exposure
E. Prevention for hepatitis B: for exposed persons HBV hyperimmune globulin and then hepatitis B vaccination after antibody testing
F. Prevention for hepatitis D: hepatitis B vaccination
G. HAV recovery not aided by activity limitation; isolate food handlers with HAV; prevention for HAV HAVRIX® or VAQTA® vaccine

VIII. Complications
A. Hepatitis A: rarely fatal, no chronic form, fulminant hepatitis, relapse
B. Hepatitis B: death; chronic disease in 5–10% of victims; of these, 50% get chronic liver disease leading to hepatocellular carcinoma in half of the cases; fulminant hepatitis, transmission to fetus 10–85%

---

*Research on Hepatitis C with combination treatment Rebetron®, Rebetrol® (ribavirin) and Introl® (interferon alfa-26, recombinant)

C. Hepatitis C: >50% of cases become chronic; cirrhosis; hepatocellular carcinoma; perinatal transmission
D. Hepatitis D: chronic liver disease, fulminant hepatitis
E. Hepatitis E: high mortality in pregnancy (fetus and mother); no reported chronic cases
F. Hepatitis G: little information to date

IX. Consultation/Referral
A. For medical treatment and follow-up

X. Follow-up
A. As appropriate for type of hepatitis
B. Encourage hepatitis B vaccination (HBV) of those who have not had disease; schedule 3 dose administration; okay in pregnancy and lactation
C. Repeat laboratory work as indicated for monitoring liver function after illness
D. Test for chronic HBV with serum assay for HBsAg
E. Encourage HAV vaccination for persons at increased risk*
F. Note availability of TWINRIX—HAV and HAB combined 3–dose vaccine

See Bibliography; http://www.cdc.gov/ncidod/diseases/hepatitis

HIV/AIDS

PREFACE: Information on AIDS/HIV continues to increase and change. Since our role as practitioners in ambulatory settings is to identify, educate, and refer persons at high risk for the disease, the purpose of this protocol is to serve as a guide in those three areas only. Because AIDS has become the leading cause of death among young women, it has become increasingly important that women's health care providers keep abreast of current information by consulting professional journals and attending seminars on the subject

I. Definition
AIDS is the commonly used acronym for acquired immune deficiency syndrome, which is the name for a complex of health problems first reported in 1981.

---

*One state now requires HAV vaccination for school children.

II. Etiology
Caused by the human immune deficiency virus (HIV); infection mainly by sexual contact (anal, vaginal, oral), contaminated blood and blood products including needle and syringe sharing, contaminated semen used for artificial insemination, intrauterine acquisition (baby of woman with AIDS) and rarely breast milk.

III. History
A. What the patient may present with
  1. Rapid weight loss without known factor (>10%)
  2. Extreme fatigue; unexplained, increasing tiredness
  3. Chronic diarrhea (>1 month)
  4. Persistent dry cough, shortness of breath, dyspnea on exertion
  5. Prolonged fever, soaking night sweats, shaking chills
  6. Loss of appetite
  7. Purple or pink flat or raised lesions on skin or under skin, inside mouth, nose, eyelids, anus
  8. Changes in neurological and/or cognitive function
  9. Generalized adenopathy
  10. Chronic herpes simplex
  11. Recurrent herpes zoster
  12. Generalized dermatitis pruritic
  13. Oral and pharyngeal candidiasis; fungal infection of nails
  14. Persistent muscle pain
  15. Fear of exposure to AIDS through sexual partner or high-risk behavior or work-related accident (needlestick, contact with infected blood)
  16. Chronic sinusitis
  17. History of abnormal Papanicolaou smears
  18. Persistent vulvar, vaginal and anal condyloma
B. Additional information to be considered
  1. Sexual history
    a. Homosexual encounters; anal penetration
    b. Use of condoms, other methods of contraception, anal intercourse as contraception
    c. High-risk partners
    d. High-risk sexual practices
    e. History of previous sexually transmitted disease
    f. Contact with prostitute
    g. Multiple partners or partner with multiple partners
  2. Use of injectable drugs by self or partner
  3. High-risk occupation

4. History of blood transfusions or recipient of blood products particularly from 1980–1985
5. Duration and frequency of any presenting symptoms
6. Reason for fear of exposure to AIDS
7. Gynecological history
   a. Recurrent sexually transmitted diseases, vaginitis, vaginosis
   b. Widespread molluscum contagiosum ≥100 lesions
   c. Infected with several sexually transmitted diseases concurrently (may include gonorrhea, syphilis, Chlamydia)
   d. Rapidly progressing cervical dysplasia
   e. Papillomavirus on Papanicolaou smear
   f. Recurrent, recalcitrant vaginal candidiasis
   g. External condyloma unresponsive to treatment
   h. Existing pregnancy
   i. Anal discharge
   j. Pelvic, abdominal pain

IV. Physical Examination
A. As appropriate to presenting complaint

V. Laboratory Examination
A. Per protocol for presenting complaint, symptoms, risk status, exposure
B. HIV testing if indicated or requested; if setting offers testing, resources must be in place for both pretest and posttest counseling for positive or negative results and follow-up; retest as needed
C. All pregnant women should have HIV screen and encourage one for women planning a pregnancy
D. Workplace exposures

VI. Differential Diagnosis
A. Widely different depending on presenting complaint

VII. Treatment
A. General measures
   1. Counseling to avoid or minimize high-risk behaviors
      a. Instruction and counseling regarding safer sexual practices to protect self and partner from exchange of body fluids (e.g., by using latex condoms, female condoms, dental dams, Saran Wrap™); by avoiding anal intercourse and oral-genital contact; avoiding sharing sex toys such as vibrators and dildos (or clean them with bleach or alcohol)

    b. Decreased number of sexual partners; mutual monogamy; abstinence
    c. Discourage use of injectable drugs; if patient is using injectable drugs, stress the need to avoid needle, works, or cooker sharing; offer resources on drug rehabilitation programs
    d. Avoid unsafe sexual contact with persons who are injectable drug users or fall into other high-risk groups
    e. Sexual activities with partner with AIDS that do not involve direct passage of body fluids, such as light kissing, caressing, mutual masturbation
    f. Empowering women to maintain equal decision making power in their relationship(s)
    g. Avoid sharing razors, toothbrushes, nail files & clippers, other items that could be contaminated with blood
B. Specific treatment
    1. Per protocol for specific presenting complaint
    2. Refer those patients falling into high-risk groups for further counseling and appropriate testing and follow-up if setting does not offer such services
    3. Referral for exposure so prophylactic therapy can be instituted

VIII. Complications
A. Opportunistic infections
B. AIDS may be fatal to some of its victims within two years of diagnosis
C. Transmission to unborn child (infant's true HIV status based on antibody testing will not be accurate until 6–10 months); for a child <18 months, definitive tests include evidence of HIV in blood or tissues by culture, nucleic acid or antigen detection

IX. Consultations and Referral
A. All patients falling into high-risk groups in need of testing for presence of HIV virus unless setting offers testing and counseling
B. Referral for all patients testing positive to HIV antibody for appropriate treatment

X. Follow-up
A. Per referral
B. Contraceptive and gynecological services for women with AIDS
See Appendix F for self-assessment of AIDS (HIV) risk list which can be photocopied or adapted for your patients. See Bibliography. www.cdc.gov/nchstp/hiv_aids/hivinfo.htm

Safe Practices for Practitioners*

1. Dispose of all needles, scalpels, capillary tubes, glass slides, lancets, and other sharp items in puncture-resistant containers. Handle as little as possible (i.e., do not recap needles).

2. Wear gloves** *when anticipating* exposure to body fluids, including for phlebotomy and for handling specimens (urine, blood, stool, sputum, vaginal secretions), and for contact with any mucus membranes (vaginal, oral, nasal, rectal) and open wounds. Don't substitute gloves for handwashing, however.

3. Wear gloves, gowns, masks, goggles as appropriate when there is to be extensive contact with body fluids as during surgery or delivery; wear double gloves for surgical procedures when possible. Change any blood-stained clothing as soon as possible.

4. Wash thoroughly (with copious amounts of soap and water) following any skin contact with patient's body fluids.

5. Wear gloves on both hands for vaginal and rectal exams; use careful technique to keep one hand clean when handling clean materials such as fixative spray for Pap smears or examination lights; wash after examination is completed. Goggles are now recommended for vaginal examinations and phlebotomy in ambulatory as well as inpatient settings.

6. Change gloves for rectal examination after vaginal examination or for fitting a diaphragm or cervical cap after pelvic examination.

7. Avoid contamination of surfaces in the examining room or laboratory with body fluids from patients.

8. Use chlorine bleach solution 1:10*** in a spray bottle to clean examining table and other surfaces and items contaminated with body fluids.

---

*Adapted from Bennett, B. & Duff, P. (1991). The effect of double gloving on frequency of glove perforations. *Obstetrics & Gynecology, 78,* 1019–1022; Gritter, M. (1998). The latex threat. *American Journal of Nursing, 98,* 26–32; Nenstiel, R.O., White, G.L. & Aikens, T. (1997). Handwashing: A century of evidence ignored. *Clinical Reviews, 7*(1), 55–62; Yeargin, P. (1998). An important risk group: Managing occupational HIV exposure. *ADVANCE for Nurse Practitioners, 6*(11), 55–93; Youngkin, E.Q. (1988). Keeping pelvic examination technique safe. *The Nurse Practitioner, 13*(1), 40–42.

**Latex gloves are the best protection. However, be aware of the possibility of latex allergy. Symptoms can be mild to severe and are typical of anaphylactic reactions: watery eyes, itching rash, shortness of breath, decrease in blood pressure, and even death. Latex-free gloves are available. One can also wear vinyl gloves under latex gloves, or wear nylon or cloth glove liners. A new product called Nitrile is artificial latex by SafeSkin Corporation.

***Due to instability with exposure to oxygen, this must be prepared daily. Commercial products are also available in single-use packets. These maintain chemical stability.

Several other commercial products are available for this use. Wear gloves for clean-up.

9. Keep hands from becoming dry and cracked.

10. Follow Centers for Disease Control (CDC) and OSHA recommendations and updates for protection of self and patients. (CDC http://www.cdc.gov; OSHA http://www.osha.gov)

11. Assume every patient has the potential to be infected with AIDS or to be HIV positive and protect him/her and yourself with good technique.

12. Educate staff and patients about modes of infection, protection, and address myths to dispel unwarranted fears.

See Bibliography.

4

Miscellaneous Gynecological Aberrations

Bartholin's Cyst

I. Definition

Bartholin's cyst is a postinflammatory pseudocyst that forms proximally to the obstructed duct of a Bartholin's gland

II. Etiology

A. Responsible organisms include
  1. Staphylococcus aureus
  2. Streptococcus fecalis
  3. Escherichia coli (E. coli)
  4. Pseudomonas may also be cultured from abscess
  5. Gonococcus
  6. Chlamydia trachomatis

III. History

A. What the patient may present with
  1. Painful, swollen lump in vaginal area
  2. Difficulty sitting and walking due to severe pain and swelling
B. Additional information to be considered
  1. Previous infection of a Bartholin's gland; if yes, how was it treated?
  2. History of sexually transmitted disease

IV. Physical Examination

A. Vital signs
  1. Temperature   2. Blood pressure
B. Visual examination of external genitalia
  1. Cyst is characteristically located in the lower half of the labia with its inner wall immediately adjacent to the lower vaginal canal
  2. Lesions may vary in size from 1–10 cm
  3. The involved area may be painfully tender
  4. There may be no subjective symptoms

V. Laboratory Examination
A. Culture lesion at time of incision and drainage
B. Consider cervical cultures for Chlamydia and gonorrhea

VI. Differential Diagnosis
A. Lipoma
B. Fibroma
C. Hydrocele
D. Carcinoma of Bartholin's gland (extremely rare)
E. Inclusion cysts, sebaceous cysts
F. Congenital anomaly

VII. Treatment
A. Sitz baths QID x 2–3 days, then reexamine. If size has increased or there is no change, perform incision and drainage or refer to physician for possible marsupialization. If cyst is extremely painful or large, immediate physician referral
B. Antibiotics as appropriate to organism; most common ampicillin 500 mg QID x 7 days or cephalexin 250 mg QID x 7 days or 500 mg BID x 7 days

VIII. Complications
Recurrence

IX. Consultation/Referral
II. A. and B. above

X. Follow-up
At clinician's discretion after incision and drainage or marsupialization

See Bibliography.

Vulvar Conditions*

I. Definition
Primary vulvar conditions are those that arise from abnormal epithelial growth that can be inflammatory, dermatologic, or congenital in origin or from

---

*The authors are indebted to Luisa Fertitta, MS, RNC, and Mimi Secor, RNC, MS, FNP for their work in this area.

neoplastic alterations. Since the vulva includes the labia majora and minora, the mons veneris, fourchette, and vestibule, and encompasses the urethral and vaginal orifices and the ducts of the Skene's and Bartholin's glands, vulvar conditions are varied both in origin and in clinical manifestations. Please refer to separate protocols for sexually transmitted diseases that can cause clinical signs and symptoms on the vulva, and protocols for Bartholin's cyst, molluscum contagiosum, herpes, and condyloma.

II. Etiology
A. Nonneoplastic epithelial disorders
    1. squamous cell hyperplasia
    2. lichen simplex chronicus
    3. lichen sclerosis
    4. pigmented lesions
    5. systemic diseases
B. Neoplastic disorder (vulvar intracellular neoplasia—VIN)
    1. vulvar intraepithelial neoplasia
        a. low grade squamous intraepithelial lesion (SIL) mild dysplasia
        b. high grade SIL moderate to severe dysplasia
        c. carcinoma in situ
        d. VIN 2–3
        e. Invasive VIN
    2. Other neoplastic disorders
        a. Paget's versus vulvar vaginal candidiasis (VVC)
        b. Melanoma (5% is vulvar)

III. History
A. What the patient may present with
    1. Pruritus, rash
    2. Hypo- or hyperpigmentation
    3. Bullae
    4. Weeping, scaling, crusting
    5. Excoriation
    6. Maceration
    7. Thickening
    8. Hyperkeratosis
    9. Fissures
   10. Abscesses
   11. Lesions: macules, papules, vesicles, warty, pedunculated, domed, flat, plaques
   12. Lichenification
   13. Change in color of vulva

14. Dyspareunia
15. Burning
B. Additional information to be considered
  1. Type of clothing commonly worn
  2. Type of underwear: cotton, synthetic
  3. Use of feminine deodorant products
  4. Use of scented, deodorant tampons, pads, panty liners
  5. Douching; shaving of perineum
  6. Detergents, bathing soap, fabric softeners
  7. Bubble bath or oils, body washes, lotions, creams
  8. Family or personal history of diabetes
  9. Sexual partners, activity; contraception; STD history
  10. Fungal infection of hands and feet, self or partner; oral candidiasis
  11. Last menstrual period
  12. Perimenopausal symptoms
  13. History of dermatologic conditions: HPV; psoriasis, eczema, seborrheic dermatitis
  14. Fever, malaise, flulike symptoms
  15. Character and changes in lesions
  16. Partner with symptoms
  17. History of Crohn's disease; other systemic disease
  18. Genital HPV history, history of Papanicolaou smear with HPV; any abnormal Papanicolaou history
  19. Any other possible allergens: plant, make-up, nail polish, depillatories, piercings & jewelry

IV. Physical Examination
A. Vulva
  1. Skin appearance: inflammation, edema, dry or moist, thickening hyperkeratosis
  2. Lesions present
  3. Weeping, scaling, crusting
  4. Fissuring
  5. Lichenification
  6. Excoriation
  7. Hypopigmentation
  8. Hyperpigmentation
B. Adenopathy
C. Groin, inner thighs, buttocks
  1. Lesions
D. Other systems as indicated by history and drugs

V. Laboratory Examination as Indicated by History and Appearance of Lesions
A. Bacterial cultures and sensitivities
B. Wood's lamp examination
C. Grain-stain scraping from lesions
D. Scrapings in KOH
E. Punch biopsy of lesions
F. Colposcopic examination
G. Staining with 1% toluidine blue
H. Fasting blood sugar
I. HPV testing

VI. Differential Diagnosis
A. Allergic vulvitis, cellulitis
B. Inflammatory conditions and reactions
C. Bacterial, viral, fungal infections
D. Lichen sclerosis
E. Necrotizing fasciitis
F. Pigmentation disorders
   1. Hyperpigmentation
   2. Congenital hypopigmentation
G. Benign epithelial changes
H. Neoplasms: vulvar intraepithelial neoplasia, Paget's disease, melanoma
I. Lesions from Crohn's disease
J. Trauma
K. Infestation

VII. Treatment
A. Medication
   1. Contact dermatitis: Burow's compresses; 1% cortisone cream
   2. Bacterial infections: Erythromycin 250 mg QID x 14 days; tetracycline 250 mg QID x 10–14 days or until resolved
   3. Tinea: topical antifungals such as GyneLotrimin, Mycelex, or Monistat Derm
   4. Analgesics for pain
   5. Topical antibiotics
B. Lifestyle changes and self-care measures
   1. Loose cotton underwear; no underwear in bed
   2. Keep area dry and clean
   3. Discontinue use of irritant or allergen
   4. Hot packs
   5. Sitz baths

C. Teaching and reassurance

VIII. Complications
A. Secondary infection
B. Progressive disease
C. Masking more serious disease

IX. Consultation/Referral
A. Unable to identify lesion or condition
B. No response to treatment
C. Progression of disease
D. For biopsy, diagnostic work-up
E. For surgical excision or other surgical intervention
F. To specialist for systemic disease or dermatoses beyond the vulva
G. To specialist for vulvar vestibulitis and vulvodynia

X. Follow-up
As indicated by therapy or for further diagnostic work.

Appendix G gives directions for vulvar self-examination which you may want to distribute to your patients.

See Bibliography.

Acute Pelvic Pain

I. Definition
Acute pelvic pain can be defined as sudden onset of severe lower abdominal pain assessed to be gynecologic in nature

II. Etiology
A. Physiologic causes
   1. Infection from a variety of organisms resulting in pelvic inflammatory disease
   2. Extrauterine pregnancy
   3. Ovarian pathology
   4. Uterine perforation
   5. Ruptured pelvic abscess in a variety of sites
   6. Aberrant uterine leiomyomata
   7. Bladder pathology; bowel pathology
   8. Ureteral pathology
   9. Proliferate endometrium beyond the uterine corpus

10. Postsurgical sequelae
11. Mittelschmerz
12. Trauma, abuse, sexual assault
13. Age related physiologic change
14. Acute cholecystitis
15. Pancreatitis
16. Appendicitis
17. Vascular

B. Psychologic causes
   1. Secondary to pelvic surgery
   2. Secondary to pregnancy whatever the outcome
   3. Secondary to resolved pelvic pathology
   4. Primary or secondary as a focal site for stress; post-traumatic stress disorder secondary to or 2° sexual abuse, assault

III. History

A. What the patient may present with
   1. Sudden onset of symptoms
   2. Chills, fever, body aches
   3. May have nausea, vomiting, and/or diarrhea
   4. May have constipation
   5. Increased vaginal discharge
   6. Acute, continuous or intermittent cramping
   7. Urinary symptoms including frequency and pain
   8. Missed menses
   9. Menses at time of onset
   10. History of pelvic surgery
   11. History of ovarian cysts
   12. History of extrauterine pregnancy
   13. History of PID
   14. History of urinary tract infection
   15. History of endometriosis
   16. History of gonorrhea or Chlamydia infection
   17. History of rape, sexual assault, incest
   18. History of bowel disease

B. Additional information to be considered
   1. Location of pain: stay in any one place or variable; ever have this pain before
   2. Description of pain: sharp, dull, throbbing; rate pain
   3. When does pain occur; does it wake patient up

4. Does anything induce the pain such as eating, defecating, urinating, sexual intercour:e, sexual stimulation; beliefs about cause of pain
5. What if anything relieves the pain
6. Any weight gain or loss
7. Associated symptoms such as diarrhea, blood in stool or urine, increase in vaginal discharge, vaginal bleeding
8. Timing in relation to menses, if any association
9. Duration of symptoms: days, weeks, months; regularity of symptoms
10. Sexual history: exposure to sexually transmitted disease, unprotected intercourse, new partner, change in contraception methods used in recent past and currently; use of sex toys
11. Psychosocial history: unusual stressors at time of onset of when pain occurs; life changes such as moving, new job, new relationship, end of relationship
12. Pelvic surgery in the past 12–24 months such as hysterectomy, laparotomy, tubal ligation
13. Diagnostic pelvic work-up such as laparoscopy, endometrial biopsy, colonoscopy, infertility work-up
14. Change in character of menses: heavier, lighter, more or less frequent

IV. Physical Examination
A. Vital signs as appropriate
    a. Temperature   c. Pulse
    b. Blood pressure   d. Respirations
B. Abdominal examination
    1. Bowel sounds: normal, hyperactive, sluggish, absent, any adventitious sounds, any bruits
    2. Generalized or localized lower abdominal tenderness
    3. Any guarding, pulsations observed
    4. Any rebound tenderness
    5. Any old scars
    6. Any distention
    7. Patient's perception of location of pain
    8. On percussion, are liver or spleen enlarged or is bladder distended
    9. Any pain elicited with light touch; with deep palpation
    10. Any organomegaly or masses
C. Vaginal examination
    1. Examine cervix for discharge
    2. Examine vagina for lesions, discharge, and any unusual odor
D. Bimanual examination

1. Examine cervix for cervical motion tenderness
2. Examine uterus for tenderness
3. Examine adnexa for ovarian tenderness, masses, or tenderness in rest of adnexa

E. Rectal examination
1. Pain or tenderness   2. Masses   3. Melena

F. Elicit psoas sign; perform obturator maneuver

V. Laboratory Examination

A. Cultures as indicated might include gonococcus culture, Chlamydia smear; wet mount; pH of vaginal fluids; vaginal & cervical cultures
B. Complete blood count/differential
C. Sedimentation rate; C-Reactive protein
D. Urinary tract infection screen
E. Pregnancy test—urine, UCG quantitative
F. Ultrasound transvaginal, pelvic, abdominal
G. Flat plate of abdomen; renal ultra sonography
H. Other tests as symptoms and/or history indicate
I. Consider CA125 if age, history, family history, and/or physical findings indicate

VI. Differential Diagnosis

A. Septic abortion
B. Ectopic pregnancy
C. Uterine leiomyomas with hemorrhage or infarction
D. Ovarian cyst with rupture extruding blood, cyst fluid, and dermoid contents into pelvic cavity
E. Uterine perforation
F. Ruptured abscess from ovary, uterus, bowel; tubo-ovarian abscess
G. Urinary tract infection: cystitis or pyelonephritis; kidney stones; interstitial cystitis
H. Appendicitis
I. Adhesions
J. Solid ovarian tumor
K. Irritable bowel syndrome; diverticulitis, acute bowel
L. Primary dysmenorrhea, especially in women over 35
M. Pelvic inflammatory disease
N. Mittelschmerz, especially in women under 35
O. Endometriosis
P. Adenomatosis
Q. Complications of intrauterine device

R. Posttubal ligation syndrome; pelvic pain syndrome
S. Constipation
T. Lower bowel tumor
U. Uterovaginal prolapse
V. Sexual/physical abuse

VII. Treatment
A. Medication as indicated for diagnosis
B. Physician consult for suspected ectopic pregnancy, appendicitis, ovarian pathology, abscess, complications of uterine leiomyomas, suspected pelvic adhesions, irritable bowel syndrome, suspected bowel or other tumors
C. Treatment for primary dysmenorrhea per protocol
D. Removal of IUD; consult as needed for complications
E. Teaching and comfort measures for Mittelschmerz

VIII. Complications
A. Generalized sepsis
B. Hemorrhage
C. Perforation of bowel
D. Rupture of abscess
E. Rupture of site of extrauterine pregnancy
F. Shock
G. Bowel obstruction

IX. Consultation/Referral
A. Unable to find cause
B. Physician consult for medical or surgical intervention
C. For hospitalization if no admitting privileges
D. If symptoms worsen or recur after treatment
E. No response to treatment
F. Unable to remove IUD or find IUD or differentiate cause of problem with method

X. Follow-up
A. Consider reevaluation in 48 hours as warranted by clinical findings
B. Consider repeating bimanual and/or abdominal examination in one week and review status
C. Seek immediate clinical consultation if symptoms worsen
D. Follow up as appropriate for specific conditions such as PID

See Bibliography.

Chronic Pelvic Pain

I. Definition

Pain in any region of the pelvis that is long-term and unresponsive to treatment of symptoms and/or undiagnosed.

II. Etiology

A. 50% enigmatic

B. 25% endometriosis

C. 25% other pathology including subacute and chronic salpingitis

III. History

A. What the patient may present with

    1. Chronic pelvic pain with or without menstrual exacerbation

    2. Dysmenorrhea

    3. Dyspareunia

    4. Dyschezia

    5. Chronicity of symptoms

    6. Absence of chills, fever associated with pain

    7. Nausea, vomiting, and/or diarrhea associated with pain

    8. Chronic constipation

    9. Chronic intermittent cramping

IV. Additional Information to Be Considered

A. Any symptoms of chronic bowel disease; any previous assessments for such and results

B. Any symptoms of chronic urinary tract infection, urinary tract anomaly, kidney disease

C. Location of pain, duration, exacerbation, and what precedes increased symptoms

D. Description of pain: sharp, dull, aching, cramping, intermittent, continuous

E. Pain relief measures; what helps; use of over-the-counter analgesics

F. Any weight gain or loss

G. Symptoms that accompany pain

H. Sexual history including sexual responsiveness; STDs, PID; contraceptive history including IUD

I. Surgical history including hernia repair

J. Medical history

K. Pelvic surgery including laparoscopy, laparotomy, tubal ligation, hysterectomy, repair of cystocele, rectocele, urethrocele, appendectomy, myomectomy, cervical cone biopsy, LEEP, LOOP

L. Menstrual history

M. Pregnancy history including extrauterine pregnancy(ies), infertility assessments and/or treatments

N. Psychosocial history including life stressors, major life changes and timing in relation to onset of symptoms; depression, anxiety disorder, personality disorder

O. History of incest, other sexual assault or abuse

V. Physical Examination

A. Vital signs as appropriate

B. Abdominal examination
   1. Bowel sounds: normal, hypo-or hyperactive, sluggish, absent, adventitious sounds, bruits
   2. Lower abdominal tenderness, sites of acute, dull pain elicited on superficial and/or deep palpation
   3. Any guarding
   4. Any rebound tenderness
   5. Scars
   6. Distention, asymmetry
   7. Patient's perception of pain location
   8. On percussion, liver, spleen enlarged, bladder distended
   9. Organomegaly, masses, hernias

C. Vaginal examination
   1. Examine cervix for discharge
   2. Examine vagina for masses, lesions, discharge, unusual odor, color

D. Bimanual examination
   1. Examine cervix for cervical motion tenderness
   2. Examine uterus for tenderness, masses, shape, size, consistency
   3. Examine adnexa for ovarian shape, size, tenderness, masses, other adnexal masses or tenderness

E. Rectal examination
   1. Pain, tenderness
   2. Masses
   3. Melena
   4. Rectovaginal masses, fistulas, adhesions
   5. Rectocele

F. Elicit psoas sign; perform obturator maneuver

VI. Laboratory Examination

A. Cultures as indicated by history, physical findings

B. Complete blood count/differential

C. Sedimentation rate, C-reactive protein
D. Urinary tract infection screen
E. Pregnancy test
F. Ultrasound evaluation based on pelvic examination
G. Consider consultation for CAT scan and/or MRI if pelvic examination is abnormal
H. Consider psychological testing

VII. Differential Diagnosis
A. Uterine
  1. Dysmenorrhea (primary or secondary)
  2. Adenomyosis
  3. Leiomyomata
  4. Positional (prolapse)
  5. Pelvic congestion
B. Adnexal
  1. Adhesive disease (infection, postsurgical)
  2. Neoplasm
  3. Functional ovarian cysts (Mittelschmerz)
  4. Endometriosis
C. Peritoneal
  1. Endometriosis
  2. Adhesive disease
D. Gastrointestinal
  1. Irritable bowel syndrome
  2. Other bowel disease (e.g. Crohn's, inflammatory)
E. Urinary
F. Musculoskeletal
G. Psychogenic (e.g. sexual abuse, rape)
H. Congenital, anatomical
I. Neurologic (neuroma)
J. Infections

VIII. Consultation/Referral
A. For laparoscopic diagnostic examination
B. For medical evaluation of suspected GI, GU conditions as indicated by history and physical examination
C. For pelvic venography
D. To confirm a suspected diagnosis and initiate treatment as co-managers of care
E. For psychological evaluation

F. For ultrasound, MRI

IX. Treatment
A. Endometriosis
   1. Create a pseudomenopause with Danocrine 200–800 mg. bid p.o. for 6 months; or GnRH analogues for 6 months (Nafarelin nasal spray 400–800 gm daily) or Leuprolide acetate (Lupron depot) 1 mg IM daily for 6 months, Zoladex® (Goserlin Acetate) implant 3.6 mg administered subcutaneously g 28 days x 6 months
   2. Continuous monophasic oral contraceptives
B. Other pathological causes
   1. Diagnose and treat cause according to established protocols (such as salpingitis, trauma from sexual assault, incest or rape, childbirth)
C. Enigmatic pelvic pain
   1. Follow-up to diagnostic laparoscopy as appropriate to any findings
   2. Multidisciplinary approach to pain management
D. Consideration of empiric therapy
   1. Antidepressant
   2. GnRH agonist
   3. Musculoskeletal relaxant

X. Follow-up
A. As appropriate for diagnosis and treatment
B. As desired by patient if no definitive cause is found and palliative treatments are suggested
C. If symptoms continue, introduce the team approach
   1. Mental health care specialist
   2. Physical therapist
   3. Nutritionist
   4. Urogynecologist
   5. Gastroenterologist

   See Bibliography.

Abdominal Pain

I. Definition
Pain (mild to severe) in any region of the abdomen as differentiated from the pelvic area, including the area from the costal margins to the beginning of the mons pubis including but not limited to the abdominal organs and anatomical structure.

II. Etiology

A. Inflammation, ulceration, infection, irritation, referred pain
B. Space occupying lesion
C. Response to injury: intra-abdominal or extra-abdominal
D. Sequelae of surgery: adhesions, presence of foreign body, unrepaired perforation
E. Systemic; hematologic; metabolic/endocrine; infectious; inflammatory; toxic; functional

III. History

A. What the patient may present with
  1. Anorexia
  2. Vomiting
  3. Nausea
  4. Change in bowel habits, constipation
  5. Urinary symptoms; dark urine
  6. Gynecological symptoms and history (see acute and chronic pelvic pain protocols); menstrual, contraceptive history
  7. Diaphoresis
  8. Fainting, malaise, confusion, fatigue, joint pain
  9. Distension of the abdomen
  10. Dyspnea, tachycardia, bradycardia
  11. Fever
  12. Chills
B. Additional information to be considered (patient will generally complain only of abdominal pain; history must be very thorough). Specific questioning is needed to elicit information about and sequence of symptoms:
  1. Onset (sudden, gradual, chronic, and so on)
  2. Character, e.g., throbbing, aching, burning, knife-like
  3. Intensity: difficult to define, but can be likened to other pain such as toothache, cramps, labor pain
  4. Location—where did pain originate; quadrant; generalized; epigastric
  5. Radiation: does it travel elsewhere
  6. Pain relief measures: what helps, what makes it worse
  7. Any weight gain or loss
  8. Pregnancy history; infertility diagnostics or treatments
  9. Psychosocial history including life stressors, major life changes and timing in relation to onset of symptoms
  10. History of incest, other sexual assault or abuse, violence or battering in relationships
  11. History of bowel obstruction, polyps, hernias

12. History of abdominal tumors benign or malignant
13. Use of GI irritants
14. Possible contaminated drinking water source here and/or abroad; food allergies, food poisoning
15. History of pelvic and/or abdominal surgery including organ transplant
16. History of extrauterine pregnancy
17. History of ovarian cysts, rupture of cysts
18. History of chronic bowel syndrome, any bowel disease
19. History of gall bladder disease
20. History of hepatitis, jaundice, liver disease, mononucleosis, abnormal liver function
21. History of trauma to the abdomen: accident, battering
22. History of travel abroad, recent immigrant and from where
23. History of exposure to industrial toxins, pesticides
24. History of kidney anomaly or disease; other genitourinary problems
25. History of appendicitis chronic or acute
26. History of ulcers; gastric surgery
27. History of cardiovascular, respiratory problems
28. Previous care for abdominal pain

IV. Physical Examination
A. Vital signs as appropriate
B. Cardiovascular, respiratory examinations; general appearance
C. Abdominal examination
    1. Bowel sounds; normal, hypo-or hyperactive, sluggish, absent, adventitious sounds, bruits
    2. Abdominal tenderness, sites of acute, dull pain elicited on superficial and/or deep palpation
    3. Any guarding
    4. Any rebound tenderness
    5. Scars
    6. Distension, symmetry or asymmetry
    7. Patient's perception of pain location
    8. On percussion liver or spleen enlarged, other abdominal organs enlarged
    9. Organomegaly, masses
    10. Abdominal bruits
D. Vaginal and bimanual examination
    1. Examine cervix for discharge
    2. Examine vagina for masses, lesions, discharge, unusual odor, color
    3. Examine cervix for cervical motion tenderness, mucopurulent discharge

4. Examine uterus for tenderness, masses, shape, size, consistency
5. Examine adnexa for ovarian shape, size, tenderness, masses; other adnexal masses or tenderness

E. Rectal examination
1. Pain, tenderness
2. Masses
3. Melena
4. Rectovaginal masses, fistulas, adhesions
5. Rectocele

F. Psoas sign, obturator sign

V. Laboratory Examination

A. Cultures as indicated by history, physical findings
B. Complete blood count/differential, serum electrolytes
C. Liver function studies, enzymes; H. pylori culture, stool cultures
D. Urinary tract infection screen; hepatitis panel
E. Pregnancy test; cervical, vaginal smears, cultures
F. Ultrasound evaluation based on examination
G. X-ray if indicated; abdomen, chest, posterior, anterior & lateral, KUB films
H. May consider consultation for CAT scan and/or MRI if abdominal or pelvic examination is abnormal
I. Sickle cell prep if indicated
J. ESR; TB skin test, blood, sputum cultures
K. TSH
L. Toxicology screen

VI. Differential Diagnosis

A. Consider possible causes under acute and chronic pelvic pain and rule out:
1. GI and GU pathology including appendicitis, pancreatitis, bowel obstruction, ulcers, cholecystitis, cholelithiasis, renal colic, biliary colic, rupture of spleen, diverticulitis, ileitis, carcinoma, irritable bowel syndrome, ulcerative colitis, pyelonephritis, hepatitis, hernias, urinary calculus, mesenteric thrombosis, urethral syndrome, perforation, strangulation, abscess
2. Acute or chronic constipation
3. Dissecting aneurysm; embolism
4. Ectopic pregnancy
5. Acute gastritis
6. Drug or toxin reaction; toxic systemic causes

7. Injury secondary to accident, violence including organ rupture
8. Abdominal pain, undetermined etiology
9. Referred pain from thoracic pathology: coronary thrombosis, pleural pneumonia, pleurisy, herpes zoster
10. Gastritis, coronitis, ileitis secondary to parasitic infection, cholera, waterborne diseases
11. Systemic diseases: hematologic, metabolic/endocrine, infectious, inflammatory, functional

VII. Consultation/Referral
A. For laparoscopic diagnostic examination
B. For medical evaluation of suspected GI, GU conditions as indicated by history and physical examination
C. To confirm a suspected diagnosis and initiate treatment as co-managers of care
D. For surgical consultation as indicated by history and findings
E. For CAT scan, MRI

VIII. Treatment
A. As indicated by findings and history
B. Etiology undetermined, pain persists
   1. Follow-up to any diagnostic work-up
   2. Multidisciplinary approach to pain or symptom management

X. Follow-up
A. As appropriate for diagnosis and treatment
B. As desired by patient if no definitive cause is found and palliative treatments are suggested

See Bibliography.

Pelvic Inflammatory Disease (PID)

I. Definition
Pelvic inflammatory disease comprises a spectrum of inflammatory disorders of the upper genital tract. This may include any combination of endometritis, salpingitis, tuboovarian abscess, and pelvic peritonitis.

II. Etiology
Causative organisms include

A. Neisseria gonorrhoea
B. Streptococcus;
   Streptococcus agalactiae
C. Peptostreptococcus, Peptococcus
D. Bacteroides
E. Chlamydia trachomatis
F. Escherichia coli
G. Mycoplasma hominis

H. H. influenza
I. U. urealyticum
J. Gardnerella vaginalis
K. Trichomonads
L. Staphylococcus
M. Pseudomonas
N. Diphtheroids
O. Cytomegalovirus

III. History

A. What the patient may present with (wide variation in symptomatology, making diagnosis difficult)
   1. Lower abdominal pain, usually bilateral
   2. Chills, fever
   3. May have anorexia
   4. May have nausea
   5. May have vomiting
   6. Increased vaginal discharge
   7. Heavier than usual period; abnormal bleeding
   8. Urinary symptoms: frequency, pain
   9. May complain of right upper quadrant pain; also Fitz-Hugh Curtis syndrome
   10. Dyspareunia
B. Additional information to be considered
   1. Known exposure to sexually transmitted disease
   2. Previous sexually transmitted disease
   3. Previous diagnosis of pelvic inflammatory disease
   4. Previously diagnosed endometriosis
   5. History of abdominal surgery
   6. Chronic illness
   7. Sexual activity (present and recent past)
   8. Last menstrual period; birth control method; is there an intrauterine device in place or recent insertion; recent pregnancy, childbirth
   9. Medication allergy
   10. Currently taking any medication
   11. Recent pelvic surgery, i.e., therapeutic abortion or dilatation and curettage
   12. Smoking cigarettes has recently been implicated as a risk factor for PID
   13. History of douching

IV. Physical Examination
A. Vital signs
    1. Temperature   3. Pulse
    2. Blood pressure   4. Respiration
B. Abdominal examination
    1. Bowel sounds: normal, hyperactive, sluggish, absent
    2. Generalized lower abdominal tenderness
    3. Guarding
    4. Rebound tenderness
C. External genitalia
    1. Lesions
    2. Observe and palpate Skene's and Bartholin's glands
D. Vaginal examination (speculum)
    1. Profuse vaginal discharge (may be purulent)
    2. Examine cervix for
        a. Erosion, ectropion
        b. Friability
        c. Discharge in os
E. Bimanual examination
    1. Examine cervix for cervical motion tenderness
    2. Examine uterus for tenderness
    3. Examine adnexa for
        a. Tenderness   b. Mass
    4. Rectovaginal examination for tenderness; if present, describe location, i.e., cervix, uterus, adnexa

V. Laboratory Examination
A. Gonococcus culture
B. Chlamydia smear
C. Complete blood count/differential, C-reactive protein
D. Sedimentation rate
E. Urinary tract infection screen
F. Serology test for syphilis
G. Human chorionic gonadotropin if history indicates—urine, serum
H. Transvaginal ultrasound
I. Endometrial biopsy with evidence of endometritis
J. Laparoscopic abnormalities consistent with PID
K. Culdocentesis (refer to physician)

VI. Criteria for Clinical Diagnosis
A. Criteria for ambulatory treatment

   1. The three minimum criteria for diagnosis of PID are:
      a. History of uterine tenderness
      b. Cervical motion tenderness
      c. Adnexal tenderness (may be unilateral)
   2. Additional criteria that will increase the specificity of diagnosis
      a. Temperature > 101°F (> 38.3C)
      b. White blood cells on saline microscopy of vaginal secretions
      c. Abnormal cervical or vaginal mucopurulent discharge
      d. Elevated C-reactive protein
      e. Culdocentesis yielding peritoneal fluid which contains bacteria, white blood cells
      f. Presence of adnexal mass noted on bimanual examination; tubo-ovarian abscess on sonography
      g. Elevated sedimentation rate > 15 mm/hour
      h. Positive gonococcal culture from cervix
      i. Positive Chlamydia smear from cervix
B. Criteria for hospitalization
   1. Surgical emergencies such as appendicitis cannot be excluded
   2. The patient is pregnant
   3. The patient does not respond clinically to oral antimicrobial therapy
   4. The patient is unable to follow or tolerate an outpatient oral regimen
   5. The patient has severe illness, nausea and vomiting or high fever
   6. The patient has a tubo-ovarian abscess
   7. The patient is immunodeficient (i.e., has HIV infection with low counts, is taking immunosuppressant therapy), or has another disease

VII. Differential Diagnosis

A. Septic abortion
B. Ectopic gestation
C. Ovarian cyst
D. Ruptured ovarian cyst
E. Cystitis
F. Pyelonephritis
G. Peptic ulcer disease
H. Hepatitis
I. Appendicitis
J. Adhesions
K. Endometriosis/endometritis
L. Diverticular disease
M. Pelvic neoplasms
N. Irritable bowel syndrome
O. Ovarian Torsion
P. Inflammatory Bowel Disease

VIII. Treatment (CDC Recommendations) for Uncomplicated Pelvic Inflammatory Disease

A. Medication
   1. Ofloxacin 400 mg orally BID x 14 days OR Levofloxacin 500 mg orally qd x 14 days with or without Metronidazole 500 mg orally BID for 14 days

   2. Alternative regimens
      a. Ceftriaxone 250 mg IM once OR
      b. Cefoxitin 2 gm IM plus Probenecid 1 gram orally once OR
      c. Other parenteral 3rd generation cephalosporin (e.g., ceftizoxime or cefotaxime PLUS Doxycycline 100 mg orally BID for 14 days (for a, b, or c) with or without Metronidazole 500 mg orally BID x 14 days
   3. Pregnant women: Hospitalize and treat with parenteral antibiotics per CDC guidelines for hospitalization
   4. Refer to CDC guidelines if patient meets hospitalization criteria
B. General measures
   1. Bed rest
   2. Increased fluid intake
   3. General diet
   4. Stress importance of partner being examined and treated
   5. Stress use of condoms to prevent reinfection or future infections
   6. No douching
C. Management of sex partners
   1. Examine and treat if sexual contact with patient during 60 days prior to onset of symptoms

IX. Complications

A. Sterility

B. Generalized sepsis

C. Chronic pelvic pain

D. Tubal pregnancy

E. Surgical interventions

F. Dyspareunia

G. Tubo-ovarian abscess

H. Fitz-Hugh-Curtis Syndrome: perihepatitis

X. Consultation/Referral

A. If failure to improve 48 hours after starting above treatment

B. For hospitalization

C. For culdocentesis if indicated

XI. Follow-up

A. Reevaluate within 72 hours or sooner if symptoms worsen or do not improve; patients should demonstrate substantial clinical improvement within 3 days

B. After completion of medication course (no sooner than 7 days)
   1. Bimanual
   2. Cultures if indicated (i.e., positive lab results prior to treatment); some recommend rescreening for gonorrhea and Chlamydia trachomatis

regardless of prior culture results 4–6 weeks after completion of therapy
C. Male sex partners of women with PID should be examined and treated if sexual contact was 60 days or less preceding symptom onset

See Bibliography.

Pelvic Mass

I. Definition
Mass found in adnexa, cul de sac, or uterus during bimanual examination

II. Etiology
A pelvic mass may be caused by any number of factors. This protocol is meant to assist the clinician in the screening and referral process.

III. History
A. What the patient may present with
   1. May be asymptomatic
   2. Bloating
   3. Abdominal pain: generalized or localized/duration/onset
   4. Flatulence
   5. Dysfunctional bleeding—can be heavy
   6. Amenorrhea; number of weeks
   7. Vaginal discharge
   8. Low back pain and/or pressure
   9. Dyspareunia
   10. Bowel or bladder dysfunction
   11. Prior abdominal surgery
   12. Prior pelvic surgery
   13. Endometriosis
   14. Pregnancy history; assisted reproduction
B. Additional information to be obtained
   1. LMP
   2. Contraception used
   3. Menstruation, pregnancy, and infertility history
   4. Any change in bowel habits; last bowel movement
   5. History of ovarian cysts
   6. History of uterine fibroids
   7. History of pelvic inflammatory disease (PID)

8. History of Chlamydia or gonorrhea
9. History of IUD use
10. History of ectopic pregnancy
11. Family history

IV. Physical Examination
A. Abdominal exam
   1. Bowel sounds
   2. Pain
   3. Organomegaly
B. Vaginal examination
   1. Examine cervix for discharge
   2. Examine vagina for masses, lesions, discharge
C. Bimanual examination
   1. Examine cervix for cervical motion tenderness
   2. Examine uterus for tenderness, masses, shape, size, and consistency
   3. Examine adnexa for masses, attempting to differentiate between ovaries and bowel
   4. Evaluate mass for shape, consistency, size, mobility and tenderness
   5. Examine bladder
   6. Cul de sac for mass
   7. Thickening or tenderness at or near utero sacral ligaments
D. Rectal examination
   1. Pain, tenderness
   2. Masses
   3. Melena
   4. Rectovaginal masses, fistulas
   5. Rectocele/occult blood

V. Laboratory Examination
1. Cultures as indicated
2. Wet prep as indicated
3. Serum pregnancy test as indicated
4. CBC with sed rate; C-reactive protein
5. Ultrasound; transvaginal and transabdominal or with doppler as indicated
6. CA 125, ovarian cancer tumor marker as indicated
7. Endometrial biopsy as indicated

VI. Treatment
A. Adnexal masses
   1. If thought to be retained stool or intestinal gas, patient should have bowel prep and be reexamined

   2. If thought to be ovarian in origin, the following differentiation must be made
     a. Age of patient (ovulation or using ovulation inhibitor, perimenopausal or menopausal)
     b. Menstrual history
     c. Indication of infection
     d. Is pregnancy test positive
   3. If ovulation is presumed, assess size of mass if:
     a. Greater than 5–6 cm, M.D. referral is indicated
     b. Less than 5 cm and asymptomatic, reexamine after next menses; if unchanged may (i) recommend ovulatory inhibitor x 3 months and reexamine. If remaining after 3 months, refer to M.D. (ii) consider ultrasound as baseline. If functional cyst is confirmed, wait 2 months and repeate ultrasound
   4. If on ovulatory inhibitor, do appropriate work-up (i.e., ultrasound) and refer or refer immediately depending on setting
   5. Perimenopausal/menopausal
     a. Do appropriate work-up; refer for M.D. evaluation as indicated
B. Uterine mass
   1. Do ultrasound—small, nonsymptomatic fibroids may be followed and assessed on a 6–month to 12–month basis as appropriate to setting. Large fibroids or other finding refer immediately to MD
C. Ectopic pregnancy
   1. Do ultrasound; if ectopic confirmed, consult or refer for treatment. Current treatment includes:
     a. serial serum human gonadotropin levels (HCG level < 2000 milli-international units and < 50% rise in 48 hours)
     b. medical management (by protocol of clinical site)
       1) methotrexate in single dose IM 50 mg/square meter of body surface calculated on body weight
       2) monitor HCG per guidelines of clinical site and possible ultrasound monitoring
     c. consult and referral for surgical management

VII. Differential Diagnosis
A. Inflammatory
   1. tubo-ovarian abscess
   2. appendiceal abscess
   3. diverticular abscess
B. Functional
   1. ovarian cysts
     a. follicular

    b. luteal
    c. polycystic ovaries (PCO)
C. Neoplastic
    1. benign
    2. malignant
D. Anatomic anomalies
    1. pelvic kidney
    2. bicornuate uterus
E. Other
    1. ectopic pregnancy
    2. endometrioma
    3. paratubal/ovarian cyst
    4. hydrosalpinx

VIII. Complications
A. Complication of individual entity as listed in differential diagnosis

IX. Consultation and Referral
A. As indicated by laboratory work-up and physical findings indicated in VI treatment

X. Follow-up
A. As indicated by diagnosis

    See Bibliography.

Uterine Leiomyomata

I. Definition
Often referred to as uterine fibroids, fibromyomas, myomas, or fibromas, leiomyomas are benign uterine tumors arising from the smooth muscle and having some connective tissue elements as well.

II. Etiology
A. Physiology
    1. Appear to arise from single (monoclonal) neoplastic smooth muscle cells (4th and 5th decades) within the myometrium
    2. May be single or multiple
    3. May range in size from microscopic to more than 20 cm (filling the abdomen)

4. May occur within the uterine wall (intramural) or extend externally from the serosal surface (subserosal) internally into endometrial cavity (submucous); have both estrogen & progesterone receptors
5. Can also be broad ligament, ovarian, or cervical
6. Occur most commonly during a woman's fertile years—35–50
7. Usually undergo regression with menopause; rare before menarche
8. Sometimes increase in size with oral contraceptives or pregnancy

III. History
A. What the patient may present with
   1. May be asymptomatic
   2. Pelvic pain (acute or chronic) 1:3 women
   3. Abnormal vaginal bleeding (30%)
   4. Urinary frequency, retention, incontinence, urgency
   5. Constipation
   6. Pelvic pressure
   7. Dyspareunia
   8. Backache
B. Additional information to be considered
   1. Menstrual history
   2. History of infertility
   3. Habitual spontaneous abortions
   4. Menopausal symptoms
   5. Last menstrual period; methods of birth control; intrauterine device in place; ever use intrauterine device
   6. Any pelvic surgery
   7. Pregnancy history; parity
   8. Use of hormones: oral contraceptives, hormone therapy, infertility drugs
   9. Family history; ethnic background
   10. Obesity ($\uparrow$ BMI)

IV. Physical Examination
A. Vital signs as indicated
B. Abdominal examination
   1. Any abdominal guarding or tenderness
   2. Location of any pain
   3. Bladder palpable or distended
C. Vaginal examination
   1. Examine cervix for any extraneous tissue, distortion of configuration
   2. Palpate vagina for any masses
   3. Examine any bleeding or discharge

D. Bimanual examination
  1. Examine uterus for tenderness, masses
  2. Examine adnexa for masses, tenderness
  3. Locate any pain if possible
E. Rectovaginal examination for tenderness, masses

V. Laboratory Examination
A. Ultrasound
B. Pregnancy test if pre-or perimenopausal
C. CBC
D. MRI
E. Endoscopic visualization
F. Hysterosalpingography
G. Sonohysterography

VI. Differential Diagnosis
A. Uterine pregnancy
B. Malignant uterine tumor
C. Ovarian cyst or tumor
D. Extrauterine pelvic mass
E. Bowel tumor
F. Bladder tumor
G. Tumor of ureter, kidney
H. Pelvic abscess
I. Extrauterine pregnancy
J. Bicornuate uterus

VII. Treatment
A. As indicated by ultrasound
  1. Watch size of leiomyomata with bimanual examination and repeat ultrasound
  2. Consultation for medical management: progestins, gonadotropin releasing hormone (GnRH) agonists (e.g. leuprolide 3.75 mg 1x/month)
  3. Consultation for surgical management: hysterectomy, myomectomy, hysteroscope, resectoscope, laser ablation; myolysis or myoma coagulation; cryomyolysis; fibroid embolization

VIII. Complications
A. Torsion of pedunculated leiomyomata resulting in necrosis
B. Uterine abscess
C. Infarction
D. Hemorrhage
E. Degeneration: hyalinization, cystic, calcification, fatty

IX. Consultation/Referral
A. Rapid change in size

B. Signs of complications
C. Menorrhagia
D. Compromise of adjacent organs
E. Intractable pelvic pressure or pain

X. Follow-up
A. Reevaluate every 6–12 months or as indicated
B. As indicated under medical management with medication
    1. Long term GnRH agonists > 6 months add estrogen for osteoporosis, menopausal symptoms

    See Bibliography.

Scabies

I. Definition
A highly contagious papulofollicular skin rash whose chief symptom is pruritus. Rash and itching are thought to be hypersensitivity reactions to the mites and are not confined to the locations of mite burrows. Scabies among adults may be sexually transmitted.

II. Etiology
Sarcoptes scabieimite. The mite burrows into skin, deposits eggs along a tunnel. Larvae hatch in 3–5 days and gather around hair follicles. Newly hatched female burrows into the skin, maturing in 10–19 days, then mates and starts a new cycle. Crusted scabies (Norwegian scabies) is an aggressive infestation.

III. History
A. What the patient may present with:
    1. Pruritus—worse at night or at times when body temperature is raised, i.e., after exercise. Pruritus exists prior to physical manifestations
    2. Lesions are usually on interdigital webs of hands, flexor aspects of wrists, extensor surfaces of the elbows, areas surrounding the nipples, anterior axillary folds, umbilicus, belt line, lower abdomen, genitalia and gluteal cleft; male genitals; can be all over body especially with immunosuppression
B. Additional information to be considered
    1. Known contact with scabies. Incubation period in persons without previous exposure is usually 4–6 weeks (mean 3 weeks). Persons who

were previously infected develop symptoms 1–3 days after repeat exposure to the mite. These reinfections are usually milder

2. Lifestyle. Persons living in close proximity with others, dormitories, crowded living conditions, shared clothing, shelters, are at increased risk for nonsexual exposures
3. History of atopic dermatitis, +HIV, or other immunosuppressed condition; hematologic malignancies
4. At high risk for crusted scabies

IV. Physical Examination
A. Skin: Thorough examination of lesions and of those areas most frequently involved
   1. Linear burrows about 1.5 to 2 cm. in length terminating in a papule or vesicle
   2. Lesions: papules or vesicles
   3. Scaling, crustation lesions, furuncles, excoriations may be present with secondary infection
B. Lymph nodes—generalized lymphadenopathy

V. Laboratory
A. KOH prep of scraping from several of the excoriated lesions, examined under low power. It may be difficult to find mite. Application of water, alcohol, or mineral oil to the skin facilitates collection of the scraping
B. Diagnosis is usually made on the basis of clinical presentation

VI. Differential Diagnosis
A. Atopic dermatitis   B. Impetigo   C. Urticaria
D. Psoriasis   E. Drug-induced eruption   F. Insect bites

VII. Treatment
A. Medication
   1. 5% permethrin cream (Elimite®), applied to all areas of the body from neck down and washed off after 8–14 hours OR
   2. 1% lindane (Kwell®, Scabene®), applied to the entire body from the neck down, left on for 8 hours, and washed off thoroughly. Lindane applications should not be used immediately after a bath or shower and should not be in excess of these recommendations to avoid the possibility of neurotoxicity from absorption through the skin. Lindane should not be used during pregnancy, lactation, by persons with extensive dermatitis and by kids < 2

3. OR Ivermectin 200 ug/Kg orally, repeated in 2 weeks (safety in children < 15 Kg not determined)
4. In pregnancy and lactation and for children under 2 use only permethrin. Do not use lindane or ivermectin.

B. Symptomatic treatment
1. Antihistamines may be given to relieve pruritus
2. Patient should be informed that pruritus may persist for several weeks. If patient does not respond to therapy and itching is still persistent after one week, she/he should be instructed to contact health care provider to decide if further therapy is necessary

C. General measures
1. Clothing, towels, bed linens should be laundered at 60° C (hot cycle) or dry cleaned on the day of treatment
2. If clothing items can't be washed or dry cleaned, these should be separated from washed clothes and not worn for at least 72 hours. Mites cannot exist for more than 2–3 days away from the body
3. Sexual partners and close personal or household contacts within the past month should be informed, examined, and treated if necessary
4. Patient should be instructed to follow treatment regimen carefully
5. Although fumigation of living areas is not necessary, some patients may wish to decontaminate mattresses, sofas, and other inanimate objects that cannot be washed. OTC sprays and powders are available for this purpose

VIII. Complications
A. Secondary infection (may require systemic antibiotics)
B. Reaction to lindane (Kwell®, Scabene®)
   1. Dermatitis   2. CNS toxicity

IX. Consultation and Referral
A. Secondary infection
B. Generalized widespread inflammatory response
C. Failure to respond to therapy
D. Reaction to lindane (Kwell®, Scabene®))
E. Patients with coexisting dermatitis or other dermatologic condition
F. Patients with coexisting HIV infection or who are otherwise immunosuppressed; those with crusted scabies

X. Follow-up
A. Failure to respond to therapy. Some experts recommend retreatment after 1–2 weeks for patients who are still symptomatic; others recommend

retreatment only if live mites can be observed. Retreatment should be with an alternative regimen

B. Recurrence

Appendix A may be copied/adapted for your patients.

Pediculosis

I. Definition

Pediculosis is the state of being infested with lice that may be found on the skin, particularly the hairy areas such as the scalp and pubis, and may cause intense pruritus.

II. Etiology

A. Two species that look like each other but have different feeding habits are:
  1. Pediculus humanus var capitis: inhabits the skin of the head or body; transmitted by shared clothing, towels, brushes, combs, batting helmets, stuffed animals, car seats, bedding, headphones, hats; P. humanus var corporis body louse lives in clothes
  2. Phthirus pubis ("crab louse," pubic louse); inhabits the genital area but may colonize other areas including axillae, eyelashes, head hair; transmitted by close personal contact, bedding
B. Nits hatch in 5–10 days incubation; adult pubic lice probably survive no more than 24 hours off their host; nits can survive in hot and humid climates up to 10 days

III. History

A. What the patient may present with
  1. Pruritus
  2. Visual identification of the parasite or feces on bed pillow
  3. Known exposure to household member or intimate partner with head, body, or pubic lice
  4. Rarely lymphadenopathy at back of neck—allergic reaction to saliva & feces of lice
B. Additional information to be considered
  Lifestyle: shared clothing, towels, beds, pillows; shag rugs or carpets, upholstered furniture

IV. Physical Examination

A. Pediculosis capitis (infestation with head lice); examine for

1. The parasite
2. Greenish-white oval attachments to hair shaft (nits)
3. Secondary impetigo and furunculosis
4. Cervical lymphadenopathy

B. Pediculosis corporis (infestation with body lice): examine for
   1. Parallel linear scratch marks on back, shoulders, trunk, buttocks (areas easily reached for scratching)
   2. Impetigo lesions and furuncles associated with scratch marks secondary to scratching
   3. Lice on clothing, especially the seams, as lice are very rarely found on the body

C. Pediculosis pubis (infestation with pubic (crab) lice): examine for
   1. The parasite (rarely found)
   2. Oval attachments on pubic hair (nits)
   3. Black dots (representing excreta) on surrounding skin and underclothing
   4. Nits in eyebrows, eyelashes, scalp hair, axillary hair, and other body hair
   5. Crusts or scabs in pubic area

V. Laboratory Examination
None

VI. Differential Diagnosis
See Etiology

VII. Treatment
A. General measures
   1. Wash with hot water, dry clean, or run through a dryer on heat cycle all contaminated clothing, hats, towels, bedclothes, etc., to destroy nits and lice; wash combs and hairbrushes in hot soapy water letting them soak for at least 15 minutes
   2. Spray couches, chairs, car seats and items that can't be washed or dry cleaned with over-the-counter product (A-200 Pyrinate® (pyrethrin), Triplex®, or RID (permethrin); alternative is to vacuum carefully to pick up living lice and nits

B. Specific treatment*
   1. Pediculosis capitis (infestation with head lice)

---

*Kwell is not recommended for use in pregnancy or lactation or for children under 2 as Lindane is a neurotoxin. Pregnant and lactating women should be treated only with 1% permethrin (Nix) or with pyrethrins with piperonyl betoxide. All products are OTC except Kwell; permethrin is available as a generic product. In a large review of efficacy, permethrin was the only product to show sufficient efficacy (cure rate measured as nit free after 14 days)

    a. Thoroughly wet hair with Kwell®* (lindane) shampoo (1% gamma benzene hexachloride) or Triplex Kit (pyrethrins + piperonyl butoxide); Pronto (piperonyl), RID (permethrin) shampoo or R&C shampoo (pyrethrins and piperonyl butoxide) or End Lice (pyrethrins** and piperonyl); work up lather, adding water as necessary; shampoo thoroughly leaving shampoo on head for 5 minutes; rinse, or use Nix® (permethrin 1% cream rinse), leave on 10 minutes and rinse thoroughly; or use Pronto shampoo/conditioner (piperonyl butoxide); or Clear® lice killing shampoo (pyrethum-based) and lice egg remover (permethrin-based) per directions on product or Klout® (nonpesticide—ingredients include isopropanol, methylparaben, propylparaben) per directions on product

    b. Rinse thoroughly, towel dry

    c. Remove remaining nits with fine-tooth metal comb or tweezers (use of vinegar solution and hair conditioner or olive oil make combing easier)

2. Pediculosis corporis (infestation with body lice)

    a. Bathe with soap and water if no lice are found

    b. Wash with hot water and dry in dryer all clothing, bedclothes, towels, etc.

    c. Dry clean items that cannot be washed; for items that cannot be washed or dry cleaned, seal in a plastic bag for 1 week: lice will suffocate (in cold climates put bags outside for 10 days; temperature change kills lice)

    d. If evidence of lice is found or patient is not relieved by a. and b. above, Kwell (lindane) Lotion® may be applied, allowed to remain 8–10 hours, and thoroughly rinsed off

3. Pediculosis pubis (infestation with pubic lice)

    a. Permethrin 1% cream (NIX) rinse applied to affected area and washed off after 10 minutes OR

    b. Lindane 1% (generics) applied for 4 minutes to affected area and thoroughly washed off OR

    c. Pyrethrins with piperonyl butoxide (RID, Clear, A-200, Pronto, generics) applied to affected area and washed off after 10 minutes

    d. Pregnancy, lactation: use permethrin or pyrethrins with piperonyl butoxide, not lindane

    e. Treat sexual partners within past month

    f. Wash in hot water and thoroughly dry on heat cycle all clothing, bed linen, towels, etc.

---

*Evidence accumulating of resistance to pediculicides

**Pyrethrins are extracted from chrysanthemums. Permethrins are synthetic pyrethroids.

C. Stress importance of careful checking of family and household members and close contacts; no treatment is needed unless there is evidence of contamination
D. Put nonwashable items in hot dryer; or spray with permethrin (RID, NIX)—check safety with children and pets
E. Screen patients with pediculosis pubis for other STDs

VIII. Complications
A. Secondary infection
B. Sensitivity reactions to treatment
C. Excoriations
D. Resistance of lice to pediculicides

IX. Consultation/Referral
A. Lice found in eyelashes: since shampoo cannot be used, occlusive ophthalmic ointment is applied to the eyelid margins
B. Treatment failures
C. Coexisting dermatologic conditions

X. Follow-up
A. Evaluate in 1 week if symptoms persist
B. Instruct patient to return for repeat treatment if symptoms or parasites recur

See Appendix A and Bibliography.

5
Breast Conditions

Breast Mass

I. Definition
A breast mass is a thickening or lump which is felt in a woman's breast which may or may not have the following characteristics:

A. Nipple retraction
B. Dimpling
C. Inflammation
D. Palpable axillary or supraclavicular nodes
E. Tenderness
F. Discharge from nipple

II. Etiology
A. "Fibrocystic disease"—catch-all term for nonmalignant conditions
B. Fibroadenoma
C. Carcinoma
D. Mammary duct ectasia
E. Intraductal papilloma
F. Normal premenstrual breast tissue, i.e., with tenderness and prominent breast tissue secondary to hormone levels—physiologic nodularity, mastoplasia
G. Mastalgia (mastodynia) chronic or cyclic
H. Mastitis: cellulitis, skin boils, abscess
I. Cysts
J. Fat necrosis
K. Superficial phlebitis
L. Phyllodes tumors—painless, solid, smooth, lobular, bulky, stromal hyperplasia
M. Paget's disease

III. History
A. What woman may present with
1. Lump
2. Pain
3. Swelling
4. Redness; bruised area that doesn't resolve
5. Discharge from nipple
6. Nipple retraction
7. Change in appearance of skin and areola
8. Dimpling, scaliness

B. Additional information to be considered
   1. Family history of breast disease
   2. History of previous breast lumps or breast disease; biopsy (type) or aspiration; breast surgery including reduction, enlargement; implants and type
   3. Last menstrual period (has patient noticed a relationship to menses?)
   4. Birth control method(s) used; hormone therapy (type, dose, duration) & when after menopause
   5. Diet
   6. Adolescents' most common complaint
      a. Trauma (sports or sexual activity)
   7. Recent pregnancy, lactation
   8. Risk factors
      a. Hormonal
         1) Early menarche (11 or younger) or late menopause (55 or older)
         2) First full-term pregnancy after 30; nullipara
         3) Obesity in postmenopausal women (produce more estrogen); high levels of abdominal fat
         4) Breast feeding—may be protective but data are not conclusive
      b. Genetic (70% of breast cancer = no known family history)
         1) Risk increases with 1st or 2nd degree relatives— maternal or paternal—with breast cancer—mother, daughter, sister, aunt, grandmother— and number of these relatives
         2) BRCA 1 or BRCA2 gene mutation; in some ethnic/cultural groups
      c. External
         1) Diet (areas under investigation): fat—low fat diet may be beneficial; increased risk with high animal fat diet
         2) Low vitamin A intake may increase breast cancer risk
         3) Alcohol even in moderate amounts (3–9 drinks a week) may increase risk esp. if on hormone therapy
         4) Radiation—risk in moderate doses (10–500 rads) (level of radiation in an up-to-date mammogram = 1/4 rad)
         5) Exogenous hormones
            □ DES exposure in utero or as a DES mother
            □ Postmenopausal hormone therapy: possible increased risk with progestin plus estrogen versus estrogen* relative risk
            □ possibility that organochlorines (pesticides) can act like estrogen in the body
         6) Exercise—strenuous exercise in adolescence and continued exercise in adulthood may have a protective effect
         7) Other: Previous diagnosis of breast cancer or atypical hyperplasia

*Per Women's Health Initiative (WHI); WHI study of estrogen only continues.

IV. Physical Examination
A. Breast Physical Examination
   1. Examine in both upright and supine positions
   2. Measurement, location, consistency of any lesion
   3. Note any skin changes such as dimpling, retraction, erythema, nipple scaling or excoriation
   4. Examine for spontaneous breast discharge
   5. Examine regional lymph nodes (axillary and suprainfraclavicular)
B. Palpation for the following:
   1. Accurate location of any detected lesion
   2. Solitary or multiple lesion(s)
   3. Consistency and extent of any mass
   4. Tenderness of mass
   5. Movable or fixed on chest wall
   6. Displacement or retraction of nipple
   7. Retraction or dimpling of skin overlying mass
   8. Palpability of regional lymph nodes (axillary or supra/ infraclavicular)
   9. Discharge expressed; color, amount, uni- or bilateral, consistency
C. Express breast for any discharge if none noted on palpation

V. Laboratory Examination
If discharge present, microscopic examination to identify fat globules

VI. Differential
See Etiology

VII. Treatment
A. Medication
   1. Appropriate antibiotic for mastitis, abscess
B. General measures
   1. If mass does not fit criteria for physician referral, have patient return 1 week after next menses for reevaluation and possible referral
   2. Dietary; discuss use of caffeine, chocolate, and salt; low fat diet
   3. Consider homeopathic remedies; herbals such as evening primrose oil, ginseng tea; vitamins A and B for cyclical mastalgia, vitamin E; green tea, antioxidants, phytoestrogens

VIII. Complications
May be grave and extensive if misdiagnosed

IX. Consultation/Referral
A. Any of the following lesions should be referred immediately to physician or breast center

1. Fixed mass
2. Mass associated with nipple retraction
3. Dimpling of skin; orange peel appearance to skin
4. Inflammation; scaling or excoriation
5. Palpable axillary or supra/infraclavicular nodes
6. Discrete mass → ultrasound to distinguish cyst from solid mass
7. Discharge that it is not fat globules: green = infection; red or brown = possible tumor; possible nipple fluid assay
8. Cystic mass; for possible aspiration
B. Refer to physician/breast center
   1. Women who do not fit above criteria but in whom mass is still found one week past next menses
   2. Women in whom mass is palpable despite negative mammogram
   3. Consider referral to breast center, specialist for evaluation with digital mammography, MRI, galactography; consideration of prophylaxis for high risk women with a selective estrogen receptor modulator (SERM)
   4. Genetic counseling & testing

X. Follow-up
A. Appropriate to VII. B. 1. and VII. B. 2.
B. Preventive measures to reduce breast cancer risk

XI. Mammogram Screening
A. All women with a breast mass (although ultrasound may be more useful for women under 35)
B. Baseline between 35 and 40
C. Earlier if family history of breast cancer in mother, sister, daughter, aunt, grandmother
D. Annually 40 and older

See Appendix A and Bibliography.
Breast Cancer and Environmental Risk Factors Program (BCERF)
www.cfe.cornell.edu/bcerf/

Abnormal Breast Discharge

I. Definition
Under certain conditions an abnormal fluid may be expressed from the breast(s) or flow spontaneously.

II. Etiology
A. Physiological cause
  1. Pregnancy, puerperium
  2. Intercourse
  3. Stimulation of the breast
  4. Chest wall surgery or trauma
  5. Exercise
  6. Emotional stress
  7. Sleep (affects measurable amounts of prolactin)
B. Pharmacological causes
  1. Numerous psychotropic drugs
  2. Cimetidine
  3. Some antihypertensives
  4. Opiates
  5. Estrogens/oral contraceptives/progestins
  6. Antiemetics
  7. Alcohol (chronic abuse)
  8. Marijuana
  9. Danazol
  10. Isoniazid (INH)
C. Pathological causes
  1. Breast tumor
  2. Pituitary tumor
  3. Hypothalamic tumor
  4. Infections
  5. Empty sella syndrome
  6. Hypothyroidism
  7. Polycystic ovaries (PCOS)
  8. Benign intraductal papilloma
  9. Bilateral ductal ectasia

III. History
A. What the patient may present with
  1. Breast discharge
  2. Amenorrhea
  3. Possibly pain
  4. Possibly localized heat and swelling
  5. Possibly, no symptoms (discharge can be an incidental finding of breast exam)
B. Additional information to be considered
  1. Last menstrual period
  2. Sexual activity
  3. Birth control method; hormone therapy
  4. Medications or illegal drugs currently being used

5. Medications recently taken
6. Recent pregnancy (within 1 year), regardless of outcome
7. Exercise program, e.g., jogging
8. Nipple stimulation, e.g., fondling, sucking
9. Recent trauma to chest or surgery
10. Description of discharge
11. Chronic illness, e.g., thyroid disease, psychiatric illness
12. Lifestyle changes, e.g., increased stress
13. Alcohol consumption (chronic abuse)
14. Family history of breast disease
15. Breast pain or tenderness
16. Breast surgery: biopsy, reduction, augmentation, implants
17. Duration of discharge

IV. Physical Examination*
A. Complete examination
  1. Palpate nipple by compressing nipple areola with thumb and index finger, gently milking the subareolar ducts from just outside the apex of the papilla. Repeat in 3 or 4 different directions, noting number of droplets that appear
  2. If discharge is expressed, is it unilateral, bilateral, clear, cloudy, dark, light, milky, bloody, thick, thin; note color

B. Thyroid: palpate for nodes, size
C. Bimanual examination
  1. Ovarian irregularity or enlargement
  2. Uterine enlargement

V. Laboratory Examination
A. Initially on all patients
  1. Microscopic examination for fat globules
  2. Prolactin level; sample should be drawn between 8 and 10 a.m. (literature indicates prolactin level is lowest between 8 and 10 a.m. but not directly after gynecological examination, intercourse, exercise, or breast stimulation including breast examination)
  3. Thyroid panel
  4. Consider mammogram, ultrasound, MRI with consultation
  5. Serum pregnancy test if indicated

---

*Per breast mass guideline.

VI. Differential Diagnosis
See Etiology

VII. Treatment
As needed according to laboratory report and etiology

VIII. Complications
Individual, according to diagnosis

IX. Consultation/Referral
A. Abnormal lab results
B. Lack of definitive diagnosis
C. Consider referral to breast center, specialist

X. Follow-up
A. If first visit was a consult visit, encourage complete physical
B. Repeat laboratory work as indicated in V.

See Appendix A, Breast Self-examination. See Bibliography.

6

Cervical Aberrations

Papanicolaou (Pap) Smear and Colposcopy

I. Definition
The Papanicolaou (Pap) test examines exfoliated cells from the endocervix to detect preinvasive lesions (e.g., dysplasia, carcinoma-in-situ) as well as invasive lesions.

II. Screening
A. History
1. DES exposure in utero
2. Smoking: exposure to passive smoke
3. Previous abnormal Papanicolaou smear; cervical treatment
4. HPV, other sexually transmitted diseases
5. Sexual practices, partners (number, partner with previous partner with abnormal Pap, partner's sexual history)
6. Family history of cervical cancer; personal history of cancer
7. Age of beginning sexual activity
8. Immunosuppressive therapy; immunosuppression
9. HIV/AIDS or risk
10. Hormone use

III. Technique
A. Cytologic specimens may be obtained prior to the bimanual pelvic exam; a nonlubricated speculum must be used (speculum can be warmed with water)
B. May do a palpation of the vagina and cervix to locate the cervix and identify the position of the os
C. The cervix and vagina must be fully visible when the smear is obtained in order to see entire squamo columnar junction
D. Vaginal discharge, when present in large amounts, should be carefully removed with a large swab prior to obtaining the smear. The presence of small amount of blood should not preclude cytologic sampling

E. The spatula is applied to the entire cervix to include the entire squamo-columnar junction. In some settings, the handle of the spatula is used to sample the vaginal pool prior to sampling the cervix. A cytobrush is inserted into the endocervix, rotated 1/2 turn, removed, and the material is rolled on a slide. If woman is pregnant, do not use cytobrush. Uniform application of the material to the slide, without clumping, both sides of spatula, roll brush on slide and with immediate fixation (within 10 seconds) to prevent drying, is required (spray from 9–12" away)

F. For DES-exposed women, additional slides are prepared using smear taken from the upper two-thirds of the vagina at its circumferences. Gentle wiping of the vaginal wall mucosa initially to remove discharge increases the diagnostic accuracy

G. With the liquid based technology (Thin Prep Pap Test™, CytoRich® Sure-Path™) the sample is collected on a broom-type cervical sampling device. This device then is rinsed in a vial of preserving solution and discarded. The vial is capped, labeled, and sent to the lab. A plastic spatula to sample the portio and cytobrush for the endocervix can be substituted for the broom

IV. Bethesda 2001 Terminology for Papanicolaou Smears
SPECIMEN ADEQUACY
  Satisfactory for evaluation (note presence/absence of endocervical/transformation zone component)
    Unsatisfactory for evaluation (specify reason)
      Specimen rejected/not processed (specify reason)
      Specimen processed and examined, but unsatisfactory for evaluation of epithelial abnormality because of (specify reason)
GENERAL CATEGORIZATION
  Negative for intraepithelial lesion or malignancy
  Epithelial cell abnormality
  Other
INTERPRETATION/RESULT
  Negative for intraepithelial lesion or malignancy
    Organisms
      Trichomonas vaginalis
      Fungal organisms morphologically consistent with Candida species
      Shift in flora suggestive of bacterial vaginosis
      Bacteria morphologically consistent with *Actinomyces* species
      Cellular changes consistent with herpes simplex virus
    Other nonneoplastic findings

Reactive cellular changes associate with inflammation (includes typical repair)
radiation
intrauterine contraceptive device
Glandular cells status posthysterectomy
Atrophy
Epithelial cell abnormalities
Squamous cell
Atypical squamous cells (ASC)
of undetermined significance (ASC-US)
cannot exclude HSIL (ASC-H)
Low-grade squamous intraepithelial lesion (LSIL)
Encompassing: human papillomavirus/mild
dysplasia/cervical intraepithelial neoplasia (CIN) 1
High-grade squamous intraepithelial lesion (HSIL)
encompassing: moderate and severe dysplasia,
carcinoma in situ; CIN 2 and CIN 3
Squamous cell carcinoma
Glandular cell
Atypical glandular cells (AGC)
(specify endocervical, endometrial, or not otherwise speci-
fied)
Atypical glandular cells, favor neoplastic
(specify endocervical or not otherwise specified)
Endocervical adenocarcinoma in situ (AIS)
Adenocarcinoma
Other (list not comprehensive)
Endometrial cells in a woman $\geq$ 40 years of age

AUTOMATED REVIEW AND ANCILLLARY TESTING (include as appropriate)

EDUCATIONAL NOTES AND SUGGESTIONS

The 2001 Bethesda system. *Journal of the American Medical Association, 287,*
2114–2119. Available online http://bethesda2001.cancer.gov/terminology/html

V. Terminology
A. AutoPap®—computer driven cytosmear evaluation technique approved by
FDA for selection of 10% of Pap smears to be manually rescreened;
selects 10% most likely to exhibit abnormalities

1. Consider offering to patients when available in lab used; can increase cost
B. PAPNET®—computerized system programmed to recognize cellular abnormalities on Pap slides prepared in the conventional way
   1. Consider offering to patients when available; can add to cost of Pap smear
C. Adjunctive screening
   1. Speculoscopy; combines with conventional Pap smear
      a. Pap smear is obtained
      b. Cervix is washed with vinegar solution and then illuminated with a chemiluminescent light attached to the upper blade of the speculum (Speculite®)—assists clinician in visualizing aceto-white areas of cervix

VI. 2001 Consensus Guidelines for Management of Cervical Cytological Abnormalities*

ATYPICAL SQUAMOUS CELLS (ASC)
ASC-US
   1. Repeat cervical cytological testing (Pap) at 4–6 month intervals until 2 consecutive "negative for intraepithelial lesions or malignancy results"; and then return to routine screening program; if any ASC-US on repeat testing, refer for colposcopy
   2. OR Repeat Pap with liquid based cytology and specify reflex HPV DNA testing
   3. OR If no liquid-based available, repeat Pap and include reflex HPV DNA testing
   4. OR Go directly to colposcopy; if no biopsy-confirmed CIN, repeat cytological testing at 12 months
   5. If positive for HPV DNA refer for colposcopy
      if colposcopy negative for CIN on biopsy, repeat cytological testing at 6 and 12 months with referral back to colposcopy if result of ASC-US or > obtained
   6. If negative for HPV DNA repeat cytological testing at 12 months
   ASC-US special circumstances
   1. Postmenopausal women: course of intravaginal estrogen and repeat cytological testing 1 week after completing regimen.
      If negative for intraepithelial lesion or malignancy, repeat test in 4–6 months; if both Paps are negative, return to routine screening.

---

*2001 Consensus guidelines for the management of women with cervical cytological abnormalities. 2002, *Journal of the American Medical Association, 287,* 2120–2139. Procedures used in the creation of the American Society of Cytopathology cervical cytology practice guidelines. *Journal of Lower Genital Tract Disease, 5,* 159–184.

If ASC-US, refer for colposcopy
2. Immunosuppressed women
   Refer for colposcopy; includes all women with HIV
3. Pregnant women manage same as nonpregnant

ASC-H
1. Refer for colposcopy
   No lesion identified, review cytology, colposcopy, histology results
   If revised interpretation, follow guidelines for this interpretation
   If no revised interpretation, cytological follow-up at 6 & 12 months
      or HPV DNA testing at 12 months
      ASC or > on repeat, refer for colposcopy

ATYPICAL GLANDULAR CELLS (AGC)
1. Colposcopy with endocervical sampling for all categories EXCEPT
2. Women with atypical endometrial cells evaluate with endometrial sampling
3. Endometrial sampling with colposcopy for women > 35 years with AGC
4. Women < 35 years with AGC and unexplained vaginal bleeding, endometrial sampling

AIS
1. Colposcopy with endocervical sampling

AGC with "favor neoplasia" and AIS without invasive disease
1. diagnostic excisional procedure—preferred cold knife conization

AGC NOS
1. with biopsy confirmed CIN of any grade
   follow 2001 Consensus Guidelines
2. no neoplasia, repeat cytological testing at 4–6 month intervals until 4 consecutive "negative for intraepithelial lesion or malignancy" results, then return to routine screening
3. IF ASC or LSIL on any follow up Pap, repeat colposcopy or referral to clinician expert in management of complex cytologic situations

LOW-GRADE SQUAMOUS INTRAEPITHELIAL LESION (LSIL)
1. Referral for colposcopy; endocervical sampling in non-pregnant women
2. Colposcopy with no cervical lesions follow up cytology at 6 and 12 months
   Referral for colposcopy with ASC-US or > or follow up with HPV DNA testing and refer for colposcopy if high-risk type of HPV

3. Unsatisfactory colposcopy:
    endocervical sampling in non-pregnant women
    failure to confirm CIN—repeat cytological testing at 6 & 12 months;
    refer for colposcopy if ASC-US or > or follow with HPV DNA
    testing at 12 months and refer to colposcopy for + result
4. Biopsy confirmed CIN manage according to 2001 Consensus Guide-
    lines for women with cervical histological abnormalities

LSIL special circumstances
1. Postmenopausal women
    Repeat cytological testing at 6 and 12 months; ASC-US or > refer
    for colposcopy or at 12 months do HPV DNA testing
    Course of intravaginal estrogen and repeat a week after completion
    of regimen; if ASC-US or > refer for colposcopy
    Negative for "intraepithelial lesion or malignancy" repeat Pap in 4–
    6 months; if negative, return to routine screening
        If ASC or >, refer for colposcopy
2. Adolescents:
    Repeat cytological testing at 6 & 12 months, ASC refer for colpos-
    copy; or do HPV DNA testing at 12 months with referral for high-
    risk types for colposcopy
3. Pregnant women:
    See HSIL special circumstances

HIGH-GRADE SQUAMOUS INTRAEPITHELIAL LESION (HSIL)
1. Colposcopy with endocervical assessment
2. Satisfactory colposcopy no lesion or only biopsy-confirmed CIN 1
    review cytology, colposcopy & histology
    Revised interpretation—follow management guidelines
    No revision—diagnostic excisional procedure in non-pregnant women
3. Unsatisfactory colposcopy review of cytologic, colposcopy and histo-
    logic results
    Revised interpretation, management by guidelines
    No revision—diagnostic excisional procedure in nonpregnant women

HSIL special circumstances
1. Pregnant women referral to clinicians experienced in colposcopy with
    pregnant women; biopsy of lesions suspected of high-grade disease or
    cancer; management per findings
    Unsatisfactory colposcopy—repeat in 6–12 weeks
    Repeat colposcopy 6 weeks postpartum or >

2. Young women of reproductive age
   Biopsy-confirmed CIN 2, 3 not confirmed, observe with colposcopy at 4–6 month intervals for 1 year assuming colposcopies are normal, endocervical sampling negative, & patient accepts risk
   Progression of lesion, diagnostic excisional procedure
Algorithm for management: www.asccp.org/pdfs/consensus/algorithms.pdf

VII. Follow-up for Any Abnormal Papanicolaou Test Finding
A. Follow-up as indicated in VI
B. Procedures for follow-up (one example)
   1. If report recommends repeat test or treatment, the patient is notified by letter and perhaps by telephone as well; also it may be useful to have a stamp with "Pap letter sent" on it to stamp the lab result sheet, and the nurse practitioner can also sign and date this sheet
   2. A file card is filled out with the patient's name and ID number, the nurse practitioners initials, and the date and results of the test. (File the card under the months of requested repeat). In some settings, a Papanicolaou book is also kept cross-referenced to the card file.*
   3. At the end of each month, the cards are pulled, attached to the patient's chart, and given to the nurse practitioner who performed the Papanicolaou smear originally and who is responsible for sending a letter to the patient reminding her of the need to repeat the test. (The card should be refiled for the next month.) If the patient still has not had a repeat test by the end of the second month, another letter is sent. If the results are less than LSIL, the nurse practitioner's responsibility ends. If results are LSIL or greater at this time, a registered letter with this information is sent to the patient. All letters and visits should be documented on charts and file cards.
   4. If test results show no abnormal cells but indicate reactive and reparative changes: inflammation, a letter should be sent to the patient stating that the laboratory findings for malignancy were negative but that there is evidence of a possible infection, and that an infection check is recommended if no check was done at the time of the Pap. No follow-up letters are necessary; no entries on cards are necessary.
   5. Some settings mark the record in some way and indicate that an annual Papanicolaou was done.

---

*Increasingly, computers are being used for this function. We recommend that a card system be continued for back-up.

VIII. Indications for Colposcopy
A. As indicated by Papanicolaou test; algorithm with ASCCP guidelines for ASCUS
B. History of physical examination that revealed possible diethylstilbestrol exposure
C. Any obvious lesions of the cervix
D. Lesions in vagina or vulva that are a diagnostic problem
E. If deemed necessary by physician or nurse practitioner

IX. Colposcopy Referral Procedure
A. Refer woman to physician of her choice or one available at same setting or to nurse practitioner or nurse midwife (increasingly being trained in colposcopy)
B. Instruct woman that she will probably be billed for procedure, which is generally covered by insurance; make any arrangements possible if she has no insurance
C. When patient chooses an outside physician or nurse practitioner or nurse midwife, a signed release form will be sent with referral sheet so a copy of the referral visit report can be returned to the original facility

X. Use of Colposcope by Nurse Practitioner
A. Use of colposcopy examination with HPV treatment
   1. A colposcopy examination of vulva, vagina, cervix done on all women found to have vulvar HPV lesions prior to beginning treatment
     a. Vulvar warts: treat according to protocol
     b. Cervical warts: refer to gynecologist or treat per nurse practitioner preparation
   2. Colposcopy examination may be done at each visit. If warts are still present after 8.-12 treatments, consult with gynecologist
   3. Colposcopy examination when warts appear to have resolved to verify treatment
B. Use of colposcope as diagnostic tool
   1. Used at discretion of nurse practitioner for closer inspection of vulva, vagina, and/or cervix
C. Procedure for colposcopy examination
   1. Explain procedure to woman
   2. Complete all necessary lab work
   3. Prepare area
     a. Swab entire vulva and vagina with acetic acid (white vinegar), applying generously

4. Examine with colposcope
5. Perform any biopsies indicated based on Pap findings

X. Follow-up
Per protocol of setting, based on Papanicolaou findings, colposcopy follow-up protocol; follow-up protocols for other evaluation methods.

AHCPR report on cervical cytology: www.ahcpr.gov/clinic/

Appendix A contains information about colposcopy which you may wish to photocopy or adapt for your patients. See Bibliography. http://cancernet.nci.nih.gov

Cervicitis

I. Definition
A. Chronic or acute inflammation of the cervix that is visible to the examiner. Causes symptoms observed by the woman and/or by cytologic examination
B. Mucopurulent cervicitis: characterized by mucopurulent exudate and easily induced cervical bleeding. CDC criteria 2002 for diagnosing indicated below by an asterisk(*)

II. Etiology
A. Bacterial
   1. Neisseria gonorrhoea
   2. Mycoplasmas
   3. Ureaplasmas
   4. Chlamydia trachomatis
B. Viral
   1. Herpes simplex
   2. Human papilloma virus (HPV)
C. Parasitic
   1. Trichomonas vaginalis
D. Nonmicrobiologic
   1. Inflammation in zone of ectopy
   2. DES exposure

III. History
A. What the patient may present with
   1. No symptoms

2. Friable cervix
3. Postcoital bleeding
4. Erythema of cervix (*if friable with first pass of swab)
5. Edematous cervix
6. Ulcerated or eroded cervix
7. Hypertrophied cervix
8. Ectropion
9. Cervical discharge; may be purulent or mucopurulent endocervical exudate on exam*
10. Vaginal discharge
11. Leukoplakia on cervix

B. Additional information to be considered
1. Onset of symptoms
2. Partner with symptoms
3. History of sexually transmitted disease
4. Sexual lifestyle; use of sex toys
5. Last Papanicolaou smear and results; any history of abnormal Papanicolaou
6. Contraception past and present
7. Colposcopy, cone biopsy, cauterization of cervix, cryo, LEEP
8. Laceration of cervix
9. Pregnancy history, infertility
10. Dyspareunia, pelvic pain
11. Urinary symptoms: frequency, urgency, dysuria
12. Menstrual history: last menstrual period
13. DES exposure

IV. Physical Examination
A. Cervix
1. Color
2. Character of any discharge: green, yellow, opaque, white, clear, cloudy, purulent, mucopurulent, serous, pH
3. Size
4. Lesions
5. Friability
6. Hood
7. Any polyps noted

B. Vagina
1. Color
2. Erythema
3. Lesions

    4. Discharge
C. Bimanual exam
    1. Masses
    2. Tenderness
    3. Cervical motion tenderness
    4. Uterine enlargement
    5. Position of organs
D. Adenopathy

V. Laboratory Examination
A. As indicated by findings
    1. Gonorrhea culture
    2. Chlamydia smear
    3. Wet prep: saline, KOH
    4. Papanicolaou smear
    5. Culture for bacteria
    6. Gram stain * > 30 polymorphonuclear (PMN) leukocytes
    7. Serology test for syphilis
    8. Herpes culture, antibodies
    9. Viratyping

VI. Differential Diagnosis
A. Condyloma acuminata
B. Chlamydia
C. Gonorrhea
D. Cervical cancer
E. Cervical infection: bacterial including mycoplasma, urea plasma
F. Ectropion
G. Leukoplakia
H. Herpetic exocervicitis
I. Trichomonas
J. Cervical ulceration (erosion) due to trauma: fingernail, cervical biopsy, postpartum, sex toys
K. Pelvic inflammatory disease (PID)
L. Infection secondary to trauma with sex toy
M. Cervical polyp

VII. Treatment
A. Medication
    1. As indicated by organism (see guidelines for gonorrhea, Chlamydia, herpes, condyloma, trichomonas, PID)

2. Bacterial (mycoplasma, urea plasma): see PID guideline
3. Mucopurulent cervicitis (women meeting CDC criteria) without confirmed organism can be treated empirically for gonorrhea and Chlamydia if
   a. prevalance of these is high in patient population,
   b. patient might be difficult to locate for treatment

B. Other measures
1. Ectropion: evaluate Papanicolaou results and follow-up as indicated; document with diagram and description for later follow-up; with persistent friability: refer or evaluate with colposcopy and biopsy
2. Leukoplakia: refer or evaluate with colposcopy and biopsy
3. Cervical cancer: refer for medical evaluation and intervention; in suspected cases in spite of negative Papanicolaou smear, refer or evaluate with colposcopy and biopsy
4. Cervical ulceration, erosion: follow-up as indicated by extent and nature of trauma; consider referral for medical evaluation and intervention
5. Consider colposcopy for all women who do not meet CDC guidelines for mucopurulent cervicitis, have a negative STD screen, and negative Papanicolaou
6. Manage sex partners appropriate for identified or suspected STD
7. Patients and sex partners abstain for course of treatment

VIII. Complications
Progression of condition to secondary or systemic infection (depending on organism) or PID; to metastatic disease; infertility; cervical stenosis

IX. Consultation/Referral
A. Unable to evaluate and diagnose
B. No response to treatment
C. For colposcopy, biopsy

X. Follow-up
A. As indicated by condition and treatment
B. Return for reevaluation if symptoms persist
   See Bibliography.

7

Menstrual Disorders

Dysmenorrhea

I. Definition
A. Primary dysmenorrhea is the occurrence of painful menses beginning within several years of menarche and in the absence of any pelvic pathology.
B. Secondary dysmenorrhea is painful menstruation due to an identifiable pathologic or iatrogenic condition, which may be readily identifiable on the basis of the history and the findings in a physical examination.

II. Etiology
A. Primary dysmenorrhea
  1. Caused by prostaglandins produced in the uterine lining and released into the bloodstream as the lining is shed, causing smooth muscle contraction, nausea, and/or diarrhea
B. Secondary dysmenorrhea
  1. Extrauterine causes
    a. Endometriosis
    b. Tumors
      1) Subserosal leiomyomata
      2) Malignancies
      3) Pelvic tumors
    c. Ovarian cysts
    d. Pelvic inflammatory disease
  2. Intrauterine causes
    a. Adenomyosis
    b. Endometriosis
    c. Intramural leiomyomata
    d. Polyps
    1) Endometrial   2) Cervical
    e. Presence of an intrauterine device
    f. Cervical stenosis
    g. Endometritis

III. History
A. What the patient may present with
   1. Recurrent pain monthly, prior to menses, sometimes with menses
      a. Abdominal pain
      b. Pelvic pain
      c. Severe backache
   2. Nausea; diarrhea or constipation
   3. Weakness
   4. Dizziness
   5. Weight gain
   6. Breast tenderness
   7. Backache
   8. Tension and nervousness
   9. Irritability and depression
B. Additional information to be obtained by asking the following questions:
   1. Relationship to menarche
   2. When does pain begin
   3. How long does it last
   4. Does anything make it feel better
   5. Last menstrual period
   6. Birth control method(s) used
   7. Any relationship to intercourse
   8. Any vaginal discharge
   9. Any fever related to pain
   10. What is menstrual flow like
   11. Is this new; is this a change in pattern
   12. Sensitivity to aspirin; nonsteroidal antiinflammatories
   13. History of chronic illness (kidney disease)
   14. Current medications (prescription and over-the-counter)
   15. Postcoital bleeding
   16. Home remedies and/or folk remedies tried; use of complementary and alternative therapies
   17. STD history, vaginitis/vaginosis

IV. Physical Examination
A. Vital signs
   1. Blood pressure
   2. Pulse
   3. Temperature, if symptoms arc present at time of visit
   4. Weight
B. Vaginal examination (speculum): cervix, cervical pathology

C. Bimanual examination

V. Laboratory Examination
A. Chlamydia (if not done within 1 year or woman has a new sexual partner), or cervical picture indicates, or if severity of symptoms has increased
B. Gonorrhea culture (same as Chlamydia)
C. Wet mount

VI. Differential Diagnosis
See Etiology

VII. Treatment
A. Medication
1. Ibuprofen (Motrin®) 400 mg, 1 QID, 200–400 mg q 4–6 hours (max 1.2 g/day)
2. Mefenamic acid (Ponstel®) 250 mg, 2 stat and 1 q 6 hours
3. Naproxen (Anaprox®) 275 mg, 2 stat and 1 q 6–8 hours (no more than 5 tabs 1.375 g per day); Aleve® 200 mg q. 8–12 hours
4. Naprosyn 500 mg q 12 hours or 250 mg q 6–8 hrs. (max. 1.25 g 1st day then 1.0 g/day)
5. Anaprox DS® 550 mg =1 q 12 hours
6. Aspirin with codeine gr ½ 1–2 tabs q 4 hours prn
7. Ibuprofen (Advil®) 200 mg, 2 tabs q 4–6 hours (max 1.2 g/day) (OTC), or
8. Flurbiprofen (Ansaid) 100 mg p.o. bid or tid
9. Meclofenamate (Meclomen®) 1 tab (100 mg) q 6 hours prn
10. Celecoxib (Celebrex®) adults 18 or older, 400 mg once then 200 mg once on 1st day, then 200 mg bid prn; not recommended under 18 years
11. Valdecoxib tablets (Bextra®) 20 mg BID; not recommend under 18 years
12. Refecoxib (Vioxx®) 50 mg qd prn
13. Other OTC analogue
14. Oral contraceptive (to produce anovulatory state)
B. Other measures
1. Reassurance
2. Refer to premenstrual syndrome protocols for diet, exercise, and vitamin recommendations
3. Heating pad; microwave pad (filled with nonpopping corn or buckwheat)

VIII. Complications
May occur with failure to recognize presence of entity as described in differential diagnosis which results in lack of appropriate treatment

IX. Consultation/Referral
A. Diagnosis of secondary dysmenorrhea
B. Failure to improve after treatment as in VII above

X. Follow-up
A. Yearly health examination and Papanicolaou smear
B. Serology test for syphilis as symptoms indicate
C. Secondary dysmenorrhea follow-up as indicated by physician or with consult
   See Bibliography.

Amenorrhea

I. Definition
A. Primary amenorrhea: failure of the menses to occur by age 15
B. Secondary amenorrhea: cessation of the menses for longer than 6 months in a woman who has established menses at least 1 year after menarche

IIA. Etiology for Primary Amenorrhea
1. Gonadal failure
2. Congenital absence of uterus & vagina
3. Constitutional delay

IIB. Etiology for Secondary Amenorrhea
A. Pregnancy; breast feeding
B. Pituitary disease or tumor; disruption of hypothalamic-pituitary axis
C. Menopause
D. Too little body fat (about 22% required for menses)
E. Excessive exercise (e.g., long-distance running, ballet dancing, gymnastics, figure skating)
F. Rapid weight loss
G. Cessation of menstruation following use of oral contraceptives, Depo-Provera, Norplant
H. Recent change in lifestyle (e.g., increase in stress)
I. Thyroid disease

J. Polycystic ovary syndrome
K. Anorexia nervosa or other eating disorders
L. Premature ovarian failure, ovarian dysgenesis, infection, hemorrhage, necrosis, neoplasm
M. Asherman's syndrome
N. Cervical stenosis—outflow tract anomaly
O. Medications including psychotropics
P. Chronic illness
Q. Tuberculosis

III. History
A. What the patient presents with
  1. Absence of menstruation
  2. Possible breast discharge
  3. Other symptoms secondary to underlying etiology
B. Additional information to be considered
  1. Careful menstrual history; pregnancy history
  2. Sexual history
  3. Contraceptive history
  4. Medications—OTC, prescription, homeopathic, herbal
  5. Sources of emotional stress
  6. Symptoms of climacteric
  7. Any current acute illness
  8. History of chronic illness
  9. Present weight, weight 1 year ago
  10. Amount of daily exercise
  11. Recent D&C or abortion
  12. History of tuberculosis
  13. Eating disorder—current or history of

IV. Physical Examination
A. Weigh patient
B. Neck: thyroid gland (look for nodes: palpable, enlarged)
C. Breast: discharge
  1. Check both breasts
  2. Milky, clear, dark, light, bloody, thick, thin, color
D. Vaginal examination (speculum): vagina may be atrophic and there may be no cervical mucus
E. Bimanual examination
  1. Uterus: may be enlarged
  2. Cervix—scarring, stenosis

   3. Adnexa: ovaries may be enlarged—cystic
   4. Recto-vaginal examination
F. Measure ratio of body fat to lean mass

V. Laboratory Examination
A. Human chorionic gonadotropin (HCG) qualitative, quantitative
B. Prolactin level
C. Thyroid stimulating hormone
D. Follicle stimulating hormone, luteinizing hormone, Dehydroepiandrosterone sulfate (DHEAS), and serum testosterone (if patient is hirsute); hemoglobin, erythrocyte sedimentation rate
E. Papanicolaou smear
F. Microscopic examination of cervical mucus
G. TB test if no history
H. Consider pituitary function assessment, ultrasound, CAT scan, MRI, hysterosalpingography, hysteroscopy after consultation with a physician
I. GnRH stimulation test

VI. Differential Diagnosis
See Etiology

VII. Treatment
A. If breast discharge is present, do not wait: do work-up as per breast discharge protocol
B. If human chorionic gonadotropin (HCG) and prolactin levels are within normal limits, pregnancy test is negative and cervical mucus positive (ferning), the nurse practitioner may give: Medroxyprogesterone acetate (Provera®) 5–10 mg x 5–10 days
   1. If no withdrawal bleed in 3–7 days after progestin, do follicle stimulating hormone and luteinizing hormone assays 2 weeks after Provera. Try oral estrogen 1.25–2.5 mg to prime the endometrium (estropipate) for 21–25 days; if no bleeding, add progestin during last 5–10 days of estrogen. If no withdrawal bleed, refer to physician
   2. If woman wishes to start oral contraceptives and has no withdrawal bleed from Provera, repeat HCG if indicated and start oral contraceptives the following Sunday regardless of brand of oral contraceptive used. If no withdrawal bleed after first cycle, consult with physician
   3. If woman wishes to start oral contraceptives and has withdrawal bleed from Provera, start oral contraceptives after start of bleed; if Provera is not completed by that time, discontinue and discard remainder (some providers have woman complete Provera)

4. If withdrawal bleed occurs with Provera, then no menses for 2 months following the bleed, possible consult with physician, then give Provera 10 mg x 10 days every 2 months. If sexually active, an HCG must be run prior to taking medication each time

5. If woman has a history of uterine infection or trauma to the uterus through multiple curettages (postpartum or postabortion), or if the work-up is negative and there is no response to Provera, referral for further evaluation (hysterosalpingography; hysteroscopy to lyse adhesions; estrogen to restore endometrium)

6. Instruct woman to complete 10 days of Provera even if withdrawal bleed begins, unless starting oral contraceptives as 3 above

VIII. Complications
Inability to conceive
Sequelae of underlying cause

IX. Consultation/Referral
A. As outlined under Treatment VII.B.5
B. After work-up for hirsutism is completed (see V.D.)
C. For all primary amenorrhea cases

X. Follow-up
A. As deemed necessary with physician consult
B. Yearly
C. Every 6 months; if taking Provera, every 2 months
    See Bibliography.

Abnormal Vaginal Bleeding

I. Definition
Any variation from a woman's usual menstrual pattern; bleeding postmenopause

II. Etiology
A. Systemic illnesses, i.e., thyroid disease, blood dyscrasias, adrenal imbalance
B. Submucous leiomyomata in uterus; polyps, liver disease, clotting disorders, kidney disease, leukemia
C. Tumor in vagina, uterus

D. Trauma to vagina, cervix; scar tissue
E. Cervical lesions
   1. Polyps
   2. Carcinoma
F. Abnormal hormone secretion (with anovulatory bleeding)
G. Change in ovarian function (perimenopause)
H. Endometrial polyps or leiomyomata in cervix, uterus
I. Pelvic malignancy—nodes, uterus, bladder, rectum, vagina
J. Ectopic pregnancy
K. Abortion
L. Placental accidents
M. Hyperplasia
N. Stress
O. Postmenopausal bleed
P. Pharmacotherapeutics
Q. STDs, PID
R. Endometriosis/adenomyosis
S. Hemorrhoids, polyps in colon, colon carcinoma mistaken for vaginal bleeding

III. History
A. What the patient may present with
   1. Midcycle bleeding
   2. Spotting
   3. Pain
   4. Sudden onset of heavy bleeding
   5. Postmenopausal bleeding
B. Additional information to be considered
   1. Is bleeding recent or since menarche
   2. Onset of bleeding
   3. Amount of flow (pads or tampons per hour); clots and size of clots
   4. Normal bleeding pattern: how does this episode differ from normal menstruation
   5. Current or recent use of medication; complementary therapies (herbals, homeopathics)
   6. Last menstrual period; previous menstrual period
   7. Last sexual contact, if sexually active
   8. Birth control method(s)
   9. Recent trauma to pelvic area or any other part of body (screen for abuse)
   10. Characteristics of present bleeding: clots, tissue

11. Any related pain
12. Any fever
13. Any dizziness; syncope
14. Symptoms of changing ovarian function (menopausal)
15. Recent pelvic surgery including tubal ligation

IV. Physical Examination
A. Vital signs
   1. Blood pressure
   2. Pulse
   3. Temperature
B. Skin: examine for evidence of bleeding disorder, e.g., petechiae or ecchymosis; pallor; fine, thinning hair
C. Neck—thyroid: examine for enlargement, palpate nodes
D. Breasts
   1. Development   4. Discharge
   2. Masses   5. Axillary nodes
   3. Tenderness, appearance of skin, nipples
E. Abdomen
   1. Tenderness
   2. Guarding
   3. Bowel sounds
   4. Distension
   5. Hepatosplenomegaly
F. Genital examination: Observe perineum for trauma
G. Vaginal examination (speculum)
   1. Observe vaginal walls for lesions or evidence of trauma
   2. Observe cervix for
      a. Polyps
      b. Lesions (evidence of trauma)
      c. Erosion or ectropion
      d. Whether os is closed or dilated; discharge in os
   3. Evaluate amount and type of bleeding
H. Bimanual examination
   1. Uterus: evaluate size, shape, position, any pain
   2. Adnexa: evaluate for possible mass, pain
   3. Recto-vaginal exam
      a. Fullness (fluid)
      b. Pain
      c. Bleeding

V. Laboratory Examination (will depend on history and assessment of bleeding)

A. Complete blood count, differential with hematocrit or hemoglobin; platelet count. Bleeding & clotting time if indicated

B. Serum pregnancy test

C. Gonococcal culture

D. Chlamydia smear

E. Thyroid studies if indicated

F. Hormone levels—LH, FSH, prolactin, GnRh, serum estradiol

G. Urinalysis

H. STD screen including HIV status

I. Wet mount

VI. Differential Diagnosis

See Etiology

VII. Treatment

A. For light flow/regular/irregular bleeding (e.g., mid-cycle)
   1. Lab work as history demands
   2. May observe 2–3 months as indicated by history and physical findings. Woman should be instructed to keep record of days that bleeding occurs.
   3. After 2–3 cycles, after normal physical exam and Papanicolaou smear with appropriate lab work, consider
      a. Provera 5–10 mg qd x 10 days or
      b. Monophasic OC x 1–3 months or 6–12 months

B. For heavy bleeding
   1. Consult/refer to physician after appropriate work-up

C. For bleeding with IUD in place see IUD protocol

D. For bleeding associated with Norplant®, consider addition of low dose oral contraceptive x 3 cycles or Premarin 1.25 mg qd until bleeding stops

E. For heavy bleeding with Depo-Provera,* consider same regimen as in D. above

F. If bleeding persists with a positive HCG
   1. Physician consultation
   2. Referral as indicated

G. If bleeding postmenopausal will need an endometrial biopsy (see Endometrial Biopsy guideline)

---

*Approach this regimen with caution remembering that menstrual changes are recognized as an early phenomenon with progestin-only contraception, decreasing with prolonged use. Also, if patient is a long-term user, the onset of new bleeding may indicate underlying pathology.

VIII. Complications
A. Severe hemorrhage
B. Shock
C. Of underlying systemic illnesses

IX. Consultation/Referral
A. After completion of all laboratory work and physical examination, nurse practitioner may consult with physician
B. Immediate referral to physician if excessive bleeding after laboratory work and work-up by nurse practitioner

X. Follow-up
As indicated by diagnosis and treatment

   See Bibliography.

Endometrial Biopsy

I. Definition
Endometrial biopsy is a method of obtaining a sample of the nonpregnant uterine lining for purposes of cytologic and histologic examination. The procedure can be done in an ambulatory setting with or without local anesthesia. The specimen obtained is glandular epithelium.

II. Etiology
Reasons for performing this diagnostic procedure may include:
A. Unexplained abnormal vaginal bleeding in the premenopausal, perimenopausal or postmenopausal woman
B. Rule out endometrial pathology prior to initiation of hormone therapy (HT) in the postmenopausal woman and periodically monitor endometrial status with unopposed estrogen use if indicated
C. Determine response of the endometrium to hormonal intervention in women experiencing infertility
D. Evaluate endometrial response during tamoxifen therapy to rule out pathologic response

III. History
A. What the patient may present with
   1. Postmenopausal bleeding

2. Unexplained abnormal vaginal bleeding in a premenopausal woman
3. Desire for hormone therapy
4. Currently taking hormone therapy with intact uterus
5. Unsuccessful attempts at pregnancy
6. Current tamoxifen therapy for breast disease

B. Additional information to be considered
   1. Hormone therapy: type, purpose, duration, dosage, side effects, bleeding history; use of hormonal contraception, IUD
   2. Gynecologic and pregnancy including STD and PID episodes; elective abortions
   3. Gynecologic surgery including previous endometrial biopsies and results, tubal ligation, cesarean section
   4. Medical conditions: cardiac, bleeding disorders, hypoglycemia
   5. Current medications including over-the-counter and botanical preparations
   6. Allergies to pharmacologics including local anesthetic agents and povidone-iodine (Betadine, similar products)
   7. Vasovagal episodes especially with pelvic examinations, uterine sounding, IUD insertion, elective abortion
   8. Symptoms of vaginitis, cervicitis, STD, PID
   9. Contraceptive methods including current method and consistency of use; any recent exposure to pregnancy risk and date
   10. Menstrual cycles, peri- and postmenopausal bleeding; LMP, PMP

IV. Physical Examination

A. Bimanual examination: uterine position, pain, flexion, size, shape; adnexal or uterine masses, cervical motion tenderness, adnexal exam; any pelvic pain, determine involution if woman is postpartum, postabortion
B. Recto-vaginal examination to determine uterine size, position, rule out pregnancy
C. Vital signs: blood pressure, temperature (rule out fever)
D. General status: last meal or snack, fluids (rule out hypoglycemia); offer juice, snack
E. Administer mild prostaglandin inhibitor 20 minutes before biopsy
F. Teach woman about the procedure and possible complications, and obtain her consent to proceed

V. Reasons to Defer Procedure

A. Pregnancy or possible pregnancy
B. PID, STD with PID as complication, cervicitis

C. Poor involution of uterus postpartum or postabortion
D. Fever
E. Blood dyscrasias, especially bleeding disorders, severe anemia
F. Extremely anteflexed or retroflexed uterus or cervical stenosis—may need to do biopsy under general anesthesia
G. Vaginitis—defer procedure until diagnosis and treatment regimen completed

VI. Laboratory
A. Pregnancy test
B. Hematocrit as indicated
C. Postprocedure biopsy specimen(s) for histologic screening
D. Other per work-up for abnormal uterine bleeding

VII. Biopsy Technique
A. Collect any routine specimens, cultures as indicated; bimanual exam to determine position of uterus
B. Visualize the cervix and inspect for any mucopurulent discharge, visual signs of cervicitis; if found, defer procedure to collect any additional specimens and treat
C. Cleanse cervix and vagina with antiseptic, considering any sensitivities, allergies
D. Administer local anesthetic agent to the cervix (lidocaine gels, other topical gel or spray products, or paracervical block) if necessary/desired depending on sampling technique and equipment to be used
E. Sound the uterus (if using curette for sampling); prior to this, grasping the cervix with a fine tenaculum is necessary (using local anesthetic gel at the site for tenaculum placement reduces pain for the woman). Having the patient cough when applying and removing the tenaculum often reduces discomfort
F. Insert the sampling device* in the os, taking care not to force the device through a resistant os; if the os is stenotic, cervical dilators may be used. Use one of the following techniques:
   1. Pipelle device (flexible sampler with a piston to create suction for sampling): insert up to fundus, pull back completely on the piston to create suction and rotate the pipelle continuously moving it from the fundus and back again several times to collect the sample completely filling the plastic tube; withdraw the pipelle and push in the piston to

---

*These include Pipelle®, Gyno Sampler®, Novak Curette®, Tis-u-trap®, Vabra aspirator®, uterine Explora currette®, Endocell®.

deposit sample into the preservative. Some devices require cutting off the tip to expel the specimen

2. Pipelle device attached to suction pump: insert as above and collect specimen by connecting the external pump, continuing suction until the device is filled

3. Suction curette that is steel and reusable or plastic and disposable: sound the uterus stabilizing the cervix with a tenaculum and then insert the curette and gently sample in a manner similar to using the pipelle devices (some are attached to a 10 cc syringe to provide the suction and some to an external pump); withdraw the curette, deposit the specimen in the preservative

G. Monitor woman's condition during and after the procedure to assess for vasovagal response, signs and symptoms of uterine perforation

H. Allow woman to rest briefly with her legs flat before getting off the examination table. Assure that she is not feeling faint and is able to get dressed safely

I. Instruct woman regarding postprocedure care

1. Signs and symptoms of complications: severe cramping or pelvic pain; bright red bleeding with or without clots; fever, chills, foul-smelling vaginal discharge—call provider and/or go to urgent care setting

2. Expect spotting for 1–2 days after the biopsy; define spotting and the difference between spotting and bleeding

3. Patient may resume vaginal intercourse in 3 days or whenever she desires

4. Prostaglandin inhibitor for mild cramping

5. Resumption of menses if premenopausal and having menstrual cycles

VIII. Referral//Consultation for Procedure

A. Women with severe cervical stenosis to consider procedure under general anesthesia

B. Women with contraindications for procedure

IX. Follow-up

A. Arrange for an opportunity to review laboratory findings

B. Care based on reason for endometrial biopsy and laboratory results

X. Referral/Consultation for Results

A. Endometrial carcinoma—referral for treatment or comanagement

B. Hyperplasia without atypia—usually means atrophic changes

1. Secretory: follow but no need for treatment unless bleeding persists and consider Provera

2. Proliferative may benefit from Provera

C. Complex hyperplasia without atypia

   1. Desires pregnancy: consider risks and co-manage with physician

   2. Does not desire pregnancy: to remove unopposed estrogen, cycle with progestins and repeat endometrial biopsy in 3–6 months

D. Complex hyperplasia with atypia—referral for D&C

   1. Co-management for pregnancy if desired and no malignancy or for surgical high risk

   2. Surgery and/or treatment per staging if malignant

   3. Hysterectomy if nonmalignant and no pregnancy desired

See Bibliography.

Premenstrual Syndrome (PMS)*

I. Definition

PMS (premenstrual syndrome) is a cluster of physical, emotional, and behavioral symptoms related to the menstrual cycle, developing or worsening during the luteal phase and clearing with the onset of the menstrual flow.

II. Etiology

No single etiology explains the various symptoms associated with PMS. A multifactorial cause is probable, involving psychosocial, genetic, hormonal, and neurotransmitter components (serotonergic dysfunction)

III. History

A. What the patient presents with (may include some or all of the following symptoms, in varying degrees)

   1. Headache, backache, migraine, syncope

   2. Edema

   3. Breast tenderness, engorgement, enlargement, heaviness

   4. Hot flashes

   5. Paresthesia of hands or feet, aggravation of epilepsy; joint or muscle pain

   6. Weight gain

   7. Fluid retention

   8. Abdominal bloating

   9. Increase in appetite and/or impulsive eating; craving for sweets and/or salt; food cravings in general

   10. Nausea, vomiting, constipation

---

*Known as periluteal phase dysphoric disorder (PPDD) in *DSM-IV* diagnosis.

11. Decreased urine output, cystitis, urethritis, enuresis
12. Exacerbation or recurrence of acne, boils, urticaria, easy bruising, herpes, rhinitis, colds, hoarseness, increased asthma, sore throat, sinusitis
13. Emotional lability (anxiety, depression, crying, fatigue, persistent & marked anger, aggression, irritability), difficulty in concentrating; decreased interest in usual activities
14. Changes in libido
15. Lethargy, fatigue, depression in mood, feeling hopeless
16. Sleep disturbances—hypersomnia, insomnia
17. Palpitations
18. Any symptoms, physical or emotional, that cluster during the same phase of menstrual cycle

B. Additional information to be considered
   1. When did these symptoms first occur in relationship to menarche
   2. When do they begin and end in relationship to menses
   3. Has there been a recent change in symptoms
   4. Do you have cramps with your period
   5. Has there been any change in your lifestyle (work, personal, family)
   6. What is your diet like
   7. How much exercise do you get
   8. Are you or have you ever been in counseling
   9. What medications are you taking
   10. Do you have a history of chronic illness; if so, which including depression
   11. When was your last menstrual period
   12. When was your last sexual contact (if sexually active)
   13. What birth control method do you use if any
   14. Have you had tubal ligation and if so, when
   15. Have you ever thought about suicide or harm to others
   16. Have you experienced depression or agitation at other times in your life

IV. Physical Examination
A. Vital signs
B. Complete physical and gynecologic exam within past year examination
C. Mental status examination

V. Laboratory Examination
A. Only as indicated medically

VI. Treatment

A. Treatment is multifaceted and diverse, aimed at symptoms which patient finds most debilitating. To aid in diagnosis and treatment, 2 months of retrospective daily logs or symptom calendars help to confirm diagnosis and guide selection of appropriate treatment

   1. Vitamin B$_6$ (pyridoxine). Begin with 50 mg to 100 mg total daily dose. Do not exceed recommended dosage. This vitamin has been shown to be toxic in large doses.
   2. Vitamin E 400 mg daily or twice a day
   3. Evening Primrose Oil. Begin with 2 capsules twice a day. May increase to 4 capsules twice a day. Improvement will occur slowly over 3–9 months. Contains vitamin E, so patient should not take both
   4. Prostaglandin inhibitors may provide relief taken during the second half of the menstrual cycle
   5. May consider
      a. Ovulation blockers
      b. Diuretics
      c. Antidepressants
      d. Antianxiety drugs
      e. Birth control pills, contraceptive patch, ring)
      f. Progesterone (synthesized, natural)
   6. Calcium 1000–1200 mg daily; magnesium 300–400 mg daily

B. General measures

   1. Lifestyle changes including stress reduction, i.e., meditation, yoga, or other relaxation techniques
   2. Diet recommendations
      a. Limit consumption of refined sugar (e.g., cookies, cakes, jelly, honey) to 5 tbs/day
      b. Limit salt intake to 3 gm or less per day (e.g., avoid using saltshaker)
      c. Limit intake of alcohol and nicotine
      d. Avoid caffeine (e.g., coffee, tea, chocolate, soft drinks)
      e. Increase intake of complex carbohydrates (e.g., fresh fruits, vegetables, whole grains, pasta, rice, potatoes)
      f. Consume moderate amounts of protein and fat (decease animal fats and increase vegetable oils)
      g. Limit red meat consumption to 2 x weekly or less
         These dietary changes should be ongoing. It is not enough to modify one's diet only on the days prior to menstruation
   3. Exercise plan recommendations: exercise three times per week for 30–40 minutes (brisk walking, jogging, aerobic dancing, swimming)

4. Consider other complementary therapies including botanicals, aroma and music therapy, acupuncture, and energy healing
5. Keep a diary of daily symptoms, diet, body temperature

VII. Differential Diagnosis
A. Sexual dysfunction
B. Chronic pelvic pain
C. Endometriosis
D. Primary dysmenorrhea
E. Post-tubal ligation syndrome
F. Prolactin-producing tumors
G. Perimenopausal symptoms
H. Fibrocystic breast disease
I. Depression
J. Psychopathology
K. Somatization of stress
L. Life stressors
M. Systemic lupus erythematosus
N. Hypertension
O. Meningioma
P. Attention-deficit disorder (residual type)
Q. Thyroid disorders

VIII. Complications
A. Serious psychological problem misdiagnosed as PMS
B. Systemic disease misdiagnosed as premenstrual syndrome

IX. Consultation/Referral
A. Referral to physician at discretion of nurse practitioner, after review of history and physical examination
B. Mental health referral if appropriate
C. Referral to nutritionist if needed/desired by woman
D. Support group referral if desired

X. Follow-up
A. Monthly x 3 checks
B. Yearly if improvement in relief of symptoms
C. If symptoms increase or change

See Complementary and Alternative therapies guideline, and Bibliography.

8

Postabortion Care

Examination After Medical or Surgical Abortion

I. Definition
An examination usually two weeks after uncomplicated therapeutic abortion to assess the patient's physical and mental status.

II. Etiology
Therapeutic abortion

III. History
A. What patient may present with
   1. surgical
      a. no unusual complaints
      b. rare complications may include
         1) excessive blood loss (typical length of light to moderate flow is 9 days)
         2) pelvic infection
         3) pelvic perforation
         4) acute hematometra
   2. Medical
      a. nausea
      b. vomiting
      c. headaches
      d. fever
      e. chills
      f. bleeding: average length of bleeding is 10–13 days; however, heavy bleeding may occur
B. Additional information to be considered
   1. Date of abortion; type of procedure
   2. Date of last menstrual period
   3. Are pregnancy symptoms gone
   4. How long after procedure did bleeding continue; any pain associated with bleeding; how much bleeding; any clots; fever

5. Results of pathological examination of products of conception (if available)
6. Any change in relationship with partner
7. Present emotional status
8. Birth control method
9. Intercourse since procedure
10. Medications taken including antibiotics, oxytocins, herbals, vitamins, homeopathic

IV. Physical Examination
A. Vital signs: blood pressure, pulse
B. Abdominal examination
C. Vaginal examination (speculum)
   1. Observe for bleeding or other discharge
   2. Cervix
      a. Os closed   b. Any lesions   c. Any discharge
D. Bimanual exam
   1. Uterus
      a. Size   b. Consistency   c. Tenderness
      d. Cervix: positive Chandelier's sign (cervical motion tenderness)
   2. Adnexa
      a. Tenderness
      b. Masses
   3. Rectovaginal: any abnormal findings

V. Treatment
A. Birth control
   1. Birth control pill, Depo-Provera®, contraceptive ring, patch
   2. Diaphragm, cap
   3. Intrauterine device
   4. Other methods (OTC): condoms, spermicides
   5. Sterilization (if desired)
B. General measures: review use and sign informed consent form for birth control method (see Appendix D)

VI. Laboratory Examination
A. Pregnancy test as indicated
B. Wet mount as indicated

VII. Differential Diagnosis
None

VIII. Complications
See Postabortion with Complications, pages 184–186

IX. Consultation/Referral
A. See Postabortion with Complications, pages 184–186
B. If unresolved issues are apparent, follow-up counseling will be recommended

X. Follow-up
A. Yearly for health examination, Papanicolaou smear, reevaluation of family planning needs
B. As per guideline for contraceptive of woman's choice

See Appendix A and Bibliography.

Postabortion With Complications

I. Definition
Any sequelae or unexpected/untoward events or conditions following a therapeutic abortion.

II. Etiology
Therapeutic abortion—medical or surgical

III. History
A. What the patient may present with
    1. Fever, body aches, chills
    2. Pelvic pain, severe cramps
    3. Bleeding; more than 1 pad an hour
    4. Passing clots larger than a quarter
    5. Abdominal pain: R or L side or bilateral; onset, duration, how relieved
    6. Nausea, vomiting
    7. Breast tenderness, discharge
    8. Foul vaginal discharge
    9. Vertigo
B. Additional information to be considered
    1. Where and when was the procedure done; has the woman spoken to that facility regarding her symptoms or follow-up care; type of procedure (medical or surgical)
    2. How much physical activity since procedure, type

3. Any intercourse since procedure
4. Anything used in vagina since procedure: contraceptive device; tampons; sex toy; douche product
5. Any exposure to flu or anyone with similar symptoms
6. Any medications taken such as analgesics, ergotrate, antibiotics, over-the-counter or prescription drugs, including herbals, vitamins
7. Urinary tract symptoms
8. Bowel symptoms
9. Still feels pregnant; symptoms of pregnancy

IV. Physical Examination
A. Vital signs

1. Temperature	3. Blood pressure
2. Pulse	4. Respirations

B. Breast examination: tender/more/less/same as before procedure (if indicated); discharge
C. Abdomen
  1. Bowel signs
  2. Guarding
  3. Rebound tenderness
  4. Referred pain (shoulder pain)
D. Vaginal examination (sterile if within 1 week after procedure):
  1. Os dilated
  2. Any tissue in os
  3. Amount of bleeding; character
  4. Any discharge present; odor
E. Bimanual examination
  1. Cervical motion tenderness: positive Chandelier's sign
  2. Uterine tenderness, enlargement; note consistency
  3. Adnexa

a. Tenderness	b. Mass	c. Fullness

  4. Rectovaginal examination: tenderness; if present, describe location

V. Laboratory Examination
A. Serum pregnancy test—quantitative
B. Gonococcal culture
C. Chlamydia smear
D. Cervical culture
E. Complete blood count with differential, sedimentation rate
F. Urinalysis and urine culture
G. Call laboratory of referring facility to get results of pathology report

VI. Differential Diagnosis
A. Retained secundae; continuation of pregnancy
B. Uterine infection, endometritis
C. Delayed involution
D. Pelvic inflammatory disease
E. Urinary tract infection
F. Uterine perforation, bowel perforation
G. Ectopic pregnancy
H. See Acute Pelvic Pain and Abdominal Pain guidelines

VII. Treatment
As indicated by symptoms and diagnosis; may include appropriate antibiotics, treatment of any urinary infection, ergotrate product to promote involution; reevacuation or evacuation if failure of medical abortion; referral for evaluation of possible ectopic pregnancy (see Pelvic Inflammatory Disease guideline and Genitourinary Tract [Urinary Tract Infection] guideline)

VIII. Complications
A. Sepsis
B. Ruptured ectopic pregnancy
C. Hemorrhage
D. Uterine perforation, bowel perforation
E. Ascherman's syndrome

IX. Consultation/Referral
Call facility or provider that performed the abortion for a consult and arrangement for return visit and further evaluation

X. Follow-up
Follow routine postabortion guideline

See Appendix A and Bibliography.

9

Abuse, Battering, Violence, and Sexual Assault

Abuse Assessment Screen*

*CONDUCT THIS SCREEN WITH THE WOMAN ALONE IN A
PRIVATE SETTING*

Inform her that
Since 1 in 6 pregnant women are abused, all women are
being asked about risks at home
This information will not be shared without her permission

1. Have you EVER been emotionally or physically abused by your
   partner or someone important to you?   YES NO
2. WITHIN THE LAST YEAR, have you been pushed, shoved, hit,
   slapped, kicked or otherwise physically hurt by someone?   YES NO
       If YES, by whom? _____
       Total number of times _____
3. SINCE YOU'VE BEEN PREGNANT, were you pushed, shoved, hit,
   slapped, kicked or otherwise physically hurt by someone?   YES NO
       If YES, by whom? _____
       Total number of times _____

Mark the areas of injury on the body map.
Score each incident according to the following scale:
1 = Threats of abuse, including use of a weapon
2 = Slapping, pushing; no injuries and/or lasting pain
3 = Punching, kicking, bruises, cuts, and/or continuing pain
4 = Beaten up, severe contusions, burns, broken bones
5 = Head injury, internal injury, permanent injury
6 = Use of weapon; wound from weapon

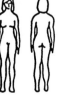

*Developed by the Nursing Research Consortium on Violence and Abuse. Readers are encouraged to reproduce and use this assessment tool. Adapted by Pregnancy Support Project, Boston College, William F. Connell School of Nursing.

(If any of the descriptions for the higher number apply, use the higher number)

4. WITHIN THE LAST YEAR, has anyone forced you to have sexual
   activities?   YES NO
           IF YES, who? _____
           Total number of times _____
5. ARE YOU AFRAID of your partner or anyone in your life?   YES NO

Note: You can use the Abuse Assessment Screen with all women by deleting the pregnancy question.

Assessment for Abuse and/or Violence*

I. Definition
Abuse and/or violence in a relationship is said to occur when one person physically, sexually, verbally and/or emotionally abuses another and/or destroys the property of the person. Experiencing fear for one's person in a relationship is characteristic of an abusive situation, regardless of whether or not there is physical violence. Fearing physical harm is enough to consider the relationship abusive. Power or control by one person over another in a relationship can constitute abuse; power and control in a relationship are hallmarks of abuse. Constant degradation damages ego, self-esteem, confidence. Dating violence affects an estimated 1.8 adolescents and domestic violence, 1:4 to 1:10 women.

II. History: Consider each woman in any setting abused until proven otherwise
A. What the patient may present with
   1. Description of abuse or violence in the relationship
   2. Unexplained symptoms inconsistent with any disease pathology
   3. Numerous psychosomatic complaints with no physical evidence
   4. Vague physical complaints

---

*Kathleen K. Furniss, RNC, MSN, a consultant for this guideline, suggests asking 2 or 3 simple questions and varying the query for the clinical situation, e.g., "Is someone physically hurting you?" Kathleen is author of many articles on abuse and is a founder of the Jersey Battered Women's Service and a principal in the Domestic Violence Prevention Project, St. Barnabas Medical Center, Livingston, NJ.

5. The woman's partner gives history and answers questions directed toward woman
6. Delay between presenting injury or problem and seeking care
7. Woman seems embarrassed or evasive in giving history
8. Woman seems fearful, withdrawn, does not name friends, family members as resources

B. Additional information to be considered (see questions on previous guideline)
1. Psychiatric, alcohol, and/or drug abuse by patient and/or partner
2. Suicide gestures or attempts; suicidal ideation
3. Many "accidents" in record, visits to emergency department
4. Any gynecologic or gastrointestinal complaints
5. Level of anxiety the woman demonstrates over the visit or the physical exam

III. Physical Examination

A. Unexplained bruises; whiplike injuries consistent with shaking; erythematous areas consistent with slapping; lacerations, burn marks, fractures, and/or multiple injuries in various stages of healing
B. Injuries on body hidden by clothing and injuries inconsistent with common accidents such as on the genitals, breasts, chest, head, face, and abdomen
C. Evidence of sexual abuse—lacerations on breasts, labia, urethra, perineum, anal area
D. Healed fractures or scars
E. Fractures inconsistent with story of accident
F. Apprehensive during examination and injuries and other findings are inappropriate to her story or inexplicable
G. Abuse can have no symptoms; well woman without visible injuries

IV. Laboratory Examination

A. As indicated by physical findings
B. May include x rays for evidence of new, healing, or old fractures

V. Interviewing the Woman

A. Provide a safe place alone and private where partner/spouse/abuser cannot hear
B. Assure her of confidentiality and safety
C. Phrase questions in a nonthreatening way conveying empathy such as: "I notice you have some bruises. Can you tell me how they happened? Have you been hit by someone?" "Has anyone hurt you in anyway?" "When

was the last time you cried?" (see also questions on Abuse Assessment Screen on page 187
D. Assess for current danger and for emotional and/or physical injuries (see Danger Assessment tool in Appendix E)

VI. Documenting Evidence
A. Data from medical records and those of other health care providers
B. Record most recent, as well as past incidents
C. Record any witnesses to abuse
D. Quote the woman's statements of abuse with, "Patient states . . ."
E. Protect patient by deleting any statements such as, "He hurt me so much I wanted to kill him"
F. If woman denies any abuse, record your assessment and suspicions for possible future use
G. Record any injuries or symptoms in detail as to size, location, duration, onset, age, pattern. Make a body map and locate injuries in as much detail as you can. Indicate any evidence of sexual abuse, restraint marks on skin
H. Collect physical evidence of injuries and label after obtaining with the woman's written permission to do so
I. Photograph all evidence of injuries with the woman's written permission

VII. Treatment
A. Assure the woman she is not alone
B. Assure the woman of confidentiality and that only she can authorize the release of evidence to the police, the release of her records, and your verbal testimony
C. Provide support that she does not deserve abuse and that no person should perpetrate any kind of abuse or violence on her
D .Show her the documentation in her record and indicate that its purpose is to protect her
E. Provide resources for her safety and for escape if she decides to do so; empower her to make her own plans and choices
F. Teach her about the patterns of violence and the laws in your state concerning abuse and violence in relationships; have copies of the state laws available
G. If she chooses to remain in the relationship, you can offer her emergency numbers of police, any domestic violence units or special forces, local emergency room(s) and shelters; help make a safety plan (money, car keys, important documents, where to go); for undocumented immigrant women who need counseling, give phone numbers of culturally sensitive programs

VIII. Referrals/Consultation
A. Medical consultation as appropriate for treatment of injuries
B. Police if woman chooses to file a complaint or police report
C. Shelters, special services for women in abusing/violent relationships
D. Mental health consultation if you believe woman is suicidal
E. Substance abuse, alcohol abuse treatment programs as appropriate and desired by the woman

X. Follow-up
A. Plan return visit so woman has another opportunity for contact with you. Women may seem fine but may be degraded, depressed, afraid, or subjugated by a powerful partner who may control finances, children's money and welfare, and may be occasionally rewarding and caring.
B. As appropriate for care of injuries, presenting concerns, contraceptive needs, treatment of STDs, vaginitis, gynecologic conditions

Appendix E on danger assessment may be photocopied or adapted for your patients.

See Bibliography on abuse, battering, and violence.

Nurses Network on Violence Against Women International www.nnvawi.org

Form for Report of Alleged Sexual Assault*

Victim's Complaint _____
Date _____ Time _____
Victim's Name _____
            Last   First   Middle
Address _____
Mode of Transportation to Facility _____

PART 1
Date and time of alleged assault _____
Month Day Year Time _____
Date and time of presentation for care _____
Month Day Year Time _____

*You may want to develop a consent form for any or all of the following: consent for treatment by nurse practitioner and/or other member of the assault crisis team to perform physical examinations, laboratory tests, evidence collection, appropriate intervention, appropriate photographs.

History of Alleged Assault
1. History as related to nurse practitioner by patient:

by _____Clinician Date: ___/___/___

Witnessed by _____ Date: ___/___/___

Make note of any comments that may be of help such as perpetrator's tech-niques, hang-ups, perversions. conversation, preoccupation with certain body parts and slang names for same.
2. Patient's report of pain (note location and bleeding, if any):

C
___Abdominal   ___Pelvic   ___Muscle
___Dysuria   ___Tenesmus   ___Skeletal
___Bleeding (indicate source)
Other (explain) _____

_____

3. Since the incident,
    has the patient changed clothing?   ___Yes ___No
    douched?   ___Yes ___No
    urinated?   ___Yes ___No
    bathed?   ___Yes ___No
    had B.M.?   ___Yes ___No
Explain _____
4. Was there penetration of the:

	Yes	No	Not Known
a. vulva	___	___	___
b. vagina	___	___	___
c. mouth	___	___	___
d. anus	___	___	___
e. ear	___	___	___
f. other	___	___	___

5. Did the alleged assailant

	Yes	No	Not Known
a. bind or tie the victim	___	___	___
b. threaten the patient	___	___	___
c. strike the patient	___	___	___
d. threaten the victim's family, friends, others	___	___	___

	Yes	No	Not Known
e. wear a condom	___	___	___
f. ejaculate	___	___	___
g. use a foreign object in any manner sexually	___	___	___
h. use a lubricant	___	___	___

6. Whom has the patient notified _____
7. Does patient wish anyone notified _____
8. Have police been notified _____
   Date _____ Time _____ a.m./p.m.
9. Does patient wish to have police notified

Medical History

1. Birthdate _____
2. Race: White___ Black___ Hispanic___ Asian___ Other___
3. Marital status:
   Single___ Married___ Separated___ Divorced___ Widowed___
4. Menstrual history
   a. Last menstrual period
   b. Last vaginal intercourse with permission within last 72 hours.
      Date: ___/___/___ Time: _____
5. Contraceptive history
   Method of birth control (if any):
   a. Birth control pill _____
   d. Tubal ligation _____
   e. Hysterectomy _____
6. Significant allergies _____
7. Medications taken by patient, including alcohol and street drugs

   _____

8. Recent injury or illness _____
9. Other relevant history _____

   _____

History obtained

by _____ Clinician. Date: ___/___/___

Witnessed by _____ Date: ___/___/___

PART 2

Physical Examination (Please note bruising, lacerations, or any other physical trauma sustained by patient.)

Vital signs: B/P _____ P_____ T_____ R_____

1. HEENT (taking careful note of pupils and nostrils):

2. Chest-lungs:

3. Breast:

4. Heart:

5. Abdomen:

6. Trunk:

7. Extremities:

8. Neurologic:

9. Pelvic Examination:
   a. vulva
   b. mons veneris, perineum
   c. urethra
   d. clitoris
   e. vagina
   f. cervix
   g. uterus
   h. adnexa, right
      left
   i. anus/rectum
   j. rectum/vagina

Other comments (describe evidence of trauma in detail)

_____

_____

_____

Impression:

_____

_____

_____

Clinician: _____

PART 3

Laboratory Evaluation
1. Slides
2. Pubic hair specimens
3. GC culture (note origin):
   Cervix_____   Urethra_____   Rectum_____   Pharynx_____
4. Serology test for syphilis
5. HCG
6. Urinalysis
7. Other (specify): _____
8. Wet mount
9. Chlamydia

Treatment Plan

1. Prophylactic antibiotic, 2002 CDC guidelines: Since not all experts agree
   with this regimen, individual clinical judgment must be exercised:
   a. Ceftriaxone 125 mg in a single IM dose PLUS Metronidazole 2 gm
      p.o. single dose plus Azithromycin 1 g. orally in single dose OR Dox-
      ycycline 100 mg p.o. BID x 7 days
   b. HBV vaccine started (if not previously vaccinated)
2. Emergency contraception (see guideline)
   a. Review options with patient
3. Tetanus toxoid
   Given_____ Refused_____ (date of last TT)_____
4. Other medications (specify): _____

_____

5. Laceration repair (specify): _____

_____

6. Other: _____
7. Consider HIV postexposure therapy (see CDC 2002)

History obtained by:_____ Clinician. Date ___/___/____

Witnessed by: _____ Date ___/___/___

Follow-up (describe, give dates and times of appointments. Give patient this information in writing)
1. Medical
2. Gynecological: including syphilis, HIV screen 6, 12, & 24 weeks after assault; repeat STD screen 2 weeks after assault
3. Mental health counseling
4. Legal
5. Clergy
6. Other (depending on lab findings, emergency contraception); for HBV vaccine #2,3 at 1–2 and 4–6 months after first dose

Facility Follow-up
1. Appointment should be made for 7–14 days for repeat STD screening and pregnancy testing at 30 days. If no STD prophylaxis, follow-up within a week for test results.
2. Pregnancy testing may be done before 30 days if menses is delayed.
3. If pregnancy test is positive, appropriate counseling will be done.
4. All patients should be contacted (whenever possible) one month after alleged assault for follow-up.
5. HIV screen and serology for syphilis 6, 12, & 24 weeks after assault.

History obtained by:
_____ Clinician Date: ___/___/___

Witnessed by: _____ Date:___/___/___

PART 4

Photographs*
All bruises,** lacerations, and other wounds, particularly in the pubic area, thigh, knees, breasts, and neck. Make notes on all photos.
Photo #:_____ Consent form to collect, store _____

Description and remarks:
_____
_____
_____

---

*Work in progress on digital photographic evidence—how to collect, store, and assure admissability of such evidence in court.
**Bruises may not show up well until a day or two after alleged assault. Victim may be asked to come back if bruises appear.

_____
_____
_____
_____
_____
_____
_____

PART 5
Victim Property and Clothing List

Victim _____ Date _____ Time _____

Item Number	Number of Articles	Description

_____
_____
_____
_____
_____
_____
_____
_____
_____
_____
_____
_____
_____
_____
_____
_____
_____
_____
_____

Clothing: If any clothing is submitted as evidence, it should be labeled and placed in a paper *(not plastic)* bag. If submitted as evidence, clothing in bag should be included with rape kit in large bag or envelope and signed again by nurse and attending officer.

The disposition of patient's clothing (sent home with family, friends, remaining with patient, or sent to police) should be noted on patient's chart and cosigned by police officer (if indicated).

The Above Listed Items Were Turned Over to _____
Of _____ On _____ At _____ (Hrs)
Signed _____
Received by _____ (Police Officer)
(Family member, friend)
(Patient)

    See Appendix E on danger assessment.
    See Bibliography on abuse, sexual assault and battering.

Patient Information Sheet

Name of Patient: _____ Date: _____

We understand that this experience has been a traumatic one and your initial response may be a wish to forget. However, follow-up care, both physical and emotional, is of utmost importance. The following is information that will be important to you during the next days and weeks.

    We recommend a pregnancy test if your menstrual period is delayed one week beyond its due date. Please call to make arrangements.

    Although we have tested you for sexually transmitted diseases, *repeat testing is necessary at 1–2 weeks and at 6, 12, and 24 weeks.* Please help yourself by returning for repeat testing.

    Listed below are the procedures that were performed during this visit plus special instructions (if any) for you.

Procedures Performed	Special Instructions

Please feel free to contact us at any time if you need further support.
_____, Clinician
Telephone Number: _____

10
Sexual Dysfunction

I. Definition
Diminished libido or lack of libido, diminished sexual response or lack of response to sexual stimulation. Vaginismus, involuntary spasm or constriction of the distal third of the vaginal musculature around the introitus on one or more occasions.

II. Etiology
A. Organic and physiologic disorders
   1. Hormonal imbalance
   2. Injuries or anomalies of the genital tract
   3. Infection of the genitalia
   4. Lesions
   5. Nerve impairment
   6. Substance abuse: alcohol, recreational drugs
   7. Recent pregnancy
   8. Effects of medications—prescription or over-the-counter
   9. Chronic illness
B. Relationship disorders
   1. Partner's and/or patient's lack of desire for sex
   2. Medical conditions
   3. Lack of privacy
   4. Fear of failure in the sexual act; lack of knowledge re: sexual response(s)
   5. Shame, guilt
   6. Expectations different from those of partner; miscommunication
   7. Rape trauma; sexual assault or abuse at any age; domestic violence
   8. Improper use of barrier or chemical contraceptives
   9. Recent gynecological event affecting sexuality, such as sterilization, pregnancy, tubal ligation, abortion, hysterectomy, mastectomy
   10. Difficulties in sexual orientation; or confusion over gender identity
   11. Clinical depression of patient and/or partner

III. History
A. What the patient may present with
   1. Lack of sexual desire

   2. Lack of response to stimulation

   3. Inability to have an orgasm

   4. Vaginal or vulvar irritation, bleeding, soreness

   5. Lack of vaginal lubrication

   6. Inability to have vaginal intercourse

   7. Dyspareunia

B. Other signs and symptoms

   1. Rectal or perineal pain

   2. Perineal lesions

   3. Abdominal pain, pelvic pain

   4. Fever

   5. Bladder, urethral pain

C. Additional information to be considered

   1. Sexual history: ever had intercourse; ever experienced orgasm; partners—men, women, both

   2. Contraceptive history and method presently using

   3. Any gynecological/obstetrical history, diethylstilbestrol exposure, perimenopausal problems

   4. Any recent contributing events: change of partner or new relationship, marriage, divorce, separation, sterilization, pregnancy, infection, surgery, or sexual assault, incest, domestic violence

   5. Any cultural or religious beliefs that relate to sexual activity

   6. Alcohol, drug use; any changes

   7. Expectations of self and partner, health of sexual partner

   8. Any problems with privacy, time together, living arrangements

   9. Use of sex toys

   10. Pattern of sexual expression; availability of sexual partner

   11. You might ask, "What do you do, how do you do it, and how does it make you feel?"

   12. Sexual fantasies, preoccupations

   13. Difficulties focusing on tactile or other sensations previously erotic

IV. Physical Examination

A. Vital signs

   1. Pulse   3. Temperature

   2. Blood pressure   4. Weight

B. General physical examination including thyroid, breasts, CVA tenderness, neurological

C. Abdominal examination with special attention to

   1. Guarding

   2. Pain

3. Masses
D. External examination
   1. Anomalies
   2. Skene's glands,
      Bartholin's glands
   3. Clitoris
   4. Status of hyman
   5. Perineum
   6. Urethra
   7. Lesions, signs of
      infection, injury
E. Vaginal examination (speculum)
   1. Vaginal walls: infection, anomalies, atrophy, injuries
   2. Discharge, lesions
   3. Cervix: lesions, signs of infection, anomalies, scarring
   4. Tolerance of speculum and size accommodated, length of vagina
F. Bimanual examination
   1. Pain on cervical manipulation
   2. Uterus: tenderness
   3. Adnexa: mass, tenderness
   4. Vaginal lesions

V. Laboratory Examination
A. Appropriate cultures when evidence of infection; wet mount; urinal-ysis
B. Consider thyroid panel, FBS, liver, renal function tests, serum corticosteroids if history and/or clinical findings warrant
C. Hormone assays as indicated

VI. Differential Diagnosis
A. Hormonal imbalance: estrogen, androgens
B. Anomaly, injury
C. Infection
D. Substance abuse: drugs, alcohol, smoking
E. Nerve impairment: spinal cord injury, neurologic diseases
F. Changes due to aging: slower responses
G. Adrenal, thyroid, liver, kidney problems
H. Diabetes, diabetic neuropathy
I. Medication side effects
J. Depression
K. Psychosocial problems, eating disorders
L. Posttraumatic stress disorder (PTSD) secondary to incest, rape, sexual assault, domestic violence
M. Vestibulitis, vulvodynia
N. Physical and/or intellectual disabilities

VII. Treatment

A. Medications: treat any infection present (see specific protocol); consider hormones especially if postmenopausal; new drugs for women—analogues to Sildennafil citrate (Viagra®) when available. Nonprescription dietary supplementy-Avilimil® (salvia rubis)

B. General measures
   1. Education about changes in sexual response that accompany aging; need for privacy, making time for intimacy
   2. Education about a woman's sexual response, how it differs from that of a man; teach Kegel (pelvic floor) exercises; positions
   3. Explore partner relationship: changes, previous responsiveness, sexual preference, communication, expectations, guilt; screen for abuse
   4. Education on techniques for stretching hymen, vagina
   5. Education regarding techniques for learning about sexual response and excitation, self and partner
   6. Emphasize role of self-care: diet, exercise, vitamins, hygiene, stress reduction
   7. Education about lubricants, nonhormonal agents to restore/maintain vaginal mucosa and moisture, other sexual aids

VIII. Complications

A. Long-term disruption of relationships
B. Exploitation in relationships: abuse, violence

IX. Consultation/Referral

A. Physician for possible hormonal imbalance, genital anomaly, nerve impairment, medical conditions underlying problem
B. Counselor for rape trauma, PTSD, exploitative relationships, abuse, depression, gender identity, sexual preferences
C. Sex therapist—single or couples
D. Support group

X. Follow-up

A. Check if infection is present; reevaluate for further treatment
B. Arrange repeat visit as appropriate for discussion of relationship problems
C. Assess success of vaginal, hymenal stretching; stimulation techniques
D. For medical/medication problems, laboratory results as appropriate

See Bibliography.

11

Peri- and Postmenopause

General Care Measures

I. Definition
The menopause is the landmark event of the climacteric, the 10-to-15-year period, beginning at about age 35 to 40, when women's bodies are changing and preparing for cessation of menses. A woman cannot say that she has gone through menopause until at least one full year has passed without any menstrual period (uterine bleeding). The postmenopausal time begins when menopause is complete and menses no longer occur. For women today, the postmenopausal years may comprise as much as three-eighths of their lives or more, the age for menopause being about 50 in the U.S. (mean 50.4 years). A woman who has had a hysterectomy (removal of uterus only) is not considered menopausal with cessation of menses.

II. Etiology
A. Physiologic: The gradual diminution of estrogens, resulting in cessation of ovulation and thus of menstruation
B. Anatomic: Surgical removal of the uterus and ovaries which results in surgical menopause, an abrupt end to ovulation and menstruation

III. History
A. What the patient presents with
  1. Changes in character of the menstrual cycle
    a. Menstrual periods that are more frequent, less frequent, of longer duration or shorter duration
    b. Scanty flow
    c. Flooding at onset of flow
    d. Gradual or abrupt cessation of menses for one or more months
    e. Irregular periods over a period of time or abrupt cessation of menstruation
  2. Changes related to menopause and/or the aging process (these changes are the presenting complaint of women with previous surgical removal of the uterus and intact ovaries)
    a. Hot flashes, hot flushes

    b. Vaginal dryness, atrophy of vaginal tissues
    c. Night sweats
    d. Dry skin and hair; skeletal pain or stiffness
    e. Graying of hair
    f. Loss of skin elasticity
    g. Alterations in sleep patterns
    h. Developmental occurrences of aging: empty nest, caring for aging parents, grandchildren, changing roles, retirement
       1) Alterations in sexual response: longer time needed for arousal, lessened vaginal lubrication
    j. Mons and vulva flatten, less fatty tissue padding, thinning of pubic hair
  3. Recent history of gynecologic surgery: hysterectomy, oophorectomy, salpingectomy, dilatation and curettage, LEEP/LOOP of cervix
B. Additional information to be considered
  1. Menstrual history, past year; previous year
  2. Contraceptive use to present
  3. Obstetrical history: pregnancies, abortions, stillbirths
  4. Gynecologic history: surgery, endometriosis, infertility, anomalies, last Papanicolaou smear, any breast problems, last mammogram, sexually transmitted disease, infections; does she do SBE; any stress incontinence
  5. Sexual history: dysfunction, unresponsiveness, recent changes, use of sex toys (see sexual dysfunction protocol); high risk sexual behaviors
  6. Life event changes: resumption of career, retirement, caring for older family members, adult children in or out of home, divorce, separation, marriage, new sexual relationship, caring for grandchildren, loss of a child
  7. Lifestyle: exercise, diet, smoking, recreation, stressors, recreational drugs
  8. Medical history: chronic disease, medications (OTC, prescription); depression, anxiety
  9. Family medical history
  10. Use of complementary therapies (botanicals, homeopathics, acupuncture, Chinese medicine, aromatherapy, etc.)
  11. Beliefs about menopause and expectations
  12. Domestic violence, elder abuse

IV. Physical Examination
A. Vital signs

1. Blood pressure	3. Height
2. Pulse	4. Weight

B. General health examination
    1. Head   4. Lungs
    2. Neck   5. Abdomen
    3. Heart   6. Extremities, joints, spine
C. External examination for lesions, infection, atrophy, anomaly
    1. Urethral orifice   3. Labia
    2. Clitoris   4. Perineum
D. Vaginal examination (speculum)
    1. Walls   4. Cervix
    2. Discharge   5. Careful inspection of
    3. Lesions   vaginal vault noting if
                                        posthysterectomy
E. Bimanual examination
    1. Adnexa
        a. Tenderness
        b. Masses
        c. Palpable tubes or ovaries, if present
    2. Uterus
        a. Size   c. Tenderness
        b. Mobility   d. Masses
    3. Cystocle, rectocele, urethrocele
F. Rectal examination: fecal occult blood

V. Laboratory Examination

A. Appropriate cultures, smears if suspicion of infection
B. Papanicolaou smear if none done in past year
C. Mammogram per American Cancer Society guidelines
(baseline at 35, annually at 40 and after); may be altered with family history or personal risk factors for breast cancer and new recommendations from ACS or NCI
D. Consider serum FSH level to assess for menopause if no menses for 12 months or on OCs, age $\geq$ 50 and/or desire to consider HT [$\geq$ 2–40 m IU/ml]. Discontinue hormones for the 2 weeks prior to blood work measuring FSH.
E. Blood glucose & lipid levels

VI. Differential Diagnosis

A. Carcinoma of genital tract
B. Pregnancy
C. Endocrine disorders
D. $\downarrow$ nutritional state; obesity
E. Marked $\uparrow$ in exercise regimen

VII. Treatment

A. Medication
   1. Perimenopausal: consider low dose oral contraceptive for contraception after assessment for risks, desire for contraceptive protection; consider cycling with Provera 10 mg x 10 days monthly if intermenstrual time decreases and/or heavy bleeding/flooding characterize menses
   2. Postmenopausal: consider nonhormonal or hormone (see hormone therapy guideline) interventions per clinical picture and patient's wishes
B. General measures
   1. Teaching about normal menopausal symptoms, changes with aging, need for more time for arousal, use of supplemental lubrication (saliva, water-soluble jelly, water soluble lubricants—these come as creams, jellies, and as vaginal inserts), non–hormonal agents to restore/maintain vaginal mucosa and vaginal moisture such as Replens®, Comfrey ointment, vitamin E supplement + 100–600 mg/day or evening primrose oil 2–4 capsules/day* (also helpful for hot flashes), Calendula, black cohosh (20–40 mg bid), changes in sexual response that accompany removal of the uterus/ovaries
   2. Teaching about self-care: diet, exercise—aerobic, weight bearing, and strengthening—prevention of osteoporosis (calcium intake 1200–1500 grains/day and 400–800 IU [20 mg] vitamin D/day in foods or supplement); breast self-examination, need for Papanicolaou smear as indicated by history and past Paps and pelvic examination yearly; regular mammograms; contraception until one full year without menses (some say 2 years); signs and symptoms of problems: postmenopausal bleeding; prevention of vaginal infections (see guidelines)
   3. Teaching re: urinary health: 6–8 glasses of water a day, ↓ caffeine, Kegel exercises; quit smoking
   4. Teaching re: triggers for hot flashes—electric blanket, alcohol, spicy foods, overheating, constrictive clothing; symptom management with evening primrose oil, kudzu, licorice root, phytoestrogens, sage or sarsaparilla
   5. Consider nonhormonal synthetic medication and bioflavonoid alternatives for symptom management; other botanicals, homeopathic medicines (for example, Sleep disorders: hops, valerian tea or tincture, melatonin, exercise, relaxation techniques; Memory: ginkgo biloba (120–240 mg/day); Irritability: anise, chasteberry, dongquai, flaxseed, ginseng, kava kava (60–120 mg), red raspberry leaf)

---

*See complementary therapies guideline.

6. Diet: low fat, avoid or ↓ caffeine, zinc 15 mg/day in foods and/or in supplements; vitamin C and B complex vitamins, ↑ fiber; ↑ phytoestrogens (soy protein isoflavone 40–160 mg/day; lignans such as flax seed, cereal bran; other isoflavones chick peas, legumes, bluegrass, clover)

VIII. Complications/Risks
A. Pregnancy
B. Carcinoma of reproductive tract
C. Breast cancer (risk is higher after menopausal years)
D. Incapacitating menopausal symptoms: hot flashes that disrupt normal life, night sweats, sleep disturbances
E. Osteoporosis
F. Possible increased risk for heart attacks
G. Interactions, adverse effects of herbals, vitamins

IX. Consultation/Referral
A. To physician or other health care professional as appropriate for complications listed above
B. Possible consultation for
   1. HT; ET   2.   Pathology
C. Sex therapist for prolonged or severe disruption in sexual relationship
D. Counseling: stresses of the middle years, depression
E. Mammogram, sigmoidoscopy or colonoscopy per protocol & risk
F. Bone mineral density
G. Consider consultation for hormonal synthetic medication and/or bioflavonoid therapies; homeopath; herbalist, naturopath, Ayurvedic practitioner

X. Follow-up
A. Annual examination, Papanicolaou smear, pelvic exam
B. Mammograms as recommended
C. As needed if problems continue or become exacerbated

See Bibliography. www.menopause.org; www.herbalgram.org; womenshealth.med.ucla.edu/community/newsletter

Hormone Therapy*

I. Definition

Hormone therapy is the use of exogenous natural or synthetic estrogen or estrogen and progestin in combination by the postmenopausal woman (whether natural or surgical menopause has occurred) to alleviate the symptoms of lower amounts of natural estrogen.

II. Etiology

A. The theca intema and granulosa cells of the ovarian follicles and the corpus luteum produce three naturally occurring estrogens: estradiol, estrone and estriol, in concert with precursors LH and FSH from the anterior pituitary and androstenedione from the adrenals. The corpus luteum and ovarian follicle produce progesterone. The stromal tissues of the ovaries produce insignificant amounts of androgens; the major sources of androgens in women are the adrenals. During the perimenopausal years, there is a gradual decrease of the production of these hormones.

III. History (see also perimenopause guideline)

A. What the patient may present with
1. Irregular menstrual cycles: longer than 35 days, shorter than 21 days
2. Changes in character of cycles: scanty, brief duration, begin with flooding, clots, dysmenorrhea
3. Sleep disturbances, night sweats
4. Experiencing hot flashes and hot flushes
5. Dyspareunia
6. Changes in vaginal tissue: dryness, itching, burning of vulva
7. Urinary urgency or frequency; urethral pain; irritation at meatus
8. No vaginal bleeding for prior 12 months or more
9. Surgical menopause: hysterectomy with oophorectomy and salpingectomy
B. Additional information to be considered
1. Age of patient and of her biological mother at menopause
2. Last Papanicolaou smear, breast self-examination, mammogram

---

*The decision about use of HT requires evaluation of the risks and benefits for each individual woman. For women currently using HT, it is important to assess their reasons for use and to evaluate potential risks, benefits, and alternatives." (ACOG Response to Women's Health Initiative Study results by the American College of Obstetricians and Gynecologists, August 9, 2002, available on the ACOG website www.acog.org).

Clinicians should keep up-to-date with ACOG guidelines, and with results from the Women's Health Initiative, the HERS study—heart and estrogen replacement study—the PEPI Trial—postmenopausal estrogen/progestin intervention, and the Nurses' Health Study.

3. Personal medical, surgical, and gynecologic/obstetric history; history of pelvic surgery
4. Family medical history, especially osteoporosis, heart disease, carcinoma, Alzheimers disease
5. Signs, symptoms of possible vaginitis, STD, cystitis
6. Lifestyle: diet, exercise, smoking, alcohol
7. Change in mood or sense of well-being
8. All medications including OTC, herbals, homeopathics

IV. Physical Examination
A. Vital signs
B. Complete physical examination
C. Pelvic examination
   1. Vulva and perineum, noting any signs of infection, atrophy, irritation; hair distribution and signs of thinning; loss of adipose tissue
   2. Vagina: color, rugae, signs of atrophy, infection or irritation, length
   3. Cervix: color, any lesions, ectropion
   4. Urethral os: signs of irritation, atrophy, urethrocele
   5. Pelvic floor integrity: cystocele, rectocele, uterine prolapse
   6. Uterus: size, shape, position, contour, mobility, presence of masses, tenderness
   7. Adnexa: masses, tenderness
   8. Rectal exam: masses, rectocele, uterine anomalies, occult blood

V. Laboratory
A. Papanicolaou smear with maturation index
B. Mammogram
C. May consider endometrial biopsy with intact uterus
D. Vaginal and/or urine cultures: HIV, STD screen as appropriate
E. Serum FSH or testosterone assay as indicated
F. Lipid profiles, thyroid function test, serum glucose
G. Hematocrit or hemoglobin as indicated
H. Bone density assays if indicated and feasible
I. Pelvic ultrasound if pelvic examination is positive for masses (vaginal probe ultrasound)
J. May consider baseline EKG
K. Per findings of physical examination and from history

VI. Considering HT
A. Contraindications*

---

*From the Women's Health Initiative Criteria, NIH.

1. Undiagnosed vaginal bleeding
2. Known or suspected pregnancy
3. History of nontraumatic pulmonary embolism (PE) or deep vein thrombosis (DVT) or PE or DVT in past 6 months
4. Known or suspected cancer of the breast or reproductive tract (estrogen-dependent carcinomas); malignant melanoma at any stage
5. Currently on anticoagulants or tamoxifen

B. Precautions: consider clinical data, risk and benefits
   1. Active gallbladder disease
   2. Family history of breast cancer
   3. Migraine headaches
   4. Elevated triglycerides, ↑ LDL, ↓ HDL

C. Weighing risks and benefits
   1. Osteoporosis in family or personal history; risk factors for osteoporosis (see osteoporosis handout in appendix)
   2. Personal and family medical history including heart and Alzheimers disease, breast cancer, ovarian cancer
   3. Presence of indicators for benefits in absence of absolute contraindications and weighing of relative risks; emerging data from the Women's Health Initiative
   4. Consideration of risks with smoking, hypertension, epilepsy, migraines, benign breast or uterine disease, endometriosis
   5. Consideration of benefits to genitourinary tract, feelings of well-being
   6. The use of hormone therapy remains a highly individualized decision and controversial issues remain
   7. Access to health care for follow-up: endometrial biopsy, mammography, monitoring for side effects, danger signs
   8. Alternatives to HT: diet, exercise, calcium from exogenous source in addition to foods, botanicals, vitamins, nonhormonal vaginal lubricants (such as Astroglide®), naturalistic interventions, homeopathic preparations (see peri- and postmenopausal general care guideline and complementary therapies guideline)

VII. Hormone Regimens

A. Absence of uterus: estrogen only or estrogen and androgen*
   1. Conjugated equine estrogen (Premarin®) 0.3–2.5 mg/day p.o.q.d. (or days 1–25)
   2. Modified estrone from plant compounds (Estratab®/Menest® 0.3–1.25 mg/day p.o.q.d. (or days 1–25)

---

*A testosterone patch is now available compounded to individual needs by Women's Health America www.womenshealth.com

3. Micronized plant estrogen, estradiol (Estrace®) 0.5–2 mg/day (or days 1–25), Gynodiol (estradiol) 1 mg, 1.5 mg, 2 mg/day

4. Estropipate (synthesized from estrone) (Ogen®, Ortho-Est® 0.625–2.5 mg/day p.o.q.d. (or days 1–25); Cenestin® synthesized conjugated estrogens 0.625–1.25 mg 1 tab/day

5. Estradiol natural plant compound transdermal patch
   (Alora®) 0.05–0.1 mg/day—apply patch twice/week
   Climara® 0.025–0.1 mg day—apply patch once/week
   Estraderm® 0.05–0.1 mg/day—apply patch twice/week
   FemPatch® 0.025 mg/day—apply patch weekly
   Vivelle® 0.0375 mg–0.1 mg/day—apply patch twice a week
   Vivelle-Dot® 0.0275–0.1 mg estradiol/day—apply patch twice weekly
   Esclim® 0.025–0.1 mg estradiol apply patch twice weekly
   FemRing®

6. Estrogen vaginal cream or suppository for dryness, atrophy: dienestrol 0.7 mg (DV) or diethylstilbestrol 0. 1 mg, 0.2 mg suppositories 1 or 2 daily; conjugated estrogens (Premarin) 0.625 mg/gm or dienestrol 0.01% (OrthoDienestrol) or dienestrol 0.01% with lactose (DV, Estroguard) or estropipate 1.5 mg/gm (Ogen) cream 1–2 applicators full per day; estradiol cream 0.1 mg/g (Estrace) 2–4 gm daily for 1–2 weeks; then 1–2 gm daily for 1–2 weeks; maintenance 1 gm 1–3x/week 3 weeks on, 1 off

7. Vagifem® estradiol vaginal tablet 25 mg 1 tab/day for 2 weeks then maintenance 1 tab vaginally 2x/week

8. Estradiol (Estring®) (2 mg) vaginal ring (rapid release for first 24 hours, then continuous low dose of 7.5 mg/24 hours). Replaced q 90 days. May be used by postmenopausal women both with and without a uterus who desire symptomatic relief from local symptoms of urogenital atrophy. Addition of progestin not necessary for woman with a uterus since adverse effects on endometrium unlikely with consistent low daily dose

9. Estradiol acetate (FemRing®) available in 2 dosages, 0.05 mg/day and 0.1 mg/day. Replace q 90 days.

10. Estratab/methyltestosterone (Estratest®) 1.25 mg esterified estrogen/ 2.5 mg testosterone or Estratest HS® 1/2 strength 0.625 mg esterified estrogen, 1.25 mg methyl-testosterone

B. Presence of uterus: add progestin

1. Medroxyprogesterone acetate (MPA) synthetic progesterone (Provera®, Cycrin®) 2.5–10 mg p.o.

   a. 10 mg MPA p.o. taken in combination with estrogen for last 12 days (days 14–25)

      b. 2.5–5 mg MPA p.o. taken in combination with estrogen on days 1–5 or q.d.

  2. Norethindrone or norethindrone acetate synthetic progesterone (Micronor®, Aygestin® 0.35–2.5 mg/day p.o. taken as in B.1a/b

  3. Micronized progesterone from plant sources (Prometrium®) 200 mg/day p.o. taken as in B.1a/b (capsules contain peanut oil; avoid for patients with peanut allergies); Promensil natural plant estrogens 40 mg/day (1 tab)

  4. Micronized progesterone from plant sources timed release intrauterine device (IUD) Mirena® (levonorgestrel-releasing intrauterine system) 20 ug/day provides continuous source of progestin for combination therapy

  5. Combination products

      a. Conjugated estrogens 0.62 mg/2.5–5 mg, 0.45 mg/1.5 mg daily p.o. (Prempro®)*

      b. Conjugated estrogens 0.625 mg p.o. alone for 14 days (Premphase®); conjugated estrogens 0.625 mg MPA p.o. for 14 days

      c. Estradiol/norethindrone acetate transdermal system (CombiPatch®). Two systems available: Continuous combined regimen 0.05 mg estradiol/0.14 or 0.25 mg norethindrone acetate continuously, changed x 2/week; continuous sequential regimen 0.05 mg estradiol patch x 14 days (Vivelle®) (replaced x2 weekly) then 0.05 mg estradiol/0.14 mg norethinrone acetate (CombiPatch®) (replaced x2 weekly)

      d. Activella™ 1 mg estradiol/0.5 mg norethindrone 1 qd

      e. Femhrt® norethindrone acetate 1 mg/1 ethinyl estradiol 0.05 mg 1 qd

      f. Orthoprefest estradiol 1.0 mg = norgestimate 0.09 mg in alternating 3–day cycles. 3 of estradiol alone, 3 of estradiol and norgestimate, repeating pattern continuously

C. Other

  1. Raloxifene hydrochloride (Evista®) synthetic selective estrogen-receptor modulator 60 mg p.o.q.d. Use daily for osteoporosis protection

  2. Custom compounded hormone therapy, oral, topical, and pellet implant (estrogen, progesterone and testosterone) may be compounded by many pharmacists and mail order pharmacies specializing in natural hormones such as:

    College Pharmacy, Colorado Springs, Colorado 1–800–888–9358

    Women's International Pharmacy, Madison, WI 608–221–7800 and Sun City, AZ 623–214–7700

---

*Precaution from Women's Health Initiative: increased risk of stroke, heart attack, breast cancer.

www.womensinternational.com

Referral to compounding pharmacists at www.iacprx.org (International Academy of Compounding Pharmacistsh)

D. Withdrawal bleeding
  1. Will occur with sequential use of progestin
  2. No bleeding should occur with continuous use

VIII. Clinical Management

A. Side effects
  1. Bleeding with hormone use
     a. with sequential use
     b. With continuous use
        1) Consider change in dosage or medication
        2) If not effective, do endometrial biopsy
     c. Unopposed estrogen use (still prescribed by some providers)
        1) Encourage combination therapy; prior to changing therapy, consider using Provera® 10 mg for 10 days. If no bleeding, begin new regimen. If bleeding does occur, do endometrial biopsy or do an ultrasound to measure lining
  2. Breast tenderness
  3. Fluid retention
  4. Weight gain (increased appetite)
  5. Dysmenorrhea with withdrawal bleed
  6. Depression
  7. Irritability or emotional lability
  8. Possible increase in size of uterine leiomyomata
  9. Allergic response to patch
  10. Virilization with androgens (rare)
B. Other clinical management strategies
  1. Short-term topical estrogen for vaginal dryness; discontinue after 6 months or when no longer necessary
  2. Alternative nonhormonal vaginal lubricants such as Astroglide®, nonhormonal products such as Replens® to maintain or restore vaginal mucosa
  3. Complementary/alternative modalities to be considered, including many botanicals as well as acupuncture, massage, and relaxation, can increase a woman's feeling of well-being.
  4. Careful teaching about modalities utilized
C. Follow-up and lifestyle on HT
  1. Reinforce need for calcium intake both from food and supplementary sources. Will also need a consistent source of vitamin D + magnesium in appropriate dose for adequate absorption

2. Regular program of exercise, strength training
3. Reinforce knowledge of risks and benefits
4. Preventive health care: annual examination, Papanicolaou smear as indicated, mammography, breast and vulvar self-examination
5. Consider periodic monitoring for bone density, lipid profile
6. Vaginal lubricants, signs of vaginal infection or cystitis versus dryness, Kegel exercises, sexuality
7. Careful use of herbals, vitamins, & isoflavones with HT

See Appendix A and Bibliography.

Osteoporosis

I. Definition
Osteoporosis, a largely preventable skeletal disease, is characterized by low bone mass and microarchitectual deterioration of bone tissue, leading to enhanced bone fragility and a consequent increase in fracture risk.

II. Etiology
Two main factors are responsible for the fragility of bone:
A. Reduced bone mass
B. Impaired repair of microdamage caused by normal wear and tear of bone, with disruption in continuity of the plates in cancellous (trabecular) bone

III. Clinical Types
A. Primary or idiopathic osteoporosis
  1. Type I bone loss occurs primarily in the trabecular compartment and is closely related to postmenopausal loss of ovarian function
  2. Type II bone loss involves cortical bone and is thought to be an exaggeration of the physiologic aging process
B. Secondary osteoporosis
  1. Medical conditions
    a. Chronic renal failure
    b. Gastrectomy and intestinal bypass
    c. Malabsorption syndrome
    d. Metastic cancer
    e. Fractures
  2. Endocrinopathies
    a. Hyperprolactinemia
    b. Hyperthyroidism
    e. Diabetes
    f. Turners syndrome

c. Hyperparathyroidism
d. Adrenocortical
   over-activity
3. Connective tissue disorder
   a. Osteogenesis imperfecta
   b. Ehlers-Danlos syndrome
4. Medications
   a. Anticonvulsants
   b. Antacids (with aluminum)
   c. Thyroid hormone therapy
   d. Excessive vitamin A
   e. Glucocorticoids—oral, inhaled
   f. Novaldex® (tamoxiphen)
   g. GNRH antagonists
   h. Lithium
   i. Long-term Depo-Provera use

g. Premature ovarian failure
h. Hypogonadism
i. Hypercalciuria

c. Homocystinuria
d. Rheumatoid arthritis

IV. History
A. Woman's medical history, including but not limited to: refer to III.B
B. Medication history
   1. Current prescription medication
   2. Current over-the-counter medication
   3. Current vitamin and botanical use
C. Ob-gyn history
   1. Age at menarche
   2. Age at menopause
   3. Months (years) of oral contraceptive, Depo-Provera use
   4. Parity
   5. Estrogen use
   6. History of menstrual dysfunction
      a. Late menarche
      b. Oligohypomenorrhea
      c. Exercise-induced amenorrhea
      d. Previous hysterectomy with oophorectomy
   7. History of extended breast feeding
D. Nutritional status
   1. Height and weight
   2. Eating habits
   3. Consumption of caffeine and alcoholic beverages
   4. History of an eating disorder
   5. Current and past exercise habits

      6. Smoker
E. Lifestyle
      1. Excessive use of alcohol   3. Caffeine ingestion
      2. Smoking   4. Inactivity
F. Family history
      1. Maternal history of osteoporosis or fractures

V. Physical Examination, Including but Not Limited to:
A. Height (compare to previous measurement), (loss of 1½")
B. Weight; body mass index
C. Observe back for dorsal kyphosis and cervical lordosis
D. Assess for physical abnormalities that interfere with mobility
E. Assess for bone pain
F. Assess for change of stature

VI. Laboratory
A. Consider one of the following screening tests
      1. X ray densitometry (DEXA) gold standard
      2. Bone ultrasound
      3. Genotyping
      4. Bone turnover markers (Urinary N-Tetopeptide) (NTX)
      5. Single Energy X ray absorptrometry (measures the bones of the wrist
         or heel)
      6. Quantitative Computed Tomography (measures the bone density of
         the spine). This test is expensive and exposes the woman to a higher
         dose of radiation than other screening tests
      7. Consider calcium and albumin (hyperparathyroidism)
      8. Consider 25 hydroxy, vitamin D (vitamin D deficiency)
      9. Consider Thyroid Stimulating Hormone (TSH) (hyperthyroidism)
     10. Consider CBC with sedimentation rate
     11. Consider liver function test

VII. Treatment
A. Medication
      1. Estrogen (see Hormone Therapy guideline)
      2. Bisphosphonates (Alendronate, Fosamax®)
      Regimen: An Alendronate regimen should include:
         a. 5 mg/10 mg a day or 35–70 mg once a week with 6–8 ounces of
            water on arising, at least a half hour before breakfast
         b. Calcium supplements and antacids interfere with absorption of Al-
            endionate; these should be taken at least a half hour later

c. To prevent GI complications, the woman must remain in an upright position for one half hour after taking medication
3. Calcitonin-Salmon
   a. Injection treatment: 100 IU subcutaneously or intramuscularly every other day
   b. Nasal spray treatment: 200 IU intranasally once a day (Miacalcin®)
4. Selective estrogen receptor modulators: Raloxifene (Evista®) 60 mg daily
5. Calcium, 1200–1500 mg with vitamin D, 400–800 IU daily (20 mg), and a multivitamin with magnesium 600 mg daily
6. Risedronate (Actonel®) 35 mg/day
7. Phytoestrogens

B. General measures
1. Increase exercise
   a. Muscle strengthening exercises concentrating on large muscle groups
   b. Aerobic exercise: walking, walking on a treadmill, climbing a Stairmaster, riding a bicycle, using a cross-country ski-type apparatus
2. Increase dietary intake of calcium, vitamin D, magnesium
3. Decrease dietary intake of caffeine and alcohol
4. Decrease or stop smoking (see smoking cessation guideline)

VIII.   Differential Diagnosis
A. Osteopenia—reduced bone mass due to inadequate osteoid synthesis
B. Arthritis
C. Paget's disease
D. Fracture

IX. Complications
A. Fracture with associated complications
B. Physical deformity

X. Referral/Consultation
A. Lack of response to treatment
B. Fractures
C. Nutritional guidance
D. Exercise program (organizations providing moderate to low cost for physical fitness)
E. Smoking cessation

See Appendix A and Bibliography.

12

Smoking Cessation

I. Definition

Smoking is the leading cause of preventable illness and premature death in the United States. An estimated 40 million Americans smoke, and it is estimated that of this number 70% want to quit. Quitting involves the process of fighting both the physical and psychological dependence of smoking. It is believed that nicotine is as addictive as cocaine, opiates, amphetamines and alcohol.

II. Etiology

A. The nicotine contained in inhaled cigarette smoke reaches the brain in approximately 10 seconds. Once received in the brain, nicotine causes the brain to release dopamine and norepinephrine. When nicotine is inhaled in a regular fashion, the brain accepts the chemicals by increasing the number of nicotine receptor sites. This mechanism is believed to underlay nicotine dependence. When inhaled nicotine binds to these receptor sites, it causes arousal, stimulation, increased heart rate and increased blood pressure. These physical reactions cause the smoker to experience mood elevation, reduced anxiety and stimulation within seconds of inhalation. Signs and symptoms of withdrawal may begin within a few hours of the last cigarette, peak at 48–72 hours and return to baseline 3–4 weeks after quitting.

B. Problems associated with smoking
   1. Pregnancy complications (low birth weight, miscarriages, preterm delivery); increased asthma risk in children, other respiratory problems
   2. Cervical dysplasia
   3. Increased risk for cancer (esophageal, bladder, kidney, pancreatic, leukemia, breast, gyn)
   4. Gastric and duodenal ulcers
   5. Premature wrinkling of the skin
   6. Decreased bone density, osteoporosis, fractures
   7. Impotence and fertility problems
   8. Lung disease
   9. Decreased HDL
   10. Peripheral vascular disease
   11. Periodontal and dental distress

12. Depression
13. Early menopause

III. Barriers to Smoking Cessation
A. Physical dependence
1. Withdrawal symptoms
   a. Depressed mood
   b. Insomnia
   c. Irritability
   d. Difficulty concentrating
   e. Increased appetite—weight gain
   f. Anger
   g. Restlessness
   h. Frustration
   i. Decreased heart rate
B. Psychological dependence
1. Behaviors associated with smoking become integrated into a person's routine
2. Smoking once integrated into routine becomes associated with pleasure and enjoyment
3. Smoking may also be used to cope with stress or lessen negative emotions

IV. History
A. Risk assessment
1. Do you smoke
2. How many cigarettes a day—for how long
3. How soon after awakening do you smoke your first cigarette
4. Do you waken at night to smoke
5. Is it difficult for you to observe "no smoking" rules
6. Which cigarette would be hardest to give up
7. Do you smoke more cigarettes in the first hours of your days than at other times
8. Have you ever attempted to stop smoking
9. If yes, what got in your way
B. What the patient may present with
1. Nagging, chronic cough
2. Sinus congestion
3. Shortness of breath
4. Fatigue
5. Elevated blood pressure
6. Inability to meet physical challenges (run for a bus, play with young children)
7. Decreased fertility
8. Osteoporosis, decreased bone density

      9. Premature wrinkling

    10. Gum disease

C. Additional questions to be asked

    1. Pregnancy complications

    2. History of abnormal Pap smears

    3. History of or presently existing cancer

    4. Fractures

    5. Cataracts/glaucoma

    6. Problems with cold hands or feet or leg pain

    7. Diabetes

    8. Gastric or duodenal ulcer

    9. Current medicines including herbals, homeopathics, vitamins

V. Physical Examination

A. Vital signs

    1. Temperature

    2. Pulse, respirations

    3. Blood pressure

B. Skin

    1. Observe for color, tone and premature wrinkling

C. ENT

    1. Thorough examination of oral cavity. Observe for dental cavities, stained teeth, tongue or buccal lesions, gum disease, foul breath

D. Lungs

    1. Listen for adventitious sounds (wheezes, rales, crackles)

E. Breast examination

F. Abdominal examination

G. Gynecologic examination (Pap, cultures, bimanual)

H. Extremities

    1. Observe extremities for signs of circulatory, peripheral vessel involvement, pulses, pedal edema

V. Laboratory Examination

A. CBC (elevated hematocrit, WBC, platelets, decreased leukocytes)

B. Lipid level (decreased HDL)

C. Consider

    1. Vitamin C level (decreased)

    2. Serum uric acid (decreased)

    3. Serum albumin (decreased)

    4. Pulmonary function tests

VI. Differential Diagnosis
A. Per physical findings   B. Depression   C. Anxiety

VII. Treatment
A. Intervention needs to be multifaceted and tailored to each patient's needs
B. Any approach needs to include information regarding the following:
 1. A clear, strong stop smoking message
 2. Risks associated with smoking
 3. Benefits of cessation
 4. Addictive components of smoking
 5. What to expect during withdrawal period
 6. Potential risk of relapse
C. Personalize the risks to each individual. Relate her current health problems or findings on physical examination to the effects of smoking
D. Emphasize how smoking cessation can reward the individual
E. If the patient indicates a willingness to quit, form a contract for a quit date. This date should be within a short time frame (1–2 weeks). A notation of this date should be made and the clinician should reinforce the contract with a phone call
F. Factors involved in successful cessation efforts include:
 1. Timely intervention and motivation by clinician
 2. Individual's desire and motivation
 3. Multifaceted program
 4. Individualization of program to patient's situation
G. Methods (may be used individually or in conjunction with each other)
 1. Behavioral
  a. Draft list of reasons to quit smoking and the rewards of quitting. This list should be kept with the person and reviewed when the urge to smoke "hits" and he or she is in need of reinforcement
  b. Inform family and friends and ask for their support and encouragement
  c. Smoker should keep a journal. In precessation stage the smoker can use the journal to record each cigarette smoked, the social cues experienced, the setting, the intensity of the craving and the time of day. This can help identify the individual's triggers and assist smoker to adapt strategies and coping skills to get past the triggers. Keeping a journal during cessation is helpful for expressing feelings and recording the steps of the journey.
  d. Patient should avoid alcohol, which weakens resolve
  e. Patient should throw out all cigarettes, ashtrays, etc.

f. Patient should avoid being around smokers

g. If possible, patient should establish a "no smoking" living space

h. Patient should increase exercise level (walking, weight lifting, yoga). Exercise assists in weight management, stress reduction, sense of well-being

i. Consider use of meditation or relaxation tapes

2. Nicotine replacement. The theory behind nicotine replacement is that by replacing the nicotine, the smoker can deal with the emotional factors and utilize behavioral changes without having to deal with the full impact of physical withdrawal at the same time

a. Gum—offers episodic satisfaction for nicotine craving as it arises

1) Nicotine Polacrilex (Nicorette™ 2 mg per piece (maximum 30 pieces per day)

2) Nicotine Polacrilex (Nicorette D.S.™ 4 mg per piece—maximum 20 pieces per (lay)

3) Adverse effects:

- mouth sores
- dyspepsia
- hiccups
- jaw ache
- 10% of those who use gum may become dependent requiring long-term use (1–2 years) to remain abstinent

b. Transdermal patches. If a patient chooses to use the patch, there should be a contract not to smoke during its use

1) Nicotine transdermal therapeutic system (Habitrol™) 21 mg/day (24 hours) for 4–6 weeks, then 14 mg/day for 2–4 weeks, then 7 mg/day for 2–4 weeks

2) Nicotine transdermal system (Nicoderm CQ™) 21 mg/day (24 hours) for 4–6 weeks, then 14 mg/day for 2–4 weeks, then 7 mg/day for 4–6 weeks

3) Nicotine transdermal system (Nicotrol™) 15 mg/day (16 hours) for 4–6 weeks

4) Nicotine transdermal system (ProStep™) 22 mg/day (24 hours) for 4–8 weeks, then 11 mg/day for 2–4 weeks

5) Adverse effects:

- skin reactions
- insomnia
- vivid dreams
- myalgia

If vivid dreams and/or insomnia are a problem, the patient may remove the patch prior to retiring and apply new patch on arising *NOTE:* If waking during the night is a problem, the 24-hour patches may provide more relief

c. Nasal spray—has the advantage of being an accelerated delivery system, delivering nicotine on demand (within 10 seconds) as a cigarette does

1) Nicotine nasal spray (Nicotrol NS™) 1 spray (0. 5 mg) in each nostril (8–40 mg/day) to a maximum of 5 times per hour or 40 times per 24 hours. Max: 3 months treatment

2) Adverse effects:
- higher incidence
- of dependence
- rhinitis
- watering eyes
- nasal irritation
- throat irritation
- sneezing
- coughing

d. Nicotrol inhaler 10 mg/cartridge (4 mg delivered) 6–16 cartridges/ day for up to 12 weeks, reduce gradually over 12 more weeks then discontinue. Max: 6 months treatment

e. Oral medication

1) Bupropion Hydrochloride (Zyban™ or Wellbutrin SR™) 150 mg every day for 2 days, then 150 mg b.i.d. for 7–12 weeks. Initiate medication one week prior to start date. This week allows the patient to initiate behavioral interventions and prepare psychologically for quitting. Bupropion Hydrochloride is an antidepressant which acts as an inhibitor of the neuronal uptake of norepinephrine, serotonin and dopamine. The mechanism of action in smoking cessation is unknown, but it may serve to mimic the neurochemical effects of nicotine that serve as the pathway to addiction

a) Contraindications

History of seizure disorder

Prior diagnosis of eating disorder

Concurrent use of monoamine oxidase inhibitor

b) Possible adverse reactions:
- rash • nausea • agitation • migraine

NOTE: If a prescription is written for Zyban Advantage Plan™ the patient receives material providing a toll-free 800 number. A phone call will enroll the patient in an individualized program providing behavioral modification and patient support materials as well as information on smoking cessation and 3 months of personal support at no additional cost

2) Nortriptyline (Pamelor™) (tricyclic antidepressant) 25 mg q.d. x 4 days, 50 mg q.d. x 4 days then 75 mg q.d. x 12 wks. For best results start medication 14 days prior to quit date

3) Citrol™ (dietary citric acid supplement). Spray 2–4 times directly on back of throat to reduce desire to smoke for approx. 1 hr. Use as needed.

f. Hypnosis

g. Plastic "cigarettes"

VII. Complications
A. Relapse—most people who return to smoking do so within a month of quitting. The longer persons have abstained, the more likely they are to continue to do so
   1. Patient may be doing well when a situation or stressor makes smoking too enticing to resist
   2. Patient may experience side effects from product used and lose resolve

VIII. Consultation
A. Question regarding possible medical contraindication to use of nicotine replacement or Bupropion Hydrochloride
B. Referral to intensive group sessions such as those offered by Nicotine Anonymous, American Cancer Society, American Lung Association, or a local hospital

IV. Follow-up
A. Telephone call to patient within 1–2 weeks of quit date
B. Office follow-up at 1 and 3 months
C. If relapse occurs
   1. Discuss and review problems and stressors that contributed to relapse
   2. Review and reinforce strategies that smoker can utilize to meet future challenges
   3. Renew smoker's commitment to total abstinence
   4. Review why patient wishes to quit; contract with patient to set another quit date
   5. Reassure patient that success is often achieved only after 5 to 6 repeated attempts; success may take several years

See Appendix A for a patient information sheet for photocopying or adapting.

See Bibliography.

13
Loss of Integrity of Pelvic Floor Structures

I. Definition
Loss of tone of pelvic floor soft tissues is often associated with childbirth and/or the general effects of aging, and may result in cystocele, rectocele, urethrocele, stress incontinence, and/or uterine prolapse. It can also result from sexual assault or abuse including incest.

II. Etiology
A. Childbirth trauma: precipitous delivery, especially of a very large baby, grand multigravida, inadequate repair of episiotomy or of lacerations
B. Aging: loss of muscle tone, relaxation of muscles, ligaments
C. Trauma due to sexual assault, incest, abuse
D. Secondary to surgery, infection especially STDs with scarring

III. History
A. What the patient may present with
1. Stress incontinence; urge incontinence; mixed incontinence
2. Feeling of pressure in pelvic area—heaviness, fullness
3. Pain on defecation, fecal incontinence
4. Inability to empty bladder completely; frequency, urgency
5. Dyspareunia
6. Lower abdominal, groin, or lower back pulling or aching
7. Bulging of organs against vaginal wall, prolapse through vagina
B. Additional information to be considered
1. Menstrual and reproductive history; pregnancies, route of delivery, any laceration, episiotomy, pelvic surgery or repair; reproductive tract cancers
2. Occurrence of present symptoms: onset, frequency, conditions under which they occur, relief measures tried
3. Contraceptive history: methods used, present method
4. History of sexual assault, abuse, incest
5. STDs, especially with tissue destruction and scarring
6. History of ritual circumcision, genital cutting
7. Caffeine intake; diet; alcohol; smoking
8. Medications including OTC and herbals, vitamins, homeopathics

IV. Physical Examination

A. Abdominal examination
    1. Masses   2. Tenderness

B. External examination
    1. Urethra
    2. Perineum
    3. Vulva
        a. Cystocele; cystourethrocele   d. Prolapsed uterus
        b. Rectocele, enterocele   e. Ritual circumcision,
        c. Urethrocele   genital cutting

C. Vaginal examination
    1. Speculum
        a. Condition of vagina: lax, good tone, any lesions, rugae
        b. Presence of cervix
        c. Integrity of vaginal walls
        d. Visible cystocele, urethrocele, and/or rectocele; uterine prolapse
    2. Digital
        a. Palpate cystocele, urethrocele
        b. Palpate rectocele both vaginally and rectally

D. Biannual examination
    1. Uterus
        a. Position   b. Tenderness   c. Masses
    2. Adnexa
        a. Masses   b. Tenderness
    3. Palpable cystocele, urethrocele, scars
    4. Rectal exam:rectocele

E. Standing evaluation: cough stress test to confirm urine loss from urethra

F. Use perineometer to measure strength of pelvic floor contractions

G. Cotton swab (Q-tip) test

V. Laboratory Examination

A. Urinalysis for stress or urge incontinence, to rule out infection

B. Postvoid residual volume test: catheterization or pelvic ultrasound

VI. Differential Diagnosis

A. Urinary tract infection   B. Genital tract mass/carcinoma

VII. Treatment

A. Medication
    1. Prescription for urinary tract infection if indicated; see urinary tract
       infection guideline

2. Consider hormone therapy—oral, patch, vaginal ring or topical
3. Treat any vaginitis, vaginosis, STD
4. Nonhormonal vaginal moisturizers such as Replens®
5. Detrol® (Tolterodine tartrate) 2 mg BID or Detrol® LA 4 mg/day can reduce to 2 mg/day for overactive bladder, urinary frequency, urgency, or urge incontinence
6. Ditropan® XL (oxybutynin chloride) 5 mg/day; or Ditropan® 5 mg BID or TID, or Oxytrol™ (oxybutynin transdermal system) 3.9 mg/d applied 2x/week

B. General measures
1. Teach Kegel (pelvic floor muscle training) exercises for stress incontinence (if there is no prolapse, cystocele, or urethrocele). (A commercial product of graduated weighted cones is available to assist in Kegel exercises; a cone is inserted in the vagina and Kegels are performed using the cone's feedback; when weight of cone can be maintained 15 minutes when walking or standing, move to next cone); also biofeedback devices available or electrical stimulation for passive exercise
2. Keep diary of occurrence of stress or urge incontinence (see Appendix A for teaching materials and diaries; bladder retraining techniques)
3. Suggestions for hygiene measures
4. Eliminate bladder irritants including milk products, sugar, chocolate, many cough medications, caffeine, nicotine, alcohol, artificial sweeteners, spicy and acidic foods
5. Improve hydration
6. Relaxation training
7. Pessary for uterine prolapse (continence ring, Mar-Land, Eva Care®, Milex® pessaries)
8. Stress incontinence devices: bladder neck support prosthesis (Introl®), the Reliance" urethral insert, the Softpatch®, FemAssist®, Impress® soft patch, FemSoft® insert, Viva® plug

VIII. Consultation/Referral
To physician for
1. Possible surgical repair, hysterectomy
2. Possible reconstruction 2° prior surgery, scarring
3. Videodynamic evaluation with anterior wall relaxation

See Appendix A, which can be photocopied or adapted for your patients. See Bibliography.

14

Genitourinary Tract

Urinary Tract Infection

I. Definition
An infection of the urethra, bladder (cystitis), ureters, or kidneys.

II. Etiology
A. Specific causes
  1. Bacteria
     a. Escherichia coli (E. coli)—80% of all infections
     b. Staphylococcus saprophyticus, second most commonly isolated organism; formerly thought to be a contaminant; now thought to be of causative significance, especially in women aged 16–25
     c. Others: Klebsiella, Enterobacteriaceae, Serratia, Proteus, Providencia, Pseudomonas, Group D Streptococcus, Staphylococcus aureus, Staphylococcus epidermidis, Staphylococcus saprophyticus, Citrobacter, Enterococcus
  2. Fungi: especially in diabetes and patients with catheters; immunocompromised persons
  3. Viruses that cause viruria: measles, mumps, herpes simplex, cytomegalo-virus, adenovirus varicella zoster leading to hemorrhage in bladder, and cystitis
B. Mechanism: most commonly ascending infection
  1. In females: gastrointestinal flora (E. coli)
  2. In males: prostate plays a role in harboring infection, constricting urethra causing urine retention
C. Other predisposing factors
  1. Size of inoculum
  2. Virulence of organism
  3. Incomplete or infrequent bladder emptying
  4. Urinary tract abnormalities: obstruction, calculi, congenital defects, prostatic hypertrophy
  5. Use of catheters
  6. Newly sexually active ("honeymoon cystitis")

7. Chemical contamination secondary to spermicidal, barrier methods of contraception

III. History

A. What the patient may present with
   1. Dysuria
   2. Frequency, urgency
   3. Suprapubic pain, ache, pressure, scorched feeling after urination
   4. Back pain; ache or pressure in genitals
   5. No systemic symptoms except occasionally a low grade fever, < 101
   6. Gross hematuria
   7. Vague abdominal discomfort
B. Additional information to consider
   1. Any previous cystitis or pyelonephritis: when, how treated, response to treatment
   2. Previous urologic work-up
   3. Any vaginal discharge
   4. Any chronic condition, diabetes, paraplegia, quadriplegia; cerebral palsy, meningomyelocele, spina bifida
   5. Duration of symptoms
   6. Possible pregnancy with high-risk complications or use of contraindicated drugs
   7. Sexual activity, especially 24–48 postvaginal intercourse
   8. Method of contraception

IV. Physical Examination

A. Vital signs: temperature
B. Abdomen: any tenderness, masses
C. Back: any costovertebral angle (CVA) tenderness or pain
D. Pelvic examination essential to rule out pelvic inflammatory disease, vaginitis, vaginosis, or sexually transmitted disease

V. Laboratory Examination

A. U/A: clean catch midstream urine; pyuria = > 5 WBC/hpf
B. Culture alone is sufficient on first time ever with urinary tract infection with no risk factor; all others should have culture and sensitivities
   1. Culture and sensitivities typically > 100,000 organisms felt to be diagnostic
   2. If between 10,000 and 100,000, probably significant if clinical symptoms support diagnosis

C. Note: Urine may be stored at room temperature for 1 hour or refrigerated up to 72 hours
D. Acute uncomplicated cystitis (nonpregnant woman)—dipstick; if + for nitrates and + leukocyte esterase or microscopic examination of urine shows increased WBCs (10 in high powered field) consider treating presumptively

VI. Differential Diagnosis
A. Upper tract disease: pyelonephritis
B. Urethritis due to
 1. Chlamydia
 2. Bacteria from urethral manipulation causing irritation; thought to be early cystitis
C. Vaginitis
D. Pelvic inflammatory disease
E. Sexually transmitted disease
F. Interstitial cystitis
G. No recognized pathology, "honeymoon cystitis"
H. Pregnancy
I. Hormonal urethral changes

VII. Treatment
A. Antibiotics
 1. For first episode of urinary tract infection in women without risk factors: institute treatment with any of the following, provided the woman is not allergic to the drug
  a. Nitrofurantoin (Macrodantin®) 50 mg QID x 7 days and, depending on repeat culture results, possibly 25 mg QID x 7 more days or Macrobid® 100 mg BID x 7 days
  b. Trimethoprim (160 mg) sulfamethoxazole (800 mg) (Septra DS®), Bactrim DS 1 BID x 10–14 days or Septra or Bactrim (80 mg trimethoprim 400 mg and sulfamethoxazole) 2 tabs BID x 10–14 days
  c. For uncomplicated first or second episodes, Trimethoprim (160 mg) and sulfamethoxazole (800 mg) 2 (Septra DS®) or Bactrim DS® STAT or BID for 3 days or trimethoprin 100 mg BID x 3 days
  d. Amoxicillin 500 mg TID x 10 days
  e. Cipro® (ciprofloxacin HCL) 100–250 mg BID x 3 days OR Floxin® (ofloxacin) 200 mg BID x 3 days OR Augmentum® (amoxicillin 400 mg/clavulantic acid 125), one BID x 3 days OR Noroxin® (norfloxacin) 400 mg BID x 3 days OR Maxaquin® (lomefloxacin) 400 mg once daily x 3 days (should be reserved for complicated UTIs only)

    f. Monurol® (fosfomycin) 3 gm in a single dose mixed in 3–4 ounces of cold water (not recommended under age 18)

2. For reinfection or urinary tract infection in women without risk factors: same as for the first episode. Important to distinguish reinfection from relapse. Reinfection occurs within weeks to months of preceding episode, and is often caused by a new organism. Relapse is a recurrence of symptoms and infection after finishing a medication course, and is caused by the same organism as the original infection

3. For relapse in women
    a. Consider retreatment with same medication, with a test of cure 24–48 hours after completion of medication
    b. Consider change of medication with test of cure 24–48 hours after completion of medication
    c. For second relapse, consult with physician

4. For patients with risk factors (past history of pyelonephritis, known urinary tract abnormality, use of catheter, diabetes): consider referral to physician

B. For pregnant women
1. The causative pathogen in pregnant women is usually E. coli. Do culture before treatment; sensitivity only if no improvement from medication
    a. First choice: Ampicillin 250 1 QID x 10 days
    b. Second choice: Nitrofarantoin (Macrodantin®) or Macrobid®
    c. Do not use Sulfa, Septra® or Bactrim® (Trimethoprim) or Ciprofloxacin (category C) in pregnancy

C. Pain relief: Phenazopyridine hydrochloride (Pyridium®, Azo-Standard, Baridium, Di-Azo, Phenazo, Urodine) 200 mg TID x 24 hours; Uristat (phenazopyridine HCL 95 mg) 2 tabs TID x no more than 2 days (available OTC) (not recommended in pregnancy)

D. General measures
1. Advise voiding before and after sex
2. Advise adequate lubrication for sex
3. Teaching re: hygiene, contamination
4. Treat as above (B.) if bacteria present
5. Consider treatment with Pyridium® Azo® Standard (Phenazopyridine hydrochloride), Uristat® or other such product only if patient symptomatic in absence of pathogenic organism
6. Cranberry juice; 6–8 glasses of water a day; ↓ bladder irritants such as caffeine, smoking; cranberry juice capsules Azo-cranberry 450 mg cranberry juice concentrate 1–4 capsules per day with meals

7. Cotton underwear, avoid tight-fitting garments
8. Consider topical or vaginal estrogen in postmenopausal woman with recurrent cystitis as adjunct

VIII. Complications
Pyelonephritis

IX. Consultation/Referral
A. Consider physician consult on
   1. Women with relapsed infections
   2. Women who are symptomatic after 3 days of treatment
   3. Women who have more than 3 episodes in a year
   4. Complicated UTIs

X. Follow-up
A. Follow-up culture if symptoms do not resolve after treatment
B. Consider test of cure up to 1 week after completion of medication

Appendix A, on cystitis, may be photocopied or adapted for your patients.

See Bibliography.

15

Preconception Care

I. Definition
Advanced planning aimed at reducing perinatal mortality and morbidity.

II. Etiology
Reasons for promoting preconception care (PCC) include
A. Maximize healthy life
B. Identify any medical condition or medications in either prospective parent
C. Identify genetic disorders
D. Review past gestational and pregnancy outcome history
E. Identify high risk exposures. Tobacco, drug and alcohol use; environmental hazards, e.g., toxins, chemicals including pesticides, gases, foods

III. History
A. Woman's medical & surgical history—including but not limited to:
    1. Diabetes   4. Lung
    2. Phenylketonuria   5. Thyroid
    3. Cardiovascular including - B/P 6. Kidney
    7. Infectious disease (e.g., HIV, hepatitis B and C, toxoplasmosis, rubella, varicella, TB, STDs, vaginosis)
    8. Autoimmune
    9. Connective tissue
    10. Eating disorders
    11. Metabolic conditions
    12. Psychiatric illness
    13. Epilepsy
    14. Thromboembolic
    15. Any surgery?
    16. DES exposure
    17. Allergies
B. Obstetrical and gynecological history
    1. Contraception   4. Pap smear history
    2. Menstrual history   5. High-risk behavior (including STDs)
    3. Gynecological history 6. Pregnancy history including SAB, TAB
C. Immune status: need to have documentation

1. Rubella
2. TB
3. Hepatitis A, B, C
4. Varicella
5. Tetanus if ≥ 10 years
6. Polio

D. Drug history
    1. Current prescription medications
    2. Current over-the-counter medications
    3. Current vitamin and botanical use
    4. "Street" drug use history

E. Nutritional status
    1. Height and weight
    2. Eating habits
    3. Food allergies
    4. Caffeine and artificial sweetener intake
    5. History of being over- or underweight
    6. History of an eating disorder
    7. Current exercise habits and other physical activities

F. Genetic history
    1. May use a Genogram, identify couples with a personal or family history of problematic diseases such as:
        a. Tay-Sachs
        b. Thalassemia
        c. Sickle-cell disease or trait
        d. Phenylketonuria
        e. Cystic fibrosis
        f. Hemophilia
        g. Mental retardation
        h. Myotonic dystrophy
        i. Adult polycystic kidney disease
        j. Birth defects
    2. Family background
        a. Related outside marriage
        b. Ethnic background: African-American, Mediterranean, Ashkenazi Jew, Asian

G. Exposure to teratogenic toxins: areas of concern include:
    1. Exposure
        a. Metals (lead)
        b. Organic solvents
        c. Gases
        d. Radiation
        e. Pollutants (e.g., second hand smoke)
        f. Pesticides
        g. Lead paint
    2. Consumption
        a. Alcohol   b. Smoking   c. Street drugs

H. Social history
    1. Age

2. Marital, partner status
3. Family structure; household composition
4. Support systems
5. Employment/financial status
6. Cultural beliefs
7. Child care issues
8. Safety issues (e.g., spousal/partner abuse)
9. Work history: exposure to chemicals, radiation; standing at work; occupational risks, such as wearing respirator, mask, special clothing

I. Partner health history
   1. Thorough health/genetic/social history should be taken on prospective fathers. Little conclusive research has been done of how partners' exposures to chemicals/toxins/drugs may affect fetal development. Recent studies have indicated that alcohol consumption in the month prior to conception contributes to low spermatogenesis
   2. Findings need to be integrated with maternal health history findings

IV. Physical Examination
A. Baseline height, weight, vital signs
B. General physical, including pelvic
C. Comprehensive exam based on medical history

V. Laboratory
A. Papanicolaou smear
B. Baseline studies may be considered, including:
   1. Blood Rh, type
   2. Hemoglobin/hematocrit
   3. Urinalysis
   4. RPR/VDRL
   5. Check status for
      a. Hepatitis B, C
      b. Varicella
      c. Rubella
      d. HIV
      e. TB
   6. Based on history, check:
      a. Toxoplasmosis
      b. CMV
   7. GC, Chlamydia, wet mount, mycoplasma & ureaplasma

VI. Education
A. Begin at least one month prior to planned conception
   1. Avoidance of environmental toxins

2. Cessation of smoking and alcohol consumption, use of street drugs
3. Begin exercise program (e.g., walking, swimming, cycling)—heart rate not to exceed 140 beats per second
4. Bring immunizations up to date. (If live vaccine used, postpone conception at least 3 months)
5. Eat a balanced diet
6. Start vitamin therapy
   a. 0.4 mg p.o. of folic acid q.d. (increase dosage for women who are at increased risk for NTD to 0.8 mg q.d.) (some sources say 5 mg/day)
   b. Increase calcium intake to an equivalent of one quart of milk daily (or 1200 mg)
7. Avoid or at least decrease caffeine intake
8. Consult with primary care provider regarding prescription medications (e.g., psychotropics, antihypertensives, anticonvulsants); botanicals, vitamins
9. Avoid hot tubs, saunas (bringing body temperature above 102° F can damage the embryo)
10. Don't empty cat litter box.
11. No raw meat or raw fish

VII. Referral/Consultation

A. For genetic consultation if indicated
B. Evaluation of prescriptive medication use with specialists
C. Substance abuse counseling if indicated
D. Nutritional counseling if indicated (e.g., obesity, gestational diabetes with prior pregnancies, vegetarian)
E. Community/federal programs for financial assistance if indicated
F. Domestic violence intervention

VIII. Follow-up

A. Refer for obstetrical care if pregnancy occurs (if setting does not provide care)
B. If conception does not occur within 1 year, return for further evaluation/ possible referral. Consider sooner if over age 30

Appendix A may be photocopied or adapted for your patients. See Bibliography.

Polycystic Ovary Syndrome (PCOS)

I. Definition

PCOS, known in the past as Stein-Leventhal Syndrome, is an endocrinological condition with complex pathophysiology and a wide variety of clinical presentations. It is one of the most common reproductive tract problems in women under 30 years of age. Typical clinical and biochemical manifestations are anovulatory cycles, infertility and hyperandrogenicity, but many women do not exhibit these characteristic signs. Some women with PCOS have ovaries with a thickened capsule and multiple follicular cysts (polycystic ovaries—PCO). Women with PCO do not necessarily have PCOS and those with PCOS do not always have PCO.

II. Etiology (unknown but posited)
A. Genetic factors
B. Possible autosomal transmission of responsible genetic sequences
C. A gene or gene series may render the ovary susceptible to insulin stimulation of androgen secretion and block follicular maturation

III. History
A. What the patient may present with (only 20–30% symptomatic)
   1. Anovulatory cycles
   2. History or presence of infertility
   3. Oligoamenorrhoea
   4. Amenorrhea
   5. Prolonged erratic menstrual bleeding
   6. Signs of hyperandrogenism including hirsutism, acne, and alopecia (especially crown pattern baldness)
   7. Galactorrhea
   8. Increased waist to hip ratio: > 0.85
   9. Hyperpigmentation: nape of neck, axillae, inguinal areas (acanthosis nigricans)
B. Additional information to be obtained
   1. Menstrual cycle history, patterns (onset, length, duration, amount of bleeding)
   2. Pregnancy history
   3. Contraceptive history
   4. History of weight gain, hirsutism
   5. Voice changes, frontal balding, increased muscle mass, acromegaly
   5. Any chronic diseases especially diabetes

    6. Family history of PCOS, infertility, diabetes
    7. Medication history

IV. Physical examination
A. Complete physical examination including height, weight, blood pressure
B. Pelvic examination—speculum and bimanual to check for enlarged PCO
C. Breast examination to rule out galactorrhea
D. Full body scan for hirsutism, acanthosis nigricans, body shape, waist to hip ratio, hair growth patterns

V. Laboratory and Other Diagnostics
A. Pregnancy test
B. Total testosterone
C. Free testosterone
D. Dehydroepiandrosterone sulfate (DHEAS)
E. Androstenedione
F. Plasma glucose, lipid
G. FSH, LH levels
H. 17–hydroxyprogesterone
I. Serum thyroid-stimulating hormone
J. 24 hour urinary free cortisol excretion
K. Prolactin level
L. Ovarian ultrasound with total testosterone > 200ng/dL
M. Adrenal imaging with DHEAS > 800 ug/dL

VI. Differential diagnosis
A. Late manifestation congenital adrenal hyperplasia
B. Adrenal adenoma
C. Adrenal carcinoma
D. Hyperthecosis
E. Ovarian carcinoma
F. Cushing's syndrome
G. Acromegaly
H. Idiopathic hirsutism
I. Hyperprolactinemias
J. Thyroid disorders
K. Disorders of adrenal and pituitary glands

VII. Treatment
A. Weight loss and exercise program

B. Low dose, low androgenic combination oral contraceptives to restore cyclic menses
C. Possibly antiandrogens for hirsutism and acne
D. Insulin-sensitizing agents: metformin, troglitazone
E. Electrolysis, depilatories
F. Ovulation induction

VIII. Complications
A. Insulin resistance and development of type 2 diabetes
B. Miscarriage
C. Infertility
D. Hysterectomy
E. Endometrial cancer
F. Ovarian cancer
G. Cardiovascular disease (atherosclerosis, hypertension, increased triglycerides)

IX. Consultation and Referral
A. For infertility treatment
B. For nonpharmacologic treatment of hirsutism

X. Follow-up
A. Education about PCOS and lifestyle alterations
B. Education about pharmacologic interventions
C. Education about fertility

16
WEIGHT MANAGEMENT

I. Definition

Obesity is an excess of body fat. The most commonly utilized method used for measuring body composition is the Body Mass Index (BMI) (see Appendix J). BMI is expressed in weight in kilograms divided by height in meters squared (Kg/m^2). Normal weight is defined as a BMI of 18.5–24.9, overweight as a BMI between 25 and 29.9, mild obesity as a BMI between 30 and 34.9, moderate obesity 35–39.9 and morbid obesity, >40. Health risks begin to surface with a BMI greater than 25, the risk increasing as the BMI increases.

II. Epidemiology

Obesity is among the most serious and prevalent health problems in the United States, second only to cigarette smoking. Over 97 million Americans are defined as having a weight problem. Of these, 58 million are obese.

Prevalence continues to rise, in the past decade rising from 25 to 35%. Research has shown that prevalence varies greatly by sex, age, race and socioeconomic status. Over 55% of the population defined as obese are women. Obesity in women is twice as common in lower socioeconomic groups than in women with higher socioeconomic status. Obesity itself is an independent risk factor for many medical conditions and negatively contributes to many others.

III. Etiology

A. Obesity is a multifactorial disorder occurring as a result of an imbalance between energy expended and food consumed and with other contributing factors such as:
  1. Metabolic (less than 1% of obese)
     a. hypothyroidism
     b. cortisol excess (Cushing's Syndrome)
     c. Stein-Leventhal Syndrome (polycystic ovary disease)
  2. Medication
     a. antidiabetics
     b. antipsychotics
     c. antidepressants
     d. antiepileptics
     e. adenergic antagonists

      f. serotonin and histamine antagonists

      g. steroids

  3. Food consumption

      a. portion size

      b. selection of foods

         1) foods high in fat

         2) foods and beverages high in sugar and complex carbohydrates

  4. Lifestyles

      a. sedentary/lack of physical activity

      b. lack of calorie burning (aerobic) exercise

      c. use of food for comfort and to reduce stress

  5. Other

      a. of lesser contribution

         1) endocrine

         2) deviant eating patterns, i.e., binge-eating, night-eating

IV. Risks Associated With Obesity

A. Obesity is associated with increased morbidity and mortality. It has been associated with over 30 illnesses, among them:

  1. Type 2 diabetes

  2. Hypertension

  3. Coronary artery disease

  4. Dislipidemia

  5. Gallstone formation

  6. Osteoarthritis

  7. Gastrointestinal disorders

  8. Sleep apnea

  9. Breast inflammation

  10. Respiratory diseases

  11. Some cancers

  12. Gynecologic conditions

  13. Increased risks in pregnancy

V. History

A. Risk Assessment

  1. Overweight and obese patients may not present with the stated desire to lose weight.

  2. Presenting complaints are most commonly those associated with the risk factors listed in IV A.

  3. A weight-loss assessment should be part of an annual exam.

  4. Weight-loss assessment

a. patient's recognition of need for weight reduction
b. patient's readiness to change
c. previous attempts at weight loss
d. dietary assessment
    1) type and amounts of food typically consumed
    2) patterns of eating
    3) meals
    4) snacks
    5) spontaneous eating
e. alcohol consumption
    1) amount
    2) frequency
f. physical activity
    1) type
    2) how often, for how long
g. presence of obesity-related problems
h. family history of weight and weight-related problems
i. signs and symptoms of depression
j. medications: prescribed, over-the-counter including herbals, homeo-pathics, and nutritional supplements
k. smoker/nonsmoker

VI. Physical Exam

A. As indicated by known problem or presenting complaint or to rule out a secondary cause of obesity
B. Regardless of above, exam should include:
    1. height
    2. weight
    3. blood pressure
C. Head and neck examination for presence of:
    1. moonfacies
    2. hirsutism
    3. goiter
    4. buffalo hump
D. Skin
    1. striae
    2. hirsutism
    3. edema
    4. dryness
E. Calculation of BMI

1. BMI may be calculated by dividing the weight in pounds, by the square of the height (square inches) and multiplying the result by 705.
2. BMI may also be assessed by consulting a BMI Table. (See Appendix J).

F. Waist circumference measurement
   1. waist circumference of >35 on women

VII. Laboratory Exam

A. As indicated by known history or physical exam
B. The following should be considered if no underlying physical problem is indicated:
   1. lipid profile
   2. TSH, free T_4
   3. FBS/2°PP
   4. CBC

VIII. Treatment

A. Intervention needs to be multifaceted and tailored to meet the patient's needs and readiness for change.
B. The need for weight loss should be presented to the patient in a nonjudgmental, nonconfrontational manner. Approach the problem as a partnership in an endeavor that will help the patient to enjoy a longer, healthier life.
C. Assessment of patient's willingness to make a change:
   1. patient may not be interested in making a change despite the identified risk and potential consequences
   2. patient may be interested, acknowledge the risk factors, but may not yet be ready to take action
   3. patient is ready to take on the challenge of weight loss
D. Assessment of the amount of weight to be lost based on physical findings and risk factors
E. Plan
   1. Assessment of caloric intake
   2. Assessment of energy expenditure and level of physical activity
   3. Assessment of limitations and/or existing factors
      a. physical limitation
      b. medications (alternatives may be considered)
      c. financial limitations
      d. cues or stimuli that affect eating
   4. Set realistic goals and expectations regarding the amount of weight to be lost

    a. short-term
      1) 5–10% loss in initial weight at 1–2 lb/week rate
    b. long-term
      1) realization of ideal weight
      2) maintaining ideal weight
  5. Contract with patient a framework for realization of goals

F. Interventions
  1. Diet/with emphasis on long range behavior changes
    a. nutritionist for evaluation and plan
    b. self-help
      1) Weight Watchers
      2) Take Off Pounds Sensibly (TOPS)
      3) Overeaters Anonymous
      4) community-based programs
      5) meal replacement programs
      6) books, magazine articles
      7) web site weight-loss programs
  2. Education in food selection and change in eating patterns (NHLBI/ NIDDK guidelines are a good source of information—see websites).
    a. low fats, ↑ omega-3 fatty acids
    b. moderate use of complex carbohydrates
    c. decrease consumption of simple carbohydrates, i.e. sugary drinks, candy
    d. moderate use of low-fat protein
    e. decrease in portion size
    f. omit late night eating
    g. eating more slowly (20 minutes should pass between first and last bites of a meal)
    h. drinking 8 (8 oz) glasses of water/day
    i. use of daily food diary to keep track of consumption
  3. Physical Activity
    a. activity needs to be tailored to the patient's needs and limitation
    b. a guideline of 30–40 min/day of aerobic exercise/ 3–4 x/week for strenuous exercise; 4–5 x/week for moderate exercise. This may be done at divided times (i.e., three 10 minute sessions)
    c. moderate-intensity physical activity provides significant health benefits, but needs to be done more often
    d. aerobic exercise may include (according to patient's ability)
      1) running/jogging
      2) brisk walking (3 mph)
      3) swimming

    4) bicycling >10 mph for strenuous exercise; <10 mph for moderate exercise

    5) cross-country skiing

    6) rowing

  e. flexibility, resistence/strength training are important components of an exercise program and provide additional health benefits. Activities include:

    1) light weight lifting

    2) resistance bands

    3) pilates

    4) Yoga

4. Pharmacotherapeutic options

  a. pharmaceutic intervention may be helpful in patients with a BMI of >30 kg/m^2. This may also be helpful in patients who are slightly less obese (i.e. BMI of 27–29.9) but who have a comorbidity.

    1) sibutramine (Meridia®). A serotonin and norepinephrine—reuptake inhibitor (in the same class that includes Prozac®/Zoloft®/Wellbutrin®).

      a) way in which sibutramine works

- Makes the patient feel full for a longer period of time, thus helping to control appetite
- Reduces food cravings
- Improves the comorbid conditions associated with being overweight, which results in improvements in triglycerides, HDL, cholesterol, uric acid and glucose.

      b) dosage

- 10 mg/qd PO
- increasing to 15 mg/qd
- may be decreased to 5 mg/qd if not tolerated at higher level

      c) minor side effects include:

- headache
- dry mouth

      d) more major side effects include

- increased blood pressure and pulse rate

      e) contraindications

- hypertension
- CHD
- history of stroke
- patients on SSRI or SSNRI

    2) Orlistat (Xenical®) a pancreatic lipase inhibitor

      a) way in which it works

- blocks absorption of about 30% of ingested dietary fats
- not an appetite suppressant
- improves comorbid conditions related to obesity especially hyperlipidemia and diabetes

b) dosage
  - 120 mg/po TID. Taken just prior to meal containing fat
  - in patients with side effects, medication may be started by taking one 120 mg tablet with the largest fat containing meal of the day and gradually titrating up to advised dosage as patient adjusts

c) side effects (are directly related to amount of fat in meal consumed)
  - soft stools
  - diarrhea (may be explosive and foul smelling)
  - anal leakage

d) additional information
  - a daily multiple vitamin should be recommended as Orlistat® inhibits absorption of fat soluable vitamins

3) Herbal or alternative medications
  a) currently not recommended as alternative medications
    - not under any regulation
    - ingredients i.e. Ma Hung, possess the potential for serious side effects

4) Behavioral
  a) stimulus control
    - identifying factors contributing to overeating and underexercising
    - identify ways in which contributory factors may be eliminated
    - structuring mechanisms for elimination of the negative stimuli
  b) stress management
    - meditation, progressive relaxation
    - guided imagery
  c) cognitive restructuring
    - identification of inner dialogue, i.e. self-talk, distorted/negative self-image
    - replacement of these negative and self-defeating cognitions with more positive ones
  d) social support
    - seek out support/educational groups as noted in VIII F1.
    - join and participate in exercise groups, and other recreation

programs geared toward physical well-being and body conditioning
- seek support systems within family or peer group
- daily journal

5) Surgical
   a) may be considered for patients who have failed trials of diet, lifestyle changes, pharmacotherapy
   b) most often used for patients under age 55 and in good health with a BMI <40 kg/m^2 and possessing a significant cofactor.
   c) prior to surgery patient should undergo assessment by multidisciplinary team. Assessment should include:
   - medical
   - surgical
   - psychological
   - nutritional
   d) patient should be well motivated and well informed about potential benefits and risks
   e) types of procedures
   - vertical banding
   - Roux-en-y gastric bypass
   f) success rates
   - Regardless of procedure, most patients lose one-half to two-thirds their excess weight within 18 months.
   g) risks
   - postoperative wound infection
   - atelectasis
   - dehiscence
   - deep vein thromboembolism
   - anastomotic leaks
   - marginal ulcers
   - pouch and distal esophageal dilation
   - persistant vomiting
   - cholecystitis
   - development of dumping syndrome
   - vitamin deficiencies, i.e. B$_{12}$, folate, iron

4) other
   a) preconception counseling
   b) preconception weight stabilization
   c) counseling of pregnant women as to micronutrient and vitamin supplementation and close monitoring for appropriate weight maintenance and weight gain

X. Consultation
A. BMI $\geq$ 40 (morbidly obese)
B. Psychiatric disorder (bulimia/depression)
C. Sleep apnea
D. Uncontrolled cofactor
   1. hypertension
   2. diabetes
   3. heart disease

X. Follow-Up
A. Weight checks on regularly scheduled contracted schedule
B. Measurements as part of above
C. Review and reassessment of goals on regular schedule
D. Review of food and exercise diaries
E. Review and assessment of problems, concerns, and side effects associated with pharmaceutical interventions

Web Sites

National Heart, Lung and Blood Institute's (NHLBI) website: www.nhlbi.gov/
National Institute of Diabetes, Digestive, and Kidney Diseases website: www.niddk.gov/
http//www.nhlbi.nih.gov/guidelines/obesity/ob_home.htm
    http://www.nhlbi.nih.gov/health/public/heart/obesity/lose_wt/index.htm
       http://www.health.gov/dietaryguidelines
       http://www.63.73.158.75
       http://www.cyberdiet.com
USDA Nutrient Data Laboratory: http://www.nalusda.gov/fnic/foodcomp

17
Complementary/Alternative Therapies (CAM*)

Increasingly, women are utilizing complementary and alternative therapy for preventative and palliative care as alternative or adjunct therapies to their traditional medical care. In the following, we will present an overview of commonly utilized therapies for peri/menopause, PMS and depression.

I. Definition
Alternative therapies refers to treatment approaches that, although utilized for many years, have not been evaluated and tested by conventional methods. The term complementary therapies is utilized to convey the concept that these therapies are often used in conjunction with conventional medically accepted treatments. When looked at in this manner, the term assumes a more holistic view of women's health care needs.

II. Types
A. The following are therapies commonly utilized by women.
1. vitamins
2. minerals
3. herbals
4. phytoestrogens (dietary)
5. natural estrogen
6. natural progesterones
7. acupuncture
8. biofeedback/hypnosis
9. homeopathy
10. therapeutic touch
11. traditional medicines
   a. Ayurveda
   b. traditional Chinese medicines
   c. Tibetan
   d. wise woman traditional
   e. herbalism
   f. these traditional methods may have
      1) complex theoretic structure

*CAM=complementary and alternative medicine

2) literature-based traditions
3) classic gynecologic texts
4) materia medica with specific herbs for reproductive and gynecologic problems
12. therapies based on oral tradition

III. Reasons for Selection/Use of CAM
A. Preference for more "natural" treatment
B. Belief in unconventional (non-Western) medicine
C. Concern about potential side effects of conventional medicines and treatments
D. Dissatisfaction with or lack of confidence in conventional methods
E. Desire to have control over their own health and health care
F. Being raised in a culture that believes in and utilizes CAM therapies

IV. Problems and Concerns
A. Lack of systemized research and well-designed studies to measure safety and efficacy
B. Self-medication based on insufficient information
C. Lack of standardization of therapeutics
D. Failure to inform health care practitioner of CAM use

V. Cautions
A. Remember "natural" isn't synonymous with safe
B. CAM should be utilized only for minor problems, not for conditions that have potential to be life-altering or life-threatening
C. CAM should not be utilized in pregnancy or breast feeding without discussion with health care practitioner
D. Use should be limited to recommended dosages for recommended time frames.
E. Users need to be knowledgeable about CAM methods. Do not use only CAM therapy that has not been personally researched and use understood. The Internet should not be the only source of research and information.
F. Use should begin with a smaller dose to observe for adverse reaction.
G. Buy therapies only from reputable manufacturers.

VI. Frequently Used/Recommended CAM Therapies
A. Menopause
   1. B Complex vitamins
      a. usual dose 50–300 mg/qd

    b. condition
        1) stress/depression
        2) water retention
    c. toxicity/adverse effects
        1) none known
  2. Vitamin C
    a. usual dose 500 mg/qd
    b. condition
        1) free radical scavenger/antioxidant
        2) linked with raising levels HDL, lowering LDL
        3) maintaining bone structures
        4) maintaining healthy connective tissues
    c. toxicity/adverse effects
        1) use with caution and medical supervision if history of compromised kidney function
        2) increased doses (5,000 mg day) associated with intestinal gas and loose stool. If history of reflux, take buffered vitamin C
  3. Vitamin D
  a. usual daily dose 400–800 IU
    b. condition
        1) osteoporosis—increase mineral absorption, bone mineralization
    c. toxicity
        1) unwise to exceed 1,000 IUs
        2) hypervitaminosis (mild), treatable
        3) hypercalcemia from extended doses of over 1,000 IUs may be irreversible
  4. Vitamin E
    a. usual daily dose 400–800 IU may be used up to 1,200 IU safely
    b. condition
        1) hot flashes
        2) cardiovascular prevention, poor circulation, atrophic vaginitis
    c. toxicity
        1) use with caution if patient is on high blood pressure medication (may decrease blood pressure)
        2) use with caution or not at all if patient is on anticoagulant therapy
        3) using more than recommended dose can result in nausea, flatulence, diarrhea, heart palpitations, fainting (all reversible with dose decrease)
  5. Calcium

    a. usual daily dose in divided doses 1,200–2,000 mg—should be used in conjunction with Vitamin D to aid in bone remineralization

    b. condition

        1) osteoporosis (prevention and treatment) provides reintegration of calcium into bones

        2) hypertension—aids in contraction and expansion of heart muscle

    c. toxicity/adverse reaction

        1) calcium has no known toxic effects (caution in use of antacids as calcium supplements. In addition to calcium many of these products contain aluminum which interferes with calcium absorption)

6. Essential fatty acids (EFAs)

    a. usual daily dose as indicated on individual preparation—no daily optimum intake

    b. conditions

        1) hot flashes, vaginal atrophy, mood swings and irritability, bloating and fluid retention, decreased libido

        2) cardiovascular disease osteoporosis. A correct balance of EFAs is essential for the rebuilding and production of new cells and to decrease inflammation and modulate hormone imbalance

        3) EFAs consist of EPA (eicosapentaenoic acid Omega 3) DHCA (docosahexaenoic acid Omega 3) and GLA (gamina linolenic acid Omega 6)

7. Coenzyme Q_{10} (ubiquinone)

    a. usual daily dose 30–100 mg

    b. conditions

        1) the name ubiquinone is appropriate because coenzyme Q_{10} is found everywhere in the body. A powerful antioxidant, it stimulates the immune system, increases tissue oxygenation and has vital antiaging effects. Extensive research has been done regarding its impact on heart disease. It is mentioned here because of its preventative effects.

8. Dong Quai (angelica sinensis)

    a. usual daily dosage—consult preparation instructions

    b. conditions

        1) hot flashes, irritability, insomnia, restlessness, night sweats, headaches, toxicity

    c. toxicity/adverse reactions

        1) no known toxicity; may cause minor GI upset (Do not use Dong Quai during menses if hypermenorrhea is a problem or with any anticoagulents)

9. Chasteberry (Vitex-agnus-castus)
   a. usual daily dosage—consult individual preparation
   b. conditions
      1) mood swings, irritability, depression, balances estrogen—progesterone levels in the body
      2) hot flashes—balances estrogen, progesterone
   c. toxicities/adverse effects
      1) usually without adverse effects—rarely causes nausea, diarrhea, weight gain, headaches, allergic rash—spontaneously disappear when discontinued
10. Black Cohosh (cimicifuga racemosa)
   a. usual daily dosage—consult individual packaging. Is frequently offered as an alternative to hormone therapy
   b. conditions addressed
      1) hot flashes
      2) fatigue
      3) irritability
      4) night sweats
      5) headaches
      6) insomnia
      7) heart palpitations
   c. toxicity/adverse effects
      1) no known adverse effects
11. Licorice (glycyrrhiza glabra)
   a. usual daily dose varies with type of preparation
   b. conditions addressed
      1) hot flashes
      2) fatigue—appears to estradiol levels while raising progesterone
   c. toxicities
      1) should not be used in patients with kidney problems, high blood pressure, patients taking potassium. Not advisable for use in persons who are on low salt diets or persons taking diuretics, corticoid treatments, cardiac glycosides or medication for hypertension.
12. Ginkgo biloba
   a. usual daily dosage—consult preparation directions
   b. conditions addressed
      1) improves circulation, helps with forgetfulness and cold hands/feet, antitoxin/antiinflammation
   c. toxicities

1) no reported toxicities or side effects
13. St. John's Wort (hypericum perforatum)
    a. usual daily dose—300 mg TID
    b. conditions
       1) depression
    c. toxicity/adverse effects
       1) gastrointestinal symptoms, tiredness, restlessness, allergic reactions. Caution: do not use with patients already on an antidepressant
14. Ginseng
    a. There are three kinds of Ginkgo—Asian (Chinese or Korean), American, Siberian. The first two are authentic Ginseng. Siberian Ginseng is not. It looks similar and has similar effects on the body.
       1) usual daily dose 200–400 mg/day
    b. conditions
       1) stress
       2) fatigue
       3) loss of libido
       4) depression (these conditions improve because Ginseng helps the body to adapt)
       5) vaginal dryness—improves because of Ginseng's direct estrogenic effects
15. Dietary phytoestrogens are naturally found in foods. These compounds may produce effects similar to estrogen; found in cereal, legumes and grasses.
    a. There are three main groups of phytoestrogens: isoflavones, lignans, and coumestans
       1) isoflavones are found in soy, garbanzo beans, and other legumes. They may be consumed in the form of soy, miso and tofu
       2) Lignans are found in seed oils such as flaxseed
       3) Coumestans are found in red clover, sunflower seeds and bean sprouts
    b. Phytoestrogens are thought to be helpful in minimizing hot flashes, maintaining bone density, and lowering cholesterol, LDLs and triglycerides
    c. Natural progesterones manufactured from wild yams—patients should be discouraged from using OTC preparations of topical progestins for their progesterone imbalance since there is no standardized compounding. Replacement hormones are usually synthesized
16. Other
    a. relaxation techniques
    b. biofeedback
    c. meditation

d. Tai Chi and Qi Gong
e. Yoga
   These techniques can be helpful in helping the body regain homeostasis, thus making it more possible to adapt to change without increasing stress
f. Ayurvedic and Chinese herbals may also be utilized. There are several preparations on the market. They include
   1) Meno-care® used to alleviate palpitations, insomnia, mood swings and hot flashes. Usual dose—2 tablets BID
   2) Geriforte® used to address the overall stress of aging. Usual dose—2 tablets BID. Source: health food store or through the manufacturer, Himalaya, USA (1–800–869–4640)
   3) Midlife for Women I®—an herbal blend designed for the perimenopausal woman. Helpful in maintaining a hormonal balance. Usual dose—1 tablet BID
   4) Midlife for Women II®—Addresses menopausal symptoms such as hot flashes, mood swings, and insomnia. To be taken in addition to Midlife I. Usual dose—1 tablet BID
      All of the above are available at health food stores, or may be ordered from manufacturer Maharishi Ayur-ued (1–800–826–8424)
   5) Nukeba Zhen Wan (Women's Precious Pills)—an herbal blend, generally used to address low estrogen levels, hot flashes, forgetfulness, confusion, insomnia, and tearfulness. Usual dose—eight small pellets three times/day
   6) Hsaio Yas Wan (Jade Empress)—helpful in alleviating symptoms of irritability, anxiety, headaches, sugar cravings and fatigue. Should not be used if experiencing break-through bleeding. Usual dose—eight small pellets three times/day
   7) Liu Wei Di Huang Wai (six mortals)—used as an antiaging tonic. Helpful for dry skin, vaginal dryness, night sweats, insomnia and loss of muscle tone
      Above herbals may be found in health food stores or ordered from Ethical Nutrients (1–800–638–2848). Although these preparations are easily available, consultation with a Ayurvedic or Chinese medicine clinician is recommended.
g. Homeopathic remedies are based on the premise that the body has the capacity to heal itself. Formulas are compounded that utilize very minute quantities of an agent to trigger the body's innate capacity to heal. Preparations specific to a symptom can be found in health food stores for self-treatment. Homeopathic practitioners are also available to work with a patient to customize preparations to fit the person's symptoms.

VI. PMS
A. B Complex
  1. usual dose 50–300 mg/d
  2. symptoms
     a. stress/depression
     b. water retention (Especially B_6)
     c. toxicity/adverse effects
        1) none known
B. Essential Fatty Acids (also helpful with dysmenorrhea)
  1. usual daily dose—as indicated on individual preparation/no daily optimum dose
  2. conditions
     a. help to reduce depression, irritability, cramps, nausea, bloating, and headaches. Correct balance of EFAs is essential for the rebuilding and production of new cells—decrease inflammation, moderate hormone imbalance
  3. Licorice (Glycyrrhiza glabra)
     a. usual daily dose varies with preparation
     b. conditions addressed—estrogen-like activity helps in irritability, mood swings, stimulates adrenal glands
     c. toxicities—should not be used by women with kidney problems, high blood pressure, patients taking potassium. Not advisable for use in persons who are on low salt diets or persons taking diuretics, corticoid treatments, cardiac glycosides or medications for hypertention.
  4. PMS—Black Cohosh (cimicifuga racemosa)
     a. usual daily dosage—as indicated on individual preparation
     b. conditions
        1) nervousness
        2) irritability
        3) sleep disturbances
        4) depressive moods
        5) headaches

VI. Depression
Consult guideline on emotional/mental health issues

Resources: CAM on PubMed www.ncbi.nlm.nih.gov/pubmed
National Center for Complementary and Alternative Medicine www.nccam.nih.gov

18

Emotional/Mental Health Issues Appropriate for Assessment and Treatment in a Women's Health Care Setting

I. Definition

A. An alteration in mood or behavior resulting in discomfort to the woman. These changes may place the woman in chronic or acute distress. Attempting to cope with this distress may alter her ability to function, causing family relationship or workplace disturbances, as well as somatic manifestations that may contribute to morbidity and mortality.

II. Psychiatric Conditions Commonly Seen in a Women's Health Care Setting:

A. In the following * indicates a condition appropriate for assessment by a clinician in an office setting. ** indicates a condition appropriate for referral for further assessment and treatment. *** indicates condition appropriate for immediate referral to a hospital emergency room or other immediate care settings.

B. Mood Disorders

    **   1. Bipolar disorder

    *   2. Dysthymia

    **   3. Major depression

    *   4. Postpartum depression

    *   5. Premenstrual dysphoric disorder—PMDD

    *   6. Seasonal affective disorder

C. Anxiety Disorders

    *   1. General anxiety disorder

    * or ** 2. Obsessive compulsive disorder

    **   3. Panic disorder

    **   4. Posttraumatic stress disorder

    *   5. Social phobia

D. Eating Disorders

    **   1. Anorexia

    **   2. Bulimia

E. Personality Disorders

257

       **   1. Borderline personality disorder
       **   2. Narcissistic
       **   3. Avoidant
       **   4. Dependent
       *   5. Self-defeating
F. Cognitive Disorders
       **   1. Dementia
       ***   2. Delirium
G. Psychotic Disorders
       /*   1. Schizophrenia
       /*   2. Other psychotic disorders
H. Sexual Disfunction   * or **
I. Sleep Disturbances
    * or **   1. Insomnia
                  a. Difficulty falling asleep
                  b. Restless/wakeful sleep
    2. Early morning awakening with inability to resume sleep
J. Substance Abuse Disorders   **
K. Suicidal Threats or Ideation ***
L. Somataform Disorders
       *   1. Body dysmorphic disorder
       *   2. Hypochondriasis
       **   3. Conversion disorder

III. Responsibilities of Clinicians

A. Knowledge of signs and symptoms indicating a psychiatric condition or a psychiatric component in a medical condition
B. Screening and assessment
C. Intervention
    1. treatment
    2. referral for further assessment
    3. emergency intervention if condition warrants

IV. History

A. What the patient may present with:
    1. Stomach pain
    2. Back pain
    3. Pain in arms, legs, joints
    4. Mood changes associated with menses
    5. Loss of libido
    6. Headaches

7. Chest pain
8. Dizziness
9. Rapid/pounding heart
10. Shortness of breath
11. Gastrointestinal complaints: pain, diarrhea, constipation, nausea, vomiting
12. Fatigue and/or low energy
13. Sleeping difficulties
14. Feeling edgy or nervous
15. Excessive worry
16. Difficulty swallowing or "lump in throat"
17. Feelings of sadness without known cause

B. Additional Information to Be Considered
1. Generalized feeling of sadness or hopelessness
2. Weight loss or weight gain. What was patient's weight 6 months ago/one year ago
3. Alcohol consumption/use of prescription or illicit drugs
4. Has partner or close associates commented on alcohol consumption
5. Does patient feel guilty about drinking
6. Does patient avoid social situations
7. Change in interest in sex or responsiveness during intimacy
8. History of depression or other psychiatric problem in biological family
9. Number of visits to health care provider in past year
10. Has patient found it difficult to concentrate or been easily distracted, finding it hard to find words, forgetting things
11. Changes in work or family environment
12. Suicidal thoughts, plan or attempt
13. Seasonal pattern
14. Prescription, OTC or herbal medication currently used
15. Information on any of the problems listed in II if not spontaneously volunteered

C. Interview Techniques
1. Nonverbal messages are important in obtaining a reliable psychiatric history
   a. patient and clinician should be seated at equal height with no furniture between them, i.e., desk
   b. establish eye contact
   c. put pen down, give patient your full attention
   d. ask clear, open-ended questions
   e. allow patient to talk
   f. be supportive

g. be watchful for important subtexts, i.e., changing the subject, avoidance, careless or exaggerated responses

h. maintain a nonjudgmental attitude; however, be open to challenge contradictory statements

V. Physical Exam

A. Appropriate to physical complaint or symptomatology

B. In addition to appropriate physical exam, clinician should be alert for the following physical manifestations of emotional distress

   1. appearance of sadness
   2. gross anxiety
   3. elevated respiratory rate and pulse
   4. excessive perspiration
   5. coldness and dampness of hands
   6. tremor
   7. inability to make eye contact

C. If indicated by information and observation of above, a general mental status exam or a mini-mental status exam should be conducted.

   1. Mini-mental status exam
      a. Appearance
         1) grooming
         2) clothing; dirty, clean, appropriate to seasonal condition, revealing
      b. Behavior
         1) are mannerisms and gestures appropriate
      c. Attitude
         1) is patient aggressive, angry, guarded, cooperative
      d. Mood
         1) anxious
         2) depressed
         3) manic or hyper
         4) alternating moods
      e. Speech
         1) quantity and quality
         2) speed; pressure
      f. Cognitive functions
         1) concentration
         2) memory
      g. Affect
         1) normal variety of facial expression
         2) blunted, flat or immobilization of facial features

VI. Differential Diagnosis

A. Mental and physical disorders are frequently overlapping; the challenge presented in diagnosis is consideration of both dimensions at the same time and ability to differentiate between the two; by the way in which both entities may be present and contributing to the symptomatology.
   1. hypothyroidism
   2. hyperthyroidism
   3. hypoglycemia
   4. mitral valve prolapse
   5. Meniere syndrome/vestibular neuronitis
   6. esophageal tumors or other obstructions
   7. asthma
   8. caffeine abuse
   9. coronary disease
   10. Alzheimer's disease or senile dementia
   11. irritable bowel syndrome
   12. Crohn's disease
   13. brain tumors

B. Signs and symptoms of conditions indicated in II as suitable for diagnosis and treatment in a primary women's health care setting.
   1. Dysthymia—milder form of depression, symptoms are not disabling but chronic, typically lasting for many years. These symptoms may be so much a part of an individual's life that they are taken for granted and patient does not complain to provider.
      a. depressed mood
      b. poor appetite
      c. insomnia
      d. hypersomnia
      e. low energy/fatigue
      f. low self-esteem
      g. poor concentration
      h. difficulty making decisions
      i. feelings of hopelessness
   2. Postpartum Depression (PPD). A self-limiting period of affective lability occurring within a few days to a week or so after childbirth. Many times PPD goes without diagnosis, which may leave the woman with lifelong feelings of guilt, fear and inadequacy. Below symptoms (a) through (d) indicate a nonpsychotic PPD and (e) through (i) indicate a psychotic illness. The psychotic and/or delusional mother may be at risk to herself and/or her child. Evaluation by a mental health

professional is indicated. Women who have experienced one episode
of PPD are at greater risk for another. Women with inadequately treated psychotic symptoms are at greater risk for future mental health
illness.
a. sleeplessness
b. weeping
c. sadness
d. guilt
e. agitation
f. prolonged sleeplessness
g. lack of personal hygiene
h. anorexia
i. preoccupation with concerns or delusions about the infant
j. untreated, the above may contribute to lack of bonding and has been
   implicated in lifelong problems for mother and infant
3. Premenstrual Dysphoric Disorder (PMDD). A cluster of symptoms
   regularly presenting during the last week of the luteal phase, beginning
   to remit within a few days of the follicular phase. Symptoms are always absent in the week following the menses. Symptoms are not
   present prior to the last week of the luteal phase. Symptoms are of
   comparable severity but not duration to those displayed in a major
   depressive episode including:
   a. sadness
   b. hopelessness
   c. anxiety/tension/feeling on edge
   d. mood instability with tearfulness
   e. persistent irritability
   f. increased anger
   g. increased interpersonal conflicts
   h. binge-eating
   i. insomnia
   j. it is helpful in making a diagnosis if the patient maintains a daily
      diary charting symptoms over a two-month period.
4. Seasonal Affective Disorder (SAD)
   a. Essential feature is that symptoms of a depressive episode occur
      seasonally, during fall or winter, remitting during spring
5. Generalized Anxiety Disorder (GAD). An essential feature is excessive
   anxiety and worry occurring more days than not during a period of 6
   months. Other symptoms include:
   a. restlessness
   b. easy fatigue

      c. difficulty concentrating
      d. irritability
      e. muscle tension
      f. disturbed sleep patterns
      g. fearfulness
      h. somatic complaints, i.e., cold hands, lump in throat, etc.

6. Body Dysmorphic Disorder (BDD). An essential feature of BDD is a preoccupation with a defect in appearance. This preoccupation must cause significant distress or impairment in lifestyle and in other areas of function. Complaints commonly include:
      a. hair thinning
      b. acne
      c. wrinkles
      d. scars
      e. vascular markings
      f. paleness or redness of complexion
      g. facial asymmetry or disproportion
      h. excessive hair on face
      i. preoccupation with a bodily part

VII. Laboratory Examination

A. The following may be considered according to presenting complaint and symptomatology
    1. CBC
    2. Urinalysis
    3. Electrolytes
    4. Blood glucose levels
    5. Thyroid function tests
    6. Liver enzymes
    7. Hormone levels
    8. EKG
    9. EEG
    10. Drug screen if indicated

VIII. Treatment

A. Medication—All of the conditions listed as suitable for office treatment usually respond well to the use of an antidepressant or antianxiety medication. Most antidepressants are effective in treating anxiety as well as depression. Included below are those medications that can be most effectively and safely used in a general practice setting. When a patient does not respond well to one choice she/he may do better with another. When switching medications, do not stop initial drug abruptly prior to starting a new one, instead cross taper over a few weeks. For pregnant women, only Prozac is currently approved.

1. Antidepressant/antianxiety medications
   a. Selective Seratonin Reuptake Inhibitors (SSRIs)
      1) Citalopram hydrobromide (Celexa®)—Starting dose: 10–20 mg/qd. Usual daily dose: 20–60 mg/qd
      2) Fluoxetine hydrochloride (Prozac®/Sarafem®)—Starting dose: 10–20 mg/qd. Usual daily dose 20–60 mg/qd. Sarafem® is used for PMDD and is generally given for the two weeks prior to menses. Usual dose is 20–40 mg/qd
      3) Fluvoxamine maleate (Luvox®)—Starting dose 50 mg/qd. Usual daily dose 50–300 mg/qd
      4) Paroxetine hydrochloride (Paxil®)—Starting dose: 10–20 mg/qd. Usual daily dose 20–60 mg/qd
      5) Sertraline hydrochloride (Zoloft®)—Starting dose: 25–50 mg/qd. Usual daily dose 50–200 mg
      6) Eszitalopram (Lexapro®) starting close 10 mg/qd. Usual daily dose 10 mg.
      7) Major side effects of SSRIs include:
         • GI disturbances
         • Sexual side effects
         • Restlessness
         • Insomnia
         • Headaches
         • Orgasmic dysfunction
         • Activation of mania in patients with bipolar disorder
   b. Dopamine—norepinephrine reuptake inhibitors (DNRIs).
      1) Bupropion hydrochloride (Wellbutrin®)—Usual starting dose: 100 mg/qd. Usual daily dose: 100 mg tid.
      2) Bupropion hydrochloride—sustained release (Wellbutrin SR®)—Starting dose 100 mg or 150 mg/qd. Usual daily dose: 300/qd (150 mg BID)
      3) Bupropion hydrochloride Wellbutrin XR 150 mg-300 mg. Starting dose: 150 mg qd x 7 days. Usual daily dose: 300 mg q/am.
      4) Major side effects of DNRIs
         a) seizures possible with high dose (450 mg/day and history of eating disorder or seizure disorder)
         b) nausea and vomiting with SR formulation
         c) headaches
         d) psychosis (use cautiously in psychotic disorders)

c. Serotonin—norepinephrine reuptake inhibitors (SNRIs)
   1) Venlafaxine (Effexor®)—Starting dose 37.5/qd. Usual daily dose 7.5 mg BID
   2) Venlafaxine extended release (Effexor XR®)—Starting dose: 37.5 mg/day. Usual daily dose 75–225 mg/day
   3) Major side effects with SNRIs
      a) hypertension
      b) nausea
      c) activation
      d) sexual dysfunction
d. Serotonin modulators (SMs)
   1) Nefazodone (Serzone®)—Starting dose: 50 mg/qd. Usual daily dose 150–300 mg/qd
   2) Trazodone (Desyrel®)—Starting dose 50 mg/qd. Usual daily dose: 75–300 mg/qd in divided doses BID
   3) Major side effects of SMs
      a) orthostatic hypotension
      b) anticholinergic symptoms
      c) sedation
      d) priapism (trazodone in males)
e. Norepinephrine—Serotonin modulators (NSMs)
   1) Mirtazapine (Remeron®)—Usual starting dose: 15 mg/qd. Usual daily dose: 15–45 mg/qd
   2) Major side effects of NSMs
      a) anticholinergic symptoms
      b) weight gain
      c) sedation
      d) increase in cholesterol levels
      e) agranulocytosis (d/c medication)
   Tricyclics and MAOs have not been included because of their side effects' profile.
2. Antianxiety Medication
   a. Benzodiazepines: Benzodiazepines should be used for short term only (i.e., specific situation known to cause anxiety/panic or sleeplessness, plane flights, recent loss) This category of drugs is habit forming and can quickly lead to dependence
      1) Alprazolam (Xanax®)—Usual dose: 0.5 mg TID
      2) Clonazepam (Klonopin®)—Usual dose: 0.5 mg BID
      3) Diazepam (Valium®)—Usual dose: 10 mg BID
      4) Lorazepam (Ativan®)—Usual dose: 1 mg TID
      5) Oxazepam (Serax®)—Usual dose: 15 mg TID

      6) Most common side effects of Benzodiazepines
- Frequent: drowsiness, ataxia
- Occasional: confusion, amnesia, disinhibition, depression, dizziness
- Withdrawal symptoms: delirium/convulsions (with abrupt discontinuation), rebound insomnia or excitement
- Discontinue by tapering dose, no more than 25%/week<

b. Other treatment

   1) psychotherapy
- cognitive therapy
- interpersonal therapy
- behavioral therapy

   2) Exposure therapy

   3) Biofeedback therapy

   4) Other medications

a. Buspirone hydrochloride (BuSpar®)—Usual starting dose: 5/10 mg/day. Usual daily dose: 10/15/30 mg BID

b. Most common side effects
- Frequent: headaches, dizziness, nausea
- Occasional: nausea, paresthesias, diarrhea
- Rare: psychosis, mania

c. Complementary therapy

   1) St. John's Wort (hypericum perforatum)—Usual daily dosage: 300 mg TID or 450 mg BID for use in depression. Interaction with all medications listed above. Serotonin syndrome of nausea, diarrhea, headaches may occur if used simultaneously.

   2) Essential fatty acids are increasingly used for mood stabilization

   3) Meditation/relaxation therapy

   4) Regular exercise program

   5) Regulation of sleep/wake patterns

   6) Dietary changes, including decrease or elimination of caffeine

   7) Light therapy with Seasonal Affective Disorder

IX. Complications

A. Untreated
1. increased risk for suicide or harm to others
2. increased risk for other impulsive and acting-out behavior
3. loss of friends, job
4. decrease in family harmony
5. exacerbation of any of the symptoms previously mentioned

B. Treated
   1. Behaviors and somatic problems listed above
C. Consultation
   1. All conditions indicated previously
   2. Failure to improve
   3. Collaboration for an appropriate medication
   4. Medication use in pregnant and lactating women

X. Follow-Up
A. Monitor response, mood relief from symptoms
B. Follow-up appointment in 3–6 weeks to monitor response to treatment, adverse reactions

XI. Web Sites: www.nimh.nih.gov; www.adaa.org; www.cognitivetherapy. com

PART II. APPENDIXES

The materials in this section include clinical forms, screening tools, and patient education information.

The sections on the cervical cap and natural family planning were developed in other settings by R. Mimi Clarke Secor and the late Eleanor Tabeek with updates by Nancy Keaveney and Mary Finnigan.

Appendix A

"For Your Information": Patient Education Handouts

Bacterial Vaginosis (BV)
Breast Self-Examination
Candidiasis (Monilia)
Cervical Cap
Chlamydia Trachomatis
Colposcopy
Constipation
Contraceptive Patch
Contraceptive Spermicides and Condoms
Contraceptive Vaginal Ring (NuvaRing)
Cystitis (Bladder Infection)
FemCap
Genital Herpes Simplex
Genital Warts (Condylomata Acuminata)
Gonorrhea
Hormone Therapy (HT)
Lice (Pediculosis)
Natural Family Planning to Prevent or Achieve Pregnancy
Osteoporosis
Polycystic Ovary Syndrome (PCOS)
Preconception Self-Care
Premenstrual Syndrome (PMS)
Scabies
Stop Smoking
Stress or Urge Incontinence (Loss of Urine)
Surgical Afterabortion Care
Syphilis
Trichomoniasis
Vaginal Discharge

For Your Information:
Bacterial Vaginosis (BV)

I. Definition
Overgrowth of a variety of anaerobic bacterial, genital mycoplasmas, and gardnerella

II. Transmission
The condition can be sexually transmitted, but it may also be identified in the nonsexually active female

III. Signs and Symptoms
A. In the female
1. Fishy, musty odor with a thin, chalk-white to gray watery vaginal discharge
2. Discharge may cause vaginal and vulvar itching and burning
3. Burning and swelling of genitals after intercourse
4. No symptoms in some women
B. In the male: no male version of BV has been identified

IV. Diagnosis
A. Female evaluation may include
1. Vaginal examination to check for bacterial vaginosis
2. Further laboratory work to rule out Candida, trichomonas, gonococcus, or Chlamydia
3. Blood test for syphilis
B. Male evaluation: Rule out other infections such as trichomonas, gonococus, or Chlamydia

V. Treatment
A. Treatment may be by mouth or with a vaginal cream or gel
B. Treatment of partners is not recommended since studies have not shown that their treatment decreases the number of recurrences unless partner is a woman also
C. It is very important to report any medical conditions you may have or medications you take regularly (especially for a seizure disorder) before taking any treatment.

VI. Patient Education

A. Sexual partners should be alerted to the diagnosis and referred for evaluation and possible treatment if the patient has other infections concurrently

B. Sexual partners should be protected by condoms until patient's treatment is over. Check with your clinician since some creams weaken the latex of condoms or vaginal diaphragms

C. Alcoholic beverages should not be consumed during or for 48 hours after oral treatment

D. Minor side effects of oral treatment may include nausea, dizziness, and a metallic taste

E. No douching with or after treatment; douching is never recommended

VI. Follow-up

Return to clinic for a reevaluation if symptoms persist or new symptoms occur.

Special notes: _____

_____

_____

_____

Practitioner: _____

For more information call: CDC STD Hotline: 1-800-227-8922: Phone numbers of free (or almost free) STD clinics are listed in the "Community Service Numbers" in the government pages of your local phone book. http://www.cdc.gov

For Your Information
Breast Self-Examination (BSE)*

Breast self-examination should be done once a month so you become familiar with the usual appearance and feel of your breasts. Familiarity makes it easier to notice any changes in the breasts from one month to another. Early discovery of a change from what is "normal" is the main idea behind BSE. The outlook is much better if you detect cancer in an early stage.

If you menstruate, the best time to do BSE is a few days after your period ends, when your breasts are least likely to be tender or swollen. If you no longer menstruate, pick a day such as the first day of the month to remind yourself it is time to do BSE.

Here is one way to do BSE:

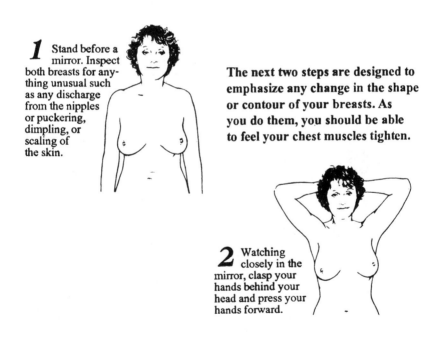

1 Stand before a mirror. Inspect both breasts for anything unusual such as any discharge from the nipples or puckering, dimpling, or scaling of the skin.

The next two steps are designed to emphasize any change in the shape or contour of your breasts. As you do them, you should be able to feel your chest muscles tighten.

2 Watching closely in the mirror, clasp your hands behind your head and press your hands forward.

*Adapted from *Breast Exams: What You Should Know.* U.S. Department of Health and Human Services, 1991; *How To Do Breast Self-Exam,* American Cancer Society, 1999. Consult your nurse practitioner or physician about having a mammogram.

3 Next, press your hands firmly on your hips and bow slightly toward your mirror as you pull your shoulders and elbows forward.

Some women do the next part of the exam in the shower because fingers glide over soapy skin, making it easy to concentrate on the texture underneath.

5 Step 4 should be repeated lying down. Lie flat on your back with your left arm over your head and a pillow or folded towel under your left shoulder. This position flattens the breast and makes it easier to examine. Use the the same circular motion described described earlier. Repeat the exam on your right breast

4 Raise your left arm. Use three or four fingers of your right hand to explore your left breast firmly, carefully and thoroughly. Beginning at the outer edge, press the pads of your fingers in small circles, moving the circles slowly around the breast. Gradually work toward the nipple. Be sure to cover the entire breast. Pay special attention to the area between the breast and the underarm, including the underarm itself. Feel for any unusual lump or mass under the skin. Repeat on your right breast.

6 Report any lumps, thickening, discharge, or changes to your clinician. Most of these are not cancer, but you won't know if you don't ask.

7 Ages 20-39; Clinical breast examination as recommended by your clinician and your personal and family history, monthly BSE. Age 40+: Annual mammogram, annual breast examination by clinician, monthly BSE. Resources: American Cancer Society, www.cancer.org

For Your Information:
Candidiasis (Monilia)

I. Definition
Candidiasis, or monilia, is a yeastlike overgrowth of a fungus called candida albicans (may also be caused by candida tropicalis or candida torulopsis glabrata and rarely by other candida species). Candida can be found in small amounts in the normal vagina but under some conditions it gets out of balance with the other vaginal flora and produces symptoms.

II. Transmission
A. Usually nonsexual
B. Some common causes of candida overgrowth are: use of oral contraceptives; antibiotics; diabetes; pregnancy; stress; deodorant tampons and other such products

III. Signs and Symptoms
A. In the female
    1. Vaginal discharge: thick, white, and curdlike
    2. Vaginal area itch and irritation with occasional swelling and redness
    3. Burning on urination
    4. Possibly, pain with intercourse
B. In the male
    1. Itch and/or irritation of penis
    2. Cheesy material under foreskin, underside of penis
    3. Jock itch; athlete's foot

IV. Diagnosis
A. Female evaluation may include vaginal examination to check for candida and rule out trichomoniasis, bacterial vaginosis, chlamydia, and gonorrhea
B. Male evaluation may include:
    1. Examination of penis to check for irritation and/or cheesy materials
    2. Culture for ruling out gonorrhea and chlamydia
    3. Urinalysis

V. Treatment
Prescription medicine: _____

VI. Patient Education
A. No intercourse until symptoms subside
B. Continue prescribed treatment even if menses occurs, but use pads rather than tampons

C. Ways to prevent recurrent candida infections
   1. Bathe daily (with lots of water and minimal soap)
   2. To minimize the moist environment Candida favors, use
      a. Cotton-crotched underwear/pantyhose (or cut out crotch of panty-hose)
      b. Loose-fitting slacks
      c. No underwear while sleeping
   3. Wipe the front first and then the back after toileting
   4. Avoid feminine hygiene sprays, deodorants, deodorant tampons/mini-pads, colored or perfumed toilet paper, tearoff fabric softeners in the dryer, etc., any of which may cause allergies and irritation
   5. Some women have found that vitamin C 500 mg 2–4 x each day helps or taking oral acidophilous tablets 40 million to 1 billion units a day (1 tablet)
D. Over-the-counter medication. Many women choose to try an over-the-counter preparation before seeking an examination. If symptoms do not subside after 1 course of treatment (1 tube or 1 set of suppositories), having an examination for diagnosis is recommended

VII. Follow-up

Return to provider for reevaluation if symptoms persist or new symptoms occur after treatment is completed.

Special Notes: _____

Practitioner: _____

For more information call: CDC STD Hotline: 1-800-227-8922; Phone numbers of free (or almost free) STD clinics are listed in the "Community Service Numbers" in the government pages of your local phone book. CDC http://www.cdc.gov

From Hawkins, Roberto-Nichols, & Stanley-Haney, *Guidelines for Nurse Practitioners in Gynecologic Settings,* 8th edition, 2004, © Springer Publishing Company.

For Your Information:
Cervical Cap

I. Definition/Mechanism of Action
The Prentif Cervical Cap is a thimble-shaped, deep-domed barrier device that fits closely over the cervix and is used with spermicidal jelly or cream. Approved by the FDA in 1988, this birth control device must be fitted by a specially trained clinician. When used consistently and carefully, the cervical cap is as effective as the diaphragm.

II. Instructions for Insertion
A. Wash your hands before handling the cap. Fill the cap 1/2 to 3/4 full of spermicidal vaginal jelly or cream. Inserting too much spermicide in the cap can interfere with the cap's suction and therefore should be avoided. Spermicide should not spill out of the cap during insertion.

B. Assume the position you plan to use when inserting the cap. Squatting shortens the vagina and lowers the cervix and may be a good position to try. Lying down may also work for you. Try different positions and remember, there is no wrong position.

C. Locate your cervix by inserting your finger into your vagina toward your tailbone. It may help to apply a small amount of lubricating jelly (like KY) to your finger before feeling for your cervix (your cervix feels like a soft nose and protrudes from the back of your vagina). Using too much lubricant may interfere with the cap's suction, so use it sparingly. The more familiar you are with your cervix, the easier inserting and removing the cap will be. Dry your fingers before handling the cap; this will make holding and inserting the cap easier. Grasp the cap and squeeze its rim together. With the other hand separate the lips (labia) of your vagina. Direct the cap into the vagina with the rim of the cap opposite from the notch going in first; this will ensure that the notch is easy to reach so you may turn the cap later. (It is thought that doing so will improve the suction of the cap.) The opening of the cap should be held up to prevent spilling the spermicide.

CERVICAL CAP

E. Once in the vagina, the cap will pop open. Quickly reposition one finger (usually the index and middle fingers work best) to either side of the thick rim and push the open part of the cap toward the cervix. (Push as far as you can until the cap stops.) Pushing the cap onto the cervix using one finger is also a good technique, but may not offer the control of the two-finger technique.

F. Check for proper placement of the cap. This is done by tracing around the rim with your finger. If the cap is over the cervix, you will not be able to locate the cervix because it is covered by the cap. Don't worry if the soft dome of the cap feels dented or wrinkled; this is normal and not significant (either regarding the quality of the suction or the location of the cap). Don't worry if you are unable to reach the underside or the very back of the cap rim.

G. Turning the cap may improve its suction; how far it should be turned is controversial. Turning may be accomplished by pushing the rim of the cap laterally with your fingers to either side. A one-quarter to one-half turn is probably adequate; however, some sources recommend one or two full turns.

H. If you are unable to rotate the cap at all, or very little, do not worry. The ability or inability to turn the cap is not necessarily an indication of cap suction or quality of fit.

I. During the first few months, use a back-up method of birth control. If you are on the pill, continue taking it for a month longer until you have tried the cap in different positions of lovemaking. If you have been using a diaphragm, consider asking your partner to use a condom initially when trying different positions with the cap. Some sources recommend use of a back-up method of birth control the first six times the cap is used.

J. If your partner is unwilling to use back-up condoms, consider the use of vaginal contraceptive film (VCF) sold over the counter at some drug stores. This is spermicidally coated gelatin paper rolled up and inserted vaginally at least five minutes before intercourse. It should not be used inside the cap as a substitute for spermicidal jelly/cream, but as an adjunct back-up method inserted after the cap is in place.

K. A diaphragm should not be used concurrently as a back-up method with the cap. However, the diaphragm may be used alternately with the cap.

L. When trying different lovemaking positions using the cap, check for proper cap placement immediately after each intercourse.

M. If you find the cap dislodged, try not to panic. Immediately insert a full applicator of spermicide high into your vagina and remain lying down for at least half an hour, preferably a full hour. Also, do not try to reposition the cap back onto the cervix, as this may cause more sperm to enter the cervical opening. Wait 8 to 12 hours to remove the cap and do not use it again until it is refitted and you have had a chance to discuss with your clinician why the dislodgement occurred.

N. Some facilities recommend use of emergency contraception if there is a possibility the cap became dislodged during intercourse, but this must be started within 72 hours of dislodgement. Contact your clinician for further information or call 1–888–NOT-2–LATE; check website http://not-2–late.com.

O. Practice using your cap. The more comfortable you are inserting and removing it, the more you will trust it as a method of contraception.

REMEMBER: Some methods of birth control should be used every time you have vaginal intercourse. There is no safe time in your cycle for unprotected intercourse (unless you have been taught and are using natural family planning).

III. Additional Points on Wearing the Cap
A. You must wear the cap for at least 8 hours after penile/vaginal intercourse.
B. The FDA has approved 48 hours as the maximum time the cap may be worn (at one time). However, your clinician may suggest a maximum time limit of 24 hours (especially if you have a history of urinary or vaginal infections).
C. During your menstrual period, do not use your cap for birth control because the menstrual flow may cause the cap to dislodge.
D. Toxic shock syndrome has not been reported in women using the cap. However, the theoretical risk exists, especially in women who wear the cap in excess of 24 hours. Please discuss this information with your clinician, especially if you have further questions. (Danger signs associated with possible toxic shock syndrome: fever (temperature 100° F and above); diarrhea, vomiting, muscle ache, rash (sunburnlike).)
E. The cap may be inserted many hours before intercourse, even a day before.
F. With initial use, the cap is best inserted within one hour of intercourse. If possible, insert the cap before foreplay because sexual stimulation may interfere with the insertion of the cap and the establishment of good suction. During the first few months do not wear the cap more than 24 hours at a time, and avoid repeated sexual acts and varied positions during this time. This will allow you to better monitor the cap and will minimize the variables you must examine if there is a problem.
G. With repeated intercourse (associated with ejaculation), while the cap is in place, you do not have to add extra spermicide.

IV. Other Considerations Related to Wearing the Cap
A. Partner complains. Most men do not feel the cervical cap. A few find, when they are able to feel it, that the sensation is unpleasant. Unfortunately, this problem is difficult to anticipate. Occasionally, it is the notch they feel and if you turn the cap's notch to the side, the problem may be eliminated. In some situations, trying a different cap size may help.
B. Sometimes, if a woman is not sufficiently stimulated, the man will feel both the cervix and the cap, in which case the solution is to increase the

amount of foreplay before actual penile intercourse is attempted. Occasionally, only certain positions pose a problem and, by avoiding them, the cap may still be used. However, if those positions are most desired, the solution may be to use a different birth control method.

C. Reinserting the cervical cap after removal. It is recommended the cap be removed a minimum of 6–8 hours before it is reinserted.

V. Removal of the Cap

A. Assume the position you used to insert the cap. Squatting while bearing down (like having a difficult bowel movement) works well for many women. This position shortens the vagina, lowering the cervix and making the rim of the cap easier to reach.

B. Using any finger, push the rim of the cap to the side (aiming for your hip). Once the cap is loosened from the cervix, reach into the dome and remove it. You may have to struggle a bit, but don't be timid. If you continue to have difficulty removing the cap, your clinician may add a loop of nylon thread through the notch of the cap to make removal easier. This is usually a temporary solution until you develop a technique that works. Consider asking your partner to assist in removing the cap.

C. If your period starts while you are wearing the cap, wait the normal 8 hours to remove it. If the cap is unable to hold the blood, it will leak out and possibly cause the cap to come off the cervix. If this happens, simply remove the cap and wait to resume using it until your period is over. A little spotting will not usually interfere with the cap fit.

VI. Care of Your Cap

A. Wash the cap with water and mild soap. You may turn the cap inside out in order to clean the inside rim more easily; some women use a fingernail or a small brush to clean the inside rim. Dry the cap thoroughly and store it in its container. If you use an airtight container, punch some small holes in it or don't seat the lid entirely because some types of bacteria grow more readily in the absence of oxygen. Do not powder your cap.

B. If your cap develops an odor, see your clinician to check for a possible vaginal infection. Some types of infection, especially bacterial vaginosis, may cause a foul cap odor without causing you symptoms. To remove the odor, try soaking the cap for 30 minutes in soapy water or rubbing alcohol. Excessive soaking may lead to cap stretching and this may affect the fit. Rinse the cap thoroughly before reinserting it. You may need a new cap if these suggestions are not effective. Some women find the cap develops an odor if it is worn for more than 24 hours.

VII. Other Special Concerns

A. For the first few months, check the cap frequently after penile intercourse, after vaginal finger activity, bowel movements, or any other time you are nervous about the cap.

B. Weight changes do not generally affect the fit of the cap. However, if your cap behaves in an odd manner and you've had more than a 15-pound weight change, have your cap resized.

C. If you give birth vaginally, you should have your cap resized 6 to 12 weeks after delivery.

D. If you have any of the following cervical procedures (biopsy, abortion, dilation and curettage, conization, laser treatment, or cryosurgery) have your cervical cap resized. Wait at least 2 or 3 weeks to do this, or until complete healing has occurred.

E. Breast feeding may alter your cap fit, so be sure to have it refitted before and after you stop breast-feeding (or any time the cap dislodges).

F. If you have been taking the birth control pill while using the cervical cap, have the cap refitted after you stop the pill. The pill may affect the cap's fit by interrupting your normal ovulatory cycle.

VIII. Follow-up

A. Within the first 3 months: follow up with your clinician to check the size and fit of the cap and your skill in using it. (You may be asked to insert the cap at home and wear it in for a visit). Do not insert your cap if you think you have a vaginal infection or if you are having problems with the cap.

B. Yearly or as recommended: a pelvic exam, Pap smear, and resizing of the cap. Bring the cap with you. According to FDA regulations, a new cap should be purchased yearly to ensure proper fit.

IX. Reasons to Temporarily Discontinue Using the Cap

A. Vaginal infection. Wait until the infection is resolved and a follow-up exam confirms this.

B. Urinary tract infection. Continuing to be sexually active while you have a urinary tract infection may slow healing and recovery.

C. Pelvic infection. Rationale is the same as for A. and B.

D. Abnormal Pap smears or conditions of the cervix such as cervicitis. The cap should not be used until your Pap smear is normal or the abnormal cervical condition is resolved.

E. Poor fit associated with such temporary situations as breast-feeding or poor vaginal tone (which may improve after Kegel practice). Refitting is essential before resumption of cap use.

X. Summary

The cap is easy to use and is very effective if the instructions provided here are followed. As with any barrier method of birth control, you may become pregnant while using the cap faithfully. If you have any questions, concerns, or problems, please be sure to contact your clinician.

If your cap slips off during intercourse, call 1–888–NOT-2–LATE or check web site http://not-2–late.com for emergency contraception information.

This guideline was developed by R. Mimi Clarke Secor, RNC, .S-FNP, MEd, MS, Certified Family Nurse Practitioner. Reprinted with permission.

For Your Information: Chlamydia Trachomatis

I. Definition
Chlamydia trachomatis is a sexually transmitted disease of the reproductive tract. It is currently believed to be the most common cause of sexually transmitted disease in males and females, more common than gonorrhea.

II. Transmission
Sexual contact with 1–3 week incubation period before symptoms present

III. Signs and Symptoms
A. In the female
  1. Often no symptoms
  2. Possibly, increased vaginal discharge
  3. Cervicitis or an abnormal Papanicolaou smear
  4. Possibly, frequent uncomfortable urination
  5. Advanced symptoms include those of pelvic infection
B. In the male
  1. Possibly, thick and cloudy discharge from the penis
  2. Possibly, painful urination and/or frequent urination

IV. Diagnosis
A. Evaluation may include tests to rule out candidiasis, trichomoniasis, bacterial vaginosis, gonorrhea, syphilis, and urinary tract infection
B. Vaginal and urethral smears are examined for the Chlamydia trachomatis organism

V. Treatment
Prescription medicine: _____

_____

Take all the prescribed medicine, even though the symptoms may decrease early in treatment. Incomplete treatment gives the causative organism a chance to lie dormant and reinfect later.

VI. Patient Education
A. Any sexual contacts should be advised to seek evaluation and treatment
B. Do not have intercourse until you and any sex partner(s) have completed treatment

C. In an untreated male or female the disease may progress to further reproductive infection with possible tissue scarring and infertility risks
D. Wash all sex toys, diaphragm, cervical cap with soap and water or soak
in rubbing alcohol or betadine scrub. Be sure to rinse thoroughly

VII. Follow-up
Return to clinic if symptoms persist or new symptoms occur.
Special notes: _____

_____

Practitioner: _____

For more information call: CDC STD Hotline: 1–800–227–8922: Phone
numbers of free (or almost free) STD clinics are listed in the "Community
Service Numbers" in the government pages of your local phone book. http:/
/www.cdc.gov

From Hawkins, Roberto-Nichols & Stanley-Haney, *Guidelines for Nurse Practitioners in Gynecologic Settings,* 8th edition, 2004, © Springer Publishing Company.

For Your Information: Colposcopy

What Is Colposcopy?

Colposcopy is a special type of diagnostic examination performed at times on women, less frequently on men. The colposcope is a microscope designed specifically for aiding the naked eye by magnifying the cervix, vagina, vulva, and anus.

Why Do You Need a Colposcopy?

You need this special examination because your practitioner suspects there may be a problem related to your cervix (the opening to your uterus), vaginal walls, vulva, or anal area based upon your initial exam. She/he may have received a report of abnormal findings from your Papanicolaou (Pap) test or may have seen some evidence of infection, inflammation, or a lesion (a sore or growth) during your exam.

If you have had an abnormal Pap smear, by using the colposcope your practitioner can examine each part of your cervix and vagina and look for abnormal appearing cells. Your cervix is made up of thousands of special cells which should have a certain pattern or structure; any changes in the expected structure require further investigation.

How Is Colposcopy Done?

It is done in much the same way as your regular gynecological exam. The only difference is that your practitioner looks at your cervix and vagina through the colposcope after inserting the vaginal speculum.

Why Else Are Colposcopies Done?

Some nurse practitioners use the colposcope for screening purposes and to identify warty lesions. She/he may need to do a more extensive exam, which may include a biopsy. She/he may also prescribe treatment if necessary.

What Is a Cervical Biopsy?

It is the removal of a small piece (or pieces) of tissue from the cervix using a specially designed instrument. This tissue is sent to the laboratory for examination.

Does the Examination Hurt?

The colposcope does not touch your body and therefore does not hurt. If your caregiver decides to perform a biopsy, you may feel a small pinch at that time only. There is no need to be tense. You will be told ahead of time if a biopsy is to be done. This procedure may be necessary to find out if there is any disease below or at the surface of your cervix.

Is There Any Vaginal Bleeding After a Biopsy?
There may be a small amount of bleeding following a biopsy. This will stop in a few minutes, with some gentle pressure. A very few patients may continue to have a small amount of bleeding afterwards, which can be easily treated. There may also be a discharge due to the medication used during the procedure.

Can a Colposcopy Be Done During Pregnancy?
Certainly. This examination is no different than the regular exam your practitioner or physician routinely performs, and it will not jeopardize your pregnancy.

How Else Can a Colposcopy Be Helpful?
With the colposcope, your care provider can identify genital warts on your cervix, in your vagina, and on your vulva. First, he/she will apply acetic acid (table vinegar) to the vulva, the walls of the vagina, and the cervix. If warts are present, they will appear white under the magnification of the colposcope, and your care provider will either locate and treat the lesions or refer you to a physician for treatment.

How Can a Colposcopy Be Helpful in Males?
Males can also have genital warts. They may be located on the shaft of the penis, at the urethral opening, on the scrotum, or around the anus. Warts are difficult to see on males with the naked eye, but with the application of acetic acid and the use of a colposcope, the most minute wart will turn white, facilitating treatment.

From Hawkins, Roberto-Nichols & Stanley-Haney, *Guidelines for Nurse Practitioners in Gynecologic Settings,* 8th edition, 2004, © Springer Publishing Company.

For Your Information:
Constipation

Constipation is a common problem and can be related to a number of factors. First, though, it is important to clarify what is meant by the term. Irregularity is another related term—it implies that there is some standard of regularity. Although many of us have been taught that daily bowel elimination (having at least one bowel movement—BM—daily) is normal, in fact for many persons normal is every two or three days.

Constipation occurs when one's regular pattern (whatever is normal for that person) changes so that the time between bowel movements lengthens, pain and/or straining are associated with them, and/or the bowel movements are very hard. Sometimes bleeding occurs because the fecal material (the stool) is hard and the person has to strain so much that there is damage to the rectum (lowest part of the bowel) or to the opening of the intestinal track (called the anal opening). There are other causes of bleeding, too, so if you ever have bleeding with a bowel movement, you should not ignore it.

Some causes of constipation are:

• *Stress.* Stress can cause "spastic constipation" meaning tightening or spasm of the muscles in the large intestine; stress can also mean not taking time to eat properly, drink enough fluids, and/or even go to the bathroom when your body signals you.

• *Diet.* More about this later, but lack of roughage or fiber in the diet can cause constipation, as can lack of sufficient fluids, notably water.

• *Lack of Exercise.* Having no active exercise on a regular basis can cause constipation.

• *Medications.* Medications such as diuretics (water pills), iron pills, and calcium pills can cause constipation in some people, so pay attention to your body and to changes in your bowel movements when taking any medication.

• *Symptoms.* Some diseases have constipation as a symptom, so be sure to tell your clinician if you continue to be constipated after trying the suggestions here.

What You Can Do About Constipation

1. *Eat right.* Select foods from the following groups, including lots of roughage or fiber in each day's diet:
2. *Time.* Take time when your body signals you; don't put off bowel evacuations.
3. *Fluids.* Fluid intake is very important to your general good health and especially for good bowel and bladder and kidney health. Six to 8

Food Group	Foods to Emphasize	Servings per Day
breads, cereals, grains	whole wheat bread, whole grains, bran cereals, rice, wheat germ, whole wheat pasta, popcorn, oats, rice cakes, granola, wheat bran	3–4 servings a day 1 cup or more
fruits, fruit juices	dates, raisins, figs, apples, berries, melons, whole oranges, pears	3 or more fresh fruits each day
vegetables	broccoli, cauliflower, peas, green and wax beans, brussels sprouts, lettuce, spinach, cabbage, celery, asparagus, artichokes, carrots, squash, turnips	3 or more; some raw vegetables each day
miscellaneous	legumes (dried peas, kidney beans, navy beans)	varies with diet
beans, nuts	seeds, nuts	some each day

glasses of water a day are recommended to prepare fecal material at the proper consistency for bowel elimination. In addition to water, add fruit juices, coffee, tea, and soda; the latter three can be irritating to your bladder or stomach or both (if caffeinated), so try to keep amounts limited and don't substitute these for water.

4. *Exercise.* Regular exercise (4 to 7 times a week) is important to general good health and also helps us to keep our regular (usual for us) bowel evacuation schedule. Walking, running, bicycling, swimming, working-out, active work routine (walking a lot, lifting and moving things), dancing, skating, sports such as tennis, soccer, touch football, basketball, volleyball, handball, racquetball, all help keep our body and its functions in shape.

5. *Flavored or Unflavored Metamucil* or store brand psyllium hydrophilic mucilloid fiber is useful if diet, exercise, and fluids don't work for you. Mix a tablespoon in 8 or more ounces of water. Metamucil also comes in wafers (cookies) in several flavors. You can also try over-the-counter stool softeners such as dialose, kasof, and colace. Follow directions carefully about use; it's best to discuss this with your health care provider. Stool softeners and sources of fiber are not harmful or habit forming, but you should try diet, fluids, and exercise first.

6. *Laxatives.* Laxatives, enemas, and drugs to cause you to evacuate your bowels can be harmful in the long run and should be used only after consulting a health care provider to rule out bowel disease as the cause of the constipation and after trying the measures discussed here.

For Your Information: Contraceptive Patch

I. Definition/Mechanism of Action

The contraceptive patch is a 3–layer transdermal polyethylene/polyester device about the size of a matchbook, with an adhesive on one side. It is impregnated by a synthetic progestin, and a synthetic estrogen, and releases 150 micrograms of the progestin and 20 micrograms of the estrogen every 24 hours. Patch is changed weekly for 3 weeks, then off for 1 week. The patch causes suppression of ovulation, changes the lining of the uterus so it is not receptive to an egg, changes the cervical mucus so sperm cannot get through, changes the transportation of the egg down the fallopian tube and possibly makes sperm less able to penetrate the egg.

II. Effectiveness

A. 99% effectiveness

III. Side Effects and Disadvantages

A. Minor side effects
  1. Local irritation from patch
  2. Dislocation of patch
  3. Breast discomfort, tenderness
  4. Nausea
  5. Spotting
  6. Decreased menstrual flow (withdrawal bleeding), no bleeding
  7. Depression, mood changes
  8. Headaches
  9. Abdominal pain
B. Risk factors
  1. Blood clots in legs, lungs, stroke
  2. Hypertension (high blood pressure)
  3. Gallbladder disease
  4. Heart attack (smokers 35 and older)
  5. Smoking increases risk associated with patch use. Women should not smoke and use the patch.

IV. Contraindications (reasons you may not be able to use the patch)

A. Women with a history of any of the following conditions may not be able to use the patch
  1. Thromboembolic disorders—blood clots in legs, lungs
  2. Coronary artery disease

3. Heart disease involving the heart valves with complications
4. Severe hypertension (high blood pressure)
5. Diabetes with vascular (blood vessel) involvement
6. Headaches, migraines with neurological symptoms
7. Major surgery on legs or with prolonged immobility
8. Cancer of the breast or reproductive system
9. Undiagnosed genital bleeding
10. Impaired liver function, liver problems
11. Known or suspected pregnancy
12. Taking certain prescription drugs
13. Smoking
14. Weight ≥ 198 pounds (90 kg); weight decreases effectiveness of patch
15. Skin disorders that may predispose to application-site reactions
16. Breastfeeding—not yet approved

V. Alternative Methods of Birth Control
A. Abstinence
B. Sterilization
C. Natural Family Planning
D. Condoms with contraceptive gel, foam, cream, jelly, suppositories, vaginal film
E. Intrauterine device
F. Diaphragm with contraceptive jelly, cream
G. Cervical cap with contraceptive jelly, cream
H. Contraceptive implant
I. Female condom
J. Depo-Provera injection
K. Oral contraceptives

VI. Explanation of Method
A. Ways in which the patch is used
   1. Apply patch on first day of menses or on the first Sunday after bleeding begins; postpartum nonnursing 4 weeks or with resumption of menses
      Apply to clean, dry, healthy skin on buttocks, abdomen, upper outer arm, or upper torso. Patch should not be applied to breasts.
   2. Do not use lotions, cosmetics, creams, powders or other topical products in area of patch or area where patch will be applied.
   3. Press down firmly on patch for at least 10 seconds and then check that the edges adhere.
   4. Check patch daily.

5. If patch detaches, immediately apply a new patch. Supplemental tapes or adhesives should not be used.
6. Apply a new patch the same day of the week 7 days after first patch. Repeat this in week 3.
7. No patch is applied in week 4.
8. Begin a new cycle on the same day of the week for week one and repeat cycle of 3 weeks on and one week off.
9. Withdrawal bleed (period) will occur during 4th week.
10. If you forget to apply a new patch and less than 48 hours have passed, you can apply a new patch as soon as you remember and then apply that next patch on the usual renewal day.
11. If more than 48 hours have elapsed, you should stop the current cycle and immediately begin a new 4–week cycle by applying a new patch. The day for patch renewal will now change. Use back-up contraception for one week.
12. If missed change day occurs at the end of the 4–week cycle, remove the patch and apply a new patch on the usual change day to begin a new cycle.

Danger Signals Associated With Patch Use
Visual problems: Loss or blurring of vision, double vision, spots before eyes, flashing lights
Numbness or paralysis in any parts of body or face, even temporary
Unexplained chest pain
Painful inflamed areas along veins or severe calf pain
Severe recurrent headaches or new headaches or worsening of migraines

Contact us at _____ if you develop any of the above problems.

From Hawkins, Roberto-Nichols, & Stanley-Haney, *Guidelines for Nurse Practitioners in Gynecologic Settings,* 8th edition, 2004, © Springer Publishing Company.

For Your Information:
Contraceptive Spermicides and Condoms

Spermicides

I. Definition/Mechanism of Action
Spermicides are a barrier method of birth control. All contain an inert base or vehicle and an active ingredient, most commonly a surfactant such as nonoxynol-9 which disrupts the integrity of the sperm membrane (acts as a spermicide).

II. Effectiveness and Benefits
A. Method: 96% effectiveness rate
B. User: 60% effectiveness rate
C. Inexpensive and readily available

III. Side Effects and Disadvantages
A. Local irritation from spermicide
B. Can necessitate interruption of lovemaking
C. Emotional difficulty with touching one's own body

IV. Types
A. Creams, jellies, gels
B. Foams
C. Foaming tablets
D. Suppositories
E. Vaginal film

V. How to Use
A. Instructions should be read prior to using any spermicide. Method of insertion, time of effectiveness, time needed prior to intercourse, etc., will vary with each type
B. Use new insertion of spermicide with each intercourse
C. After each use, wash the applicator with soap and water
D. When using a spermicide, partner should always use a condom unless you use female condom

VI. Follow-up
A. Yearly physical examination with Papanicolaou smear is recommended

Condoms

I. Definition/Mechanism of Action
Condoms are thin sheaths, most commonly made of latex (female condoms are made of polyurethane; male polyurethane condoms are now on the market) which prevent the transmission of sperm from the penis to the vagina

II. Effectiveness and Benefits
A. Method: 97–98% effectiveness rate, providing the method is used correctly
B. User: 70–94% effectiveness rate
C. Inexpensive and readily available
D. Offer protection against sexually transmitted disease. Only latex condoms provide protection against the AIDS (HIV) virus. The female condom is made of thick polyurethane so it does offer protection
E. Encourage male participation in birth control

III. Side Effects and Disadvantages
A. Allergic reaction to latex (rare). (Female condom is polyurethane as are some male condoms)
B. Use necessitates interruption of lovemaking for application
C. May decrease tactile sensation
D. Psychological impotency with male condom
E. If latex allergy is a problem, double condom use is an option. If the woman is allergic, the male can wear a latex condom with a skin or polyurethane condom covering it. If the man is allergic, he can wear a polyurethane or skin condom with a latex condom over it. Skin condoms should not be worn alone since they do not offer protection from HIV.

IV. Types
Condoms vary in color, texture (smooth, studded, or ribbed), shape and price; they come lubricated and plain; some have spermicide; some are extra strength, some sheerer and thinner, some have a unique shape; some are scented or flavored

V. How to Use Male Condom
A. Always pull the male condom on an erect penis and before there is any sexual contact. Use for every act of intercourse
B. Do not pull the male condom tightly over the end of the penis; leave

about an inch extra for ejaculation fluid and to avoid breakage; some
condoms have a reservoir tip
C. Withdraw before the penis becomes limp and hold the open end of the
condom tightly while withdrawing
D. Partner should always use a contraceptive spermicide along with condom
E. Condoms should be used only once

VI. How to Use Female Condom
The female condom comes prelubricated
A. Pinch ring at closed end of pouch and insert like a diaphragm covering
the cervix; adding 1–2 drops of additional lubricant makes insertion eas-
ier and decreases or eliminates squeaking noise and dislocation during
intercourse
B. Adjust other ring over labia
C. Can be inserted several minutes to 8 hours prior to intercourse
D. Remove before standing up by squeezing and twisting the outer ring and
pulling out gently

If the condom breaks or slips off, call 1-800-NOT-2-Late or web site http:/
/not-2–late.com for emergency contraception information.

From Hawkins, Roberto-Nichols, & Stanley-Haney, *Guidelines for Nurse Practitioners in
Gynecologic Settings,* 8th edition, 2004, © Springer Publishing Company.

For Your Information:
Contraceptive Vaginal Ring (Nuva Ring)

I. Definition of Mechanism of Action

The contraceptive vaginal ring is flexible, transparent, colorless, and about 2 inches in diameter. It is impregnated with a synthetic progestin, and a synthetic estrogen, and releases 120 micrograms of progestin and 15 micrograms of the estrogen every 24 hours over a period of 3 weeks. The ring is removed at the end of the third week and a new ring placed at the beginning of a new cycle, one week later. The ring causes suppression of ovulation, changes the lining of the uterus so it is not receptive to an egg, changes the cervical mucus so sperm cannot get through, changes the transportation of the egg down the fallopian tube and possibly makes sperm less able to penetrate the egg.

Physical Changes Occurring With Use of the Ring

II. Effectiveness

A. 98–99% effectiveness

III. Side Effects and Disadvantages

A. Minor side effects
1. Vaginal irritation from the ring
2. Dislocation of the ring
3. Sensation of something in the vagina
4. If ring is out more than 3 hours, need to use back-up contraception for 7 days

IV. Contraindications (reasons you may not be able to use the ring)

1. Blood clots in your legs (thrombosis), lungs (pulmonary embolism), or eyes now or in the past
2. Chest pain (angina pectoris)
3. Heart attack or stroke
4. Severe high blood pressure
5. Pregnancy or suspected pregnancy
6. Diabetes with complications of the kidney, eyes, nerves or blood vessels
7. Headaches with neurological symptoms
8. Need for a long period of bedrest following major surgery
9. Known or suspected cancer of the breast or cancer of the lining of the uterus, cervix, or vagina (now or in the past)

10. Unexplained vaginal bleeding
11. Yellowing of the whites of the eyes or of the skin (jaundice) during pregnancy or during past use of oral contraceptives (birth control pills)
12. Liver tumors or active liver disease
13. Disease of the heart valves with complications
14. Allergic reaction to any of the components of the rings
15. Smoking and over age 35 (15 cigarettes a day or more)
16. Weight ≥ 198 pounds (90 kg); > weight decreases effectiveness of the ring
17. A prolapsed (dropped) uterus, dropped bladder (cystocele), or rectal prolapse (rectocele)
18. Under 35 and a heavy smoker (>15 cigarettes/day)
19. Breast-feeding—not yet approved for use

IV. Alternative Methods of Birth Control
A. Abstinence
B. Sterilization
C. Natural Family Planning
D. Condoms with contraceptive gel, foam, cream, jelly, suppositories, vaginal film
E. Intrauterine device
F. Diaphragm with contraceptive jelly, cream
G. FemCap
H. Female condom
I. Depo-Provera
J. Contraceptive Patch
K. Oral contraceptives

V. Explanation of Method
A. Ways in which the ring is used
   1. Insert ring into vagina between day 1 and day 5 of menstrual cycle and note start day
   2. Keep ring in place for 3 weeks in a row
   3. Remove ring for one week for withdrawal bleeding
   4. Insert new ring on the same start day for 3 weeks, with one week out intervals
   5. If ring is removed during the 3 weeks and is out for more than 3 hours, back-up contraception is required for the next 7 days

VII. Danger Signals Associated With Patch Use
1. Visual problems
   a. Loss or blurring of vision, double vision
   b. Spots before eyes, flashing lights
2. Numbness or paralysis in any parts of body or face, even temporary
3. Unexplained chest pain
4. Painful inflamed areas along veins or severe calf pain
5. Severe recurrent headaches or new headaches or worsening of migraines

Contact us at _____ if you develop any of the above problems.

Web Site for ring information: www.organoninc.com; www.nuvaring.com

From Hawkins, Roberto-Nichols, & Stanley-Haney, *Guidelines for Nurse Practitioners in Gynecologic Settings,* 8th edition, 2004, © Springer Publishing Company.

For Your Information: Cystitis (Bladder Infection)

Cystitis, a bladder infection, is usually caused by bacteria. Women are more prone to cystitis because the urethra (connection between the bladder and the outside through which we urinate or pee) is short and the vagina and rectum are close to the opening of the urethra, called the urethral meatus. However, men can also develop cystitis.

Symptoms of cystitis include:

- Frequent urination of small amounts of urine; often you will experience urgency–a feeling of needing to urinate and then just urinating a little
- Burning, pain, or difficulty in urinating
- Blood in the urine
- Pain in the lower part of the abdomen (pelvic pain) around the pubic bone
- Chills, fever

Treatment

Treatment of cystitis is with an antibiotic. It is important that you tell your clinician if you are allergic to any antibiotics or to sulfonamides so that you are given a suitable medication.

You may be asked to give what is called a clean catch urine specimen prior to the diagnosis (as opposed to just urinating in a paper cup for the specimen). For the clean catch specimen, you will be given special wipes to use on your perineal area and instructions on collecting the urine specimen in a sterile container. This specimen will be sent to the laboratory to evaluate the bacteria in the urine and to see what sulfonamides or antibiotics will be effective against the bacteria.

It is important to take the entire prescription given to you even if symptoms disappear quickly. Follow the directions for times to take the medication and try not to skip a dose as this may allow the bacteria to increase in number. You may also be given a prescription for a bladder pain medication or information about over-the-counter medication (Aso-Standard®, Uristat®) to take away the bladder pain. These bladder pain medications are to be used with, and not instead of, the antibiotic or sulfonamide as they only relieve bladder pain and have no effect on the bacteria causing your cystitis.

Things You Can Do About Cystitis

There are several things you can do to avoid cystitis and to help your body heal if you have cystitis.

- After going to the bathroom, wipe from front to back, or wipe the front first and then the back so as not to carry bacteria from your rectal area to the vaginal area where your urethral opening is.
- If your lovemaking includes vaginal or oral contact following anal contact, you may consider washing off your genitals and those of your partner before proceeding.
- During a tub bath, it is better not to use bath oils and bubble bath because they help bacteria travel up your urethra.
- Try to empty your bladder before sex, and after sex empty your bladder as soon as you can to wash bacteria from your urethra.
- Tight clothing, especially clothes made of synthetic fabrics such as polyester, helps bacteria grow more easily by creating a warm, dark, moist environment. Cotton underpants and loose clothing help your body breathe and discourage bacterial growth.
- Always urinate when you have the urge; don't put it off until you are desperate. Bacteria grow better in urine that is sitting in your bladder for a long period of time.
- Drink 6–8 glasses of water and juice a day; cranberry juice helps to decrease cystitis. Cranberry is also available as Azo-Cranberry—cranberry juice capsules with 450 milligrams of cranberry juice concentrate; the dose is 1–4 capsules per day with meals.
- Caffeine is a bladder irritant, meaning it can cause bladder pain or spasms (cramps), so the less caffeine you take in, the less bladder irritation you will experience.
- Smoking (nicotine) is also very irritating to the bladder.
- A well-balanced diet including 6 or more servings of fresh fruits and vegetables a day and 3–4 servings of whole grain breads, cereals, and pasta, will increase your resistance to infection.

Cystitis is the least serious of the urinary tract infections. Untreated, it can lead to infection of the rest of the urinary tract including the ureters and kidneys. Prompt and correct treatment of cystitis will help you avoid having a more serious urinary tract infection. If your symptoms worsen or do not get better with the treatment prescribed by your clinician, call or return to the health care setting for further help.

From Hawkins, Roberto-Nichols, & Stanley-Haney, *Guidelines for Nurse Practitioners in Gynecologic Settings,* 8th edition, 2004, © Springer Publishing Company.

For Your Information: FemCap

I. Definition of Mechanism of Action

The contraceptive FemCap is a prescription-only contraceptive device that is used to hold spermicide and to provide a partial barrier to sperm when placed over the cervix. Available in 3 sizes: 22mm, 26mm, 30mm. Practitioner will advise on size.

II. Effectiveness

A. 96–98% effectiveness

III. Side Effects and Disadvantages

A. Minor side effects
   1. Vaginal irritation from the device
   2. Vaginal irritation from the spermicide used with the device
   3. Sensation of something in the vagina

IV. Contraindications (reasons you may not be able to use FemCap)

A. Allergy to spermicide
B. Allergy to material device is made of
C. Partner allergy to device or spermicide
D. Device is expelled repeatedly during use
E. Cannot be used during menses
F. Known or suspected uterine or cervical cancer
G. History of toxic shock syndrome
H. Current infection of vagina or cervix
I. Cannot be used during postpartum or after an abortion for 6 weeks

IV. Alternative Methods of Birth Control

A. Abstinence
B. Sterilization
C. Natural Family Planning
D. Condoms with contraceptive gel, foam, cream, jelly, suppositories, vaginal film
E. Intrauterine device
F. Diaphragm with contraceptive jelly, cream, Prentif Cervical cap
G. Female condom
H. Depo-Provera injection

I. Contraceptive Patch, Ring

J. Oral contraceptives

VI. Explanation of Method

A. Ways in which the device is used (Device comes with instructional video)
  1. Insert spermicide into the device according to directions by manufacturer and place in the vagina over the cervix before any sexual arousal
  2. Keep device in place for at least 6 hours after last act of intercourse
  3. Add additional spermicide to outside of device for each repeated act of intercourse within next 48 hours. Do not remove device to add spermicide.
  4. Remove cap by squatting and bearing down. Slip finger between the dome and the removal strap and pull gently.
  5. Wash device thoroughly with antibacterial hand soap, rinse thoroughly in clear water and allow to air dry.

Contact us at _____if you have any questions or develop any problems. You will need to return for a Pap smear after first three months of use.

Web Site for ring information: www.FemCap.com

From Hawkins, Roberto-Nichols, & Stanley-Haney, *Guidelines for Nurse Practitioners in Gynecologic Settings,* 8th edition, 2004, © Springer Publishing Company.

For Your Information:
Genital Herpes Simplex

I. Definition

The herpes simplex virus is one of the most common infectious agents of humans. It is transmitted only by direct contact with the virus from an active infected oral or genital lesion. The herpes simplex virus (HSV) is of two types:

HSV Type 1: Usually affects body sites above the waist (mouth, lips, eyes, fingers) **HSV Type 2:** Usually involves body sites below the waist, primarily the genitals.

Genital herpes may be caused by either HSV 1 or 2. If oral sex is practiced, remember that "cold sores" are herpes lesions and can be spread to the genital area. The cause, symptoms, complications, diagnosis, treatment, and patient education are the same for males and females.

II. Symptoms

A. Painful, itchy sores similar to cold sores or fever blisters, surrounded by reddened skin, that appear around the mouth, nipples or genital areas 4 to 7 days up to 4 weeks after contact
B. Fever or flu-like symptoms
C. Burning sensation during urination
D. Swollen groin lymph nodes
E. Symptoms may last 2 to 3 weeks

III. Diagnosis

A. Examination based on your clinical symptoms and history
B. Laboratory analysis of discharge from the lesions to identify virus
C. Blood test for HSV-1, HSV-2 antibodies in your blood

IV. Treatment

A. Tepid bath with or without the addition of iodine solution
B. Unrestrictive clothing
C. Prevent secondary infection
D. Medication for pain
E. There are topical and oral medications that do not cure the infection but can shorten the duration and severity of symptoms and decrease recurrence. These medications may, in some cases, be taken on a long-term basis to suppress virus

V. Complications
A. Secondary infection of herpes lesions
B. Severe systemic and life-threatening infections in infants born vaginally during an episode of herpes in the mother.

VI. Recurrences
Herpes sores may never recur after the first episode or there may be occasional flare-ups, not as painful as the initial infection, lasting up to 7 days. Recurring infections may be related to stress (physical or emotional), illness, fever, overexposure to sun, or menstruation. Recurrences are due to a reactivation of the virus already present in the nerve endings of your body.

VII. Patient Education
A. After urinating, wash the genital area with cool water
B. If urinating is difficult, sit in a tub of warm water to urinate
C. Cool, wet tea bags applied to the lesions may offer some relief
D. Avoid intercourse when active lesions are present. If intercourse does occur, condoms should be used
E. Women with chronic herpes should have a Pap smear yearly.

Medication: _____

Special notes: _____

_____

Practitioner: _____

For more information:
1. CDC STD Hotline: 1-800-227-8922: Phone numbers of free (or almost free) STD clinics are listed in the "Community Service Numbers" in the government pages of your local phone book.
2. Seek out local rap and support groups
3. Try resources on the internet: http://www.cdc.gov, alt.support.herpes (usenet news group), www.herpes.com, www.ashastd.org/herpes/hrc.html

From Hawkins, Roberto-Nichols, & Stanley-Haney, *Guidelines for Nurse Practitioners in Gynecologic Settings,* 8th edition, 2004, © Springer Publishing Company.

For Your Information:
Genital Warts (Condylomata Acuminata)

I. Definition
Genital warts, or condylomata acuminata, may occur on either the male or female genital areas. The virus causing the warts is believed to be sexually transmitted, although warts have been found on individuals whose partner has no history or sign of warts.

II. Signs and Symptoms
Warts may not appear until two weeks to many months (or even years after exposure).
A. In moist areas, the warts are small, often itchy bumps, sometimes with a cauliflowerlike top, appearing singly or in clusters.
B. On dry skin (such as the shaft of the penis), the warts commonly are small, hard, and yellowish-gray, resembling warts that appear on other parts of the body.
C. On the female, the warts are commonly found on or around the vaginal opening, vaginal lips, in the vagina, around the rectum, and on the cervix.
D. On the male, the warts can be found on any part of the penis and scrotum, rectal area.

III. Diagnosis
A. The diagnosis is usually obvious on the basis of appearance of the warts, but sometimes a microscopic examination is necessary to identify minute lesions.
B. Laboratory tests may include checking for gonorrhea, chlamydia, and syphilis, HIV/AIDS, and a Papaniolaou smear if none within a year.

IV. Treatment
A. If small, the warts may be treated by several weekly applications of medication by you or your practitioner
B. Patients with large, persistent warts or warts in the vagina or on the cervix may be referred to a physician for treatment. Some treatments include cryotherapy (freezing) and lasering the warts

V. Patient Education
A. Always advise sexual partners to see a clinician for examination
B. Having warts may increase vaginal discharge; have it checked and treated

C. Treatment medication is applied weekly by the practitioner in office or clinic. *Some of the drugs used must be rinsed off in four hours. Your nurse practitioner will advise you.* Certain treatment medication should never be used in pregnant patients. If pregnancy is suspected, tell your practitioner.
D. You may be given medication for self-treatment and separate instructions on how to do this.
E. Recurrence is possible without reinfection, as treatment does not always eradicate very small warts. Microscopic examination and treatment by a specialist may be necessary.
F. A woman with a history of warts, especially if on the cervix, is encouraged to have an annual gynecological examination with a Pap smear as recommended by her clinician (often twice a year).

Special notes: _____

_____

Practitioner: _____

For more information and/or care for friends:
CTD STD Hotline: 1-800-227-8922 Phone numbers of free (or almost free) VD clinics are listed in the "Community Service Numbers" in the government pages of your local phone book.
http://www.cdc.gov, www.nci.nih.gov=National Cancer Institute

From Hawkins, Roberto-Nichols, & Stanley-Haney, *Guidelines for Nurse Practitioners in Gynecologic Settings,* 8th edition, 2004, © Springer Publishing Company.

For Your Information:
Self-Treatment for Genital Warts
(Condylomata Acuminata)

Condylox® is a prescription treatment for genital warts that you can use at home. Fill your Condylox prescription at any drugstore or the pharmacy in a department store. The Condylox package contains directions for use of the medication.* Please read these carefully and use the medication as directed. It is important to follow these directions and those of your health care provider to assure the maximum possible effect from the medication.

Condylox works by destroying the wart tissue. This does not happen all at once, but gradually. The wart will change in color, from skin color to a dry, crusted, dead appearance, and then disappear. You may feel some pain or burning when applying the Condylox as these changes occur. You may also see some redness, have some soreness or tenderness at the wart sites, and may even see small sores in that area. These symptoms usually disappear within a week after you have completed the treatment. If any of these changes are severe or concern you, stop the treatment and contact your health care provider.

Treating Your Warts
Treat your warts twice a day with Condylox. (It is okay to do so even if you get your menstrual period during the time you are treating your warts). Plan a time in the morning and again in the evening to apply the medication. Repeat the twice-a-day treatments for 3 days and then do not treat the warts again for 4 days. You can repeat this pattern of treatment—3 days of medication and then 4 days off—for up to 4 weeks. Stop the treatment, however, as soon as the warts disappear. It is important that you not treat the warts in any week for more than 3 days as such treatment will not help them to disappear faster and may cause you to have side effects from the medication.

If you have completed 4 weeks of treatment and still have warts, return to your health care provider for further evaluation and do not use Condylox until you have this check-up.

Remove any clothing over the affected area and wash your hands before treating your warts. Open the bottle of Condylox and place it on a flat surface so it will not spill while you are treating your warts. It may be helpful to use a hand mirror to locate the warts so that you can treat them. Good light is also important so that you do not get medication on skin that is free of warts.

---

*Adapted from manufacturer's literature Oclassen Pharmaceuticals, 1990; Watson Laboratories, 1998.

Holding onto the bottle to steady it, dip the tip of one cotton tip applicator (Q-tip) into the medication. The tip should be wet with the medication, but not dripping. Remove any excess medication by pressing the applicator tip against the inside of the bottle. Apply the Condylox only to those areas you and your health care provider have identified as warts.

Try not to get any Condylox on any area of your skin that is not a wart. If the wart is on a skin fold, gently spread the skin with one hand to flatten out the wart and touch the medication applicator to the area with the other hand. Allow the Condylox to dry before letting skin folds relax into normal position and before putting clothing over the affected area.

After application, throw away the Q-tip. Close the bottle tightly to prevent evaporation of the medication and wash your hands carefully when you are finished with the treatment.

If you are using Condylox® gel, follow the same treatment schedule as for the liquid. Wash your hands before treating your warts. Squeeze out a small amount of gel (about half the size of a pea) onto your fingertip. Dab a small amount of the gel onto the warts or the areas your clinician has instructed you to treat. Try not to get any of the gel on normal skin areas. For warts in skin folds, spread the folds apart and apply the gel to the wart, letting the area dry before you return the skin folds to their normal position. Wash your hands carefully after completing the treatment.

The area you have treated may sting when you apply the gel. It may also become red, sore, itchy or tender after treatment.

Precautions in Self-Treatment
Condylox is intended only for treatment of venereal warts and only on the outside of the body. It is not safe to use Condylox on any other skin condition. If you have severe pain, bleeding, swelling, or itching, stop the treatment and contact your health care provider. Do not get this medication in your eyes. If you do so accidentally, flush your eyes immediately with running water and call your health care provider. The effects of Condylox on pregnancy are unknown, so it is not safe to use this medication during pregnancy.

Follow-up Care
It is important to return for a check-up as suggested by your health care provider or if you have completed 4 weeks of treatment and still have warts. If the warts reappear after you have completed treatment, contact your health care provider prior to restarting treatment. Your partner should also be checked and treated for any warts; otherwise, you can be reinfected.

Self-treatment With Imiquimod Cream 5% (Aldara®)*

Aldara® is a prescription treatment for genital warts that you can use at home. Fill your Aldara prescription at any drugstore or pharmacy in a department store. The Aldara package contains directions for use of the medication. Please read these carefully and use the medication only as directed.

Aldara probably works by boosting your body's immune response to the wart virus (there are over 100 types of wart virus, called human papilloma virus or HPV). Aldara should be used only on warts outside the vagina, on the labia and the area around your anus.

Treating Your Warts

Careful handwashing before and after application of the cream is recommended so that you do not experience a secondary bacterial infection in the wart area and get the cream on other parts of your body. Apply Aldara three times a week just prior to your normal sleeping hours. Apply a thin layer of the cream to all external genital warts and rub it in until it is no longer visible. Leave Aldara on the skin for 6–10 hours. Don't cover the treated area. Following this treatment period, remove the cream by washing the treated area with mild soap and water. Continue treatment until the warts disappear. Do not continue treatment past 16 weeks without consulting your health care provider.

Precautions in Treatment

Aldara cream may weaken condoms and vaginal diaphragms, so do not use these while you are treating your warts. Sexual (genital contact) should be avoided while the Aldara cream is on the skin. Common reactions to Aldara include redness, burning, swelling, itching, rash, soreness, stinging and tenderness. If any of these occur, wash the cream off with mild soap and water. Do not retreat until these symptoms are gone. For any questions, call your health care provider. A very small percentage of persons have flu-like symptoms, fever, fatigue, headache, diarrhea, and/or achy joints. If you experience any of these, call your health care provider.

From Hawkins, Roberto-Nichols, & Stanley-Haney, *Guidelines for Nurse Practitioners in Gynecologic Settings,* 8th edition, 2004, © Springer Publishing Company.

---

*Adapted from the Aldarat manufacturer's literature, 3M Pharmaceuticals, 1998.

For Your Information:
Gonorrhea

I. Definition
Gonorrhea is an acute infection which is spread by sexual contact and involves the genitourinary tract, throat, and rectum of both sexes. It is caused by the organism Neisseria gonorrhoea.

II. Important Information
A. The highest incidence of gonorrhea occurs in males between the ages of 20 and 24 and in females from 18 and 24. Gonorrhea is usually contracted from an infected person who has ignored symptoms or has no symptoms. This source can reinfect the patient, or possibly infect others unknowingly.
B. Incubation: 1–13 days. Symptoms can occur 3–30 days after sexual contact; average is 2–5 days after exposure

III. Usual Signs and Symptoms
A. Females
   1. Up to 80% have no symptoms
   2. Abnormal, thick green vaginal discharge
   3. Frequency, pain on urination
   4. Urethral discharge
   5. Rectal pain and discharge
   6. Unilateral labial pain and swelling
   7. Abnormal menstrual bleeding; increased dysmenorrhea (menstrual cramps)
   8. Lower abdominal discomfort
   9. Sore throat
B. Males
   1. 4–10% have no symptoms
   2. Frequency, pain on urination
   3. Burning sensation in the urethra
   4. Whitish discharge from the penis (early); may appear only as a drop during erection
   5. Yellow or greenish discharge from the penis (late)
   6. Sore throat

IV. Diagnosis (for Both Sexes)
A. History of sexual contact with a person known to be infected with gonorrhea

B. Smears and cultures taken from infected areas (cervix, penis, rectum, and throat)

V. Treatment for Males and Females

Antibiotics will be prescribed and are effective if taken according to directions. Be sure to tell your clinician if you are allergic to any antibiotic.

VI. Complications

A. *Females:* If gonorrhea goes untreated, it may lead to pelvic inflammatory disease (PID). PID involves severe abdominal cramps, pelvic pain, and high fever that will lead to scarring and possible blockage of the fallopian tubes, the risk of tubal pregnancy, and infertility.
B. *Males:* If gonorrhea goes untreated, scar tissue may form on the sperm passageway causing pain and sterility.
C. *Females and males:* The infection may spread throughout the body causing arthritis, sometimes with skin lesions.

VII. Patient Education (for Both Sexes)

A. All medication must be taken as directed.
B. No intercourse until treatment of self and partner(s) is completed.
C. Return to the clinic for reevaluation if symptoms persist or new symptoms occur after treatment is complete.
D. **Important:** The responsible lover informs all partners immediately upon finding out about exposure to sexually transmitted disease so that all persons involved can be evaluated adequately and treated immediately.

Special notes: _____

_____

Practitioner: _____

For more information and for care of friends: CDC STD Hotline, 1-800-227-8922. For phone numbers of free (or almost free) STD clinics see the "Community Service Numbers" in the government pages of your local phone book. http://www.cdc.gov

From Hawkins, Roberto-Nichols, & Stanley-Haney, *Guidelines for Nurse Practitioners in Gynecologic Settings,* 8th edition, 2004, © Springer Publishing Company.

For Your Information:
Hormone Therapy (HT)

I. Definition

Hormone therapy is the use of synthetic hormones (estrogen, progesterone, and/or testosterone) by postmenopausal women. Now known as HT, the use of hormones after menopause was once known as estrogen therapy (ET) because women were given synthetic estrogen only.

II. Reasons for Taking HT

A woman's body produces declining amounts of estrogens, progesterones and androgens during the perimenopausal period, culminating in the cessation of menstrual cycles (ovulation and bleeding). After 12 months without any bleeding (periods), you can consider that you are postmenopausal. A woman is said to have gone through surgical menopause if she has had her tubes, ovaries, and uterus removed.

Some natural estrogen production does continue after natural menopause; heavier women produce more estrogen since fat cells convert body chemicals called precursors to estrone, the most common form of natural estrogen in menopause.

Decline in natural estrogen production contributes to such menopausal symptoms as loss of elasticity of the vagina, a less lush vaginal lining causing a feeling of itching or burning or dryness, and pain around the urethra (the opening to the urinary bladder). Hot flashes or hot flushes, including night sweats, characterize menopause for some women. There may also be a relationship between menopause and loss of bone density leading to osteoporosis.

III. What You Should Know When Considering HT

HT should never be taken by women who have vaginal bleeding after menopause until the cause of the bleeding is discovered. Pregnant women or perimenopausal women who suspect pregnancy cannot take HT. If you have ever had a stroke, heart attack, or a blood clot in your legs or lungs, liver disease or any problems with the function of your liver, you may not be an HT candidate. Women with known or suspected cancer of the breast, ovaries, uterus, or cervix may not be good candidates for HT.

A number of conditions require special evaluation to determine if taking HT will be safe. These include undiagnosed vaginal bleeding, known or suspected pregnancy, a history of blood clots in your lungs or legs, known or suspected cancer of the breast or reproductive tract or malignant melanoma, history of bleeding disorder treated with blood transfusion, active gallbladder disease, family history of breast cancer, migraine headaches, elevated triglycerides and a ratio of good to bad cholesterol that is concerning, and endometriosis.

Considering HT is a decision that is yours to make if you and your clinician decide you have no contraindications to its use. To make the best decision, you and your clinician will discuss whether you are at greater risk of loss of bone density leading to osteoporosis because of your family or personal history, whether you have risk factors for developing osteoporosis, and your personal and family medical history including heart disease. Your desire for taking HT as well as your access to health care for monitoring HT will be considered. Some clinicians recommend that a sample of the lining of your uterus be analyzed before beginning HT, with a repeat of this test, called an endometrial biopsy, every year. An annual mammogram for women 40 and older as well as a Pap smear as indicated are important to your well-being.

IV. Evaluating Your Physical Risks and Benefits in Taking HT
In addition to a careful personal and family history, your clinician will recommend that you have a complete physical exam including a pelvic (internal) exam and Pap smear, and testing for infections such as vaginitis, sexually transmitted diseases, and bladder infection (cystitis) if you have any signs or symptoms. Testing might also include: a mammogram if you have not had one in the past year, examination of hormone levels, an endometrial biopsy, a lipid profile to determine your cholesterol level and the ratio of low density lipids (LDL—the bad ones) to high density lipids (HDL—the good ones), a hematocrit and/or hemoglobin to see if you are anemic, a bone density scan, and an electrocardiogram (EKG) if you have never had one and/or have a family history of heart disease. Other testing will depend upon findings from the physical exam and your personal and family health history.

For some women, the benefits of taking HRT outweigh the risks. For others, the risks and benefits balance, and for still others, the risks outweigh the benefits.

V. Taking HT
If your uterus has been removed (hysterectomy) you will take estrogen only without progestin. You and your clinician will decide the estrogen that you will take, both the amount and the way you take it (in pill form, the patch, or as a vaginal cream, suppository, or vaginal ring). If you still have your uterus, you may take both estrogen and a progestin patch or pill. Some women bleed when taking progestin, so you and your clinician will need to decide what is best for you.

As androgen levels drop with menopause, some women also take a small amount of male hormone (androgen), which may help women whose menopausal symptoms arc not resolved with estrogen or estrogen and progestin alone, have a decreased sense of well-being, a lower libido (sex drive), and/ or generalized loss of energy (lethargy).

VI. Consider Alternatives and Adjuncts to HT

All women need a diet with at least 6–8 servings of fruit and vegetables a day, several servings of complex carbohydrates such as breads and pasta, sources of protein including diary products, eggs, meat, fish and poultry, legumes such as beans, peas, and calcium. Women also need to decrease fat to 30% or less of total calories daily through using nonfat dairy products (rich in protein and calcium), limiting red meat, and eating lean meat, poultry, and fish. Whole grain pastas, cereals and breads, bran, vegetables and fruit add roughage to the diet. Most women need calcium supplements. Postmenopausal women need a total of 1500 milligrams each day of calcium as well as 400–800 international units of vitamin D. Six to eight 8-ounce glasses of water daily will help keep all tissues healthy and promote both bowel and bladder health. Consider adding phytoestrogens to diet and essential fatty acids in recommended amounts.

Regular weight-bearing exercise and strength training is critical to maintenance of bone density; 30 to 45 minutes four to six times a week is recommended. Botanicals, Chinese remedies, vitamins, nonhormonal vaginal lubricants such as KY jelly, KY liquid, Lubrin®, Vagisil®, Replens®, and Astroglide®, naturalistic interventions, and homeopathic preparations can be helpful supplements to or alternatives to HT. Because herbs and homeopathic remedies can interact with each other and with prescription and over-the-counter medications, it is best to consult a practitioner who specializes in their use. Your local library, health food store, bookstore, and health care providers are all sources of information about caring for yourself after menopause.

Menopause: Another change of life http://www.ppfa.org.ppfa/menopub/html
National Institute on Aging: http://www.pueblo.gsa.gov/cic-text/health/other/menopause.txt
Power Surge: http://www.dearest.com/refer.htm
www.allwise.com

From Hawkins, Roberto-Nichols, & Stanley-Haney, *Guidelines for Nurse Practitioners in Gynecologic Settings,* 8th edition, 2004, © Springer Publishing Company.

For Your Information:
Lice (Pediculosis)

I. Definition
Pediculosis means having the skin infested with lice, particularly on hairy areas such as the scalp, underarms, and the pubic area. Three types of lice prey on humans: head lice (*p. capitis*), body lice (*p. corposis*), and pubic lice or "crab lice" (*p. pubis*).

II. Transmission
Lice are transmitted by lice-infected shared clothing, bedding, brushes, towels, pillows, and upholstered furniture, or by close personal contact with an infected person. Head lice move from head to head. Adult pubic lice probably survive no more than 24 hours off their host.

III. Signs and Symptoms
A. Intense itching
B. Observing the lice or, more easily, their nits (eggs), which are greenish-white ovals attached to hair shafts—in eyebrows, eyelashes, scalp hair, pubic hair, and other body hair.
C. Known exposure to household member or intimate partner with lice
D. Crusts or scabs on body from scratching
E. Enlargement of lymph nodes (swollen glands) in the neck, an allergic response to lice
F. Body lice found on clothing, especially in the seams, as lice are rarely found on the body
G. Black dots (representing excreta) on skin and underclothing

IV. Diagnosis
See Signs and Symptoms above. Lice can best be detected by using a magnifying glass or microscope

V. Treatment
A. General measures
   1. Wash clothing, towels, etc., with hot water, or dry clean contaminated items or run them through a dryer on heat cycle to destroy nits and lice; wash combs and hairbrushes in hot, soapy water. Items can also be sealed in a plastic bag for 2 weeks; lice will suffocate. Or items can be put outside in cold weather for 10 days.
   2. Spray couches, chairs, car seats, and items that can't be washed or dry cleaned with over-the-counter products (A-200 Pyrinate®, Triplex®, RID,

    or store brand products); alternative is to vacuum carefully to pick up lice and nits.

B. Specific measures

  1. Head lice

    a. Thoroughly wet hair with Lindane (Kwell®), Triplex Kit, Clear, Klout, Pronto, RID, R&C, or End Lice shampoo; work up lather, adding water as necessary. Shampoo thoroughly, leaving shampoo on head for 5 minutes. Pronto shampoo/conditioner can be used as an alternative to these. *OR* use Nix®, leave on 10 minutes. Lindane (Kwell®) cannot be used by women who are pregnant or breastfeeding or for children under 2 years of age (and it requires a prescription)

    b. Rinse thoroughly, towel dry

    c. Remove remaining nits with fine-tooth metal comb or tweezers. Putting olive oil on the hair can help make running the comb through the hair easier

  2. Body lice

    a. Bathe with soap and water even if no lice are found

    b. If evidence of lice is found, Lindane (Kwell Lotion®) may be may be applied, allowed to remain 8–10 hours, and thoroughly rinsed off

  3. Pubic lice

    a. Apply Lindane (Kwell®) shampoo to affected area, leave on 4 minutes, or apply A-200 Pyrinate Gel® as directed to hair and skin of pubic area and leave on for 10 minutes

    b. Rinse thoroughly

    c. Repeat application if symptoms persist

    d. Treat any sexual partner of the past month as in a., b., c.

VI. Patient Education

A. Carefully check family and household members and close contacts for evidence of lice contamination and if found, treat as above.

B. Call your health care provider if signs of infection from scratching occur (redness, swelling of skin, discharge that looks like pus, bleeding, fever)

C. Stop using the treatment and call your health care provider if you or your family members experience sensitivity to the treatment (pain, swelling, rash)

D. Consult with your health care provider if you have lice on the eye lashes as the treatments cannot be used near eyes. Ophthalmic (eye) ointment must be applied to the eyelashes twice a day × 10 days.

VII. Follow-up

Contact your health care provider if itching, redness or other problems listed above persist or recur,

Special notes: _____

Practitioner: _____

For Your Information:
Directions for Using Natural Family Planning to Prevent or Achieve Pregnancy

Modern natural family planning methods use normally occurring signs and symptoms of ovulation for both the prevention and achievement of pregnancy. No drugs or devices are used. The couple that uses one of the natural methods to prevent pregnancy makes the choice not to have intercourse during the method defined fertile phase. Natural methods of family planning are 75%-99% effective in preventing pregnancy, depending on the method used and on how well the information is taught and applied. The monitoring of fertility signs also provides invaluable information for couples seeking pregnancy or struggling with infertility. Successful use of natural methods depends on competent instruction and follow up, correct and consistent charting and client compliance with rules.

Commonly Used Methods of Natural Family Planning
1. Cervical mucus method—based on detectable changes in cervical mucus throughout the cycle
2. Basal body temperature method—based on changes in the temperature of the woman's body at rest
3. Symptothermal method—based on the changes in the body temperature, cervical mucus, and other bodily signs
   To become knowledgeable about natural family planning methods requires instruction and can be a pleasant, healthy way to learn to avoid or achieve pregnancy and be aware of your individual fertility pattern.

Terminology Used In a Natural Family Planning Class
abstinence—not having vaginal sexual intercourse
fertile days—the days in the menstrual cycle when pregnancy (conception) is possible
genitals or genitalia—organs of the reproductive system in both male and female
genital-to-genital contact—penis *touching* or coming into close contact with the vaginal area
hormone—a substance that causes special changes in the body; may be naturally occurring or synthetically produced

---

By the late Eleanor Tabeek, RN, PhD, CNM, updated by Mary Finnigan, BA, MA. Reprinted with Dr. Tabeek's family's permission.

infertile days—the days in the menstrual cycle when pregnancy (conception) cannot occur

menstruation—bleeding that occurs when the lining of the uterus breaks down and is released; this happens about 12–16 days after ovulation

menstrual cycle—the time from the first day of menstrual bleeding to the day *before* the next menstrual bleeding begins; may vary normally from 21 to 40 days in length

ovulation—release of the egg (ovum) from the ovary about 12 to 16 days *before* the onset of the next menstrual period (the day bleeding begins)

ovum—female sex cell, egg

sperm—male sex cell (spermatozoa) found in the semen of a man

Review of the Menstrual Cycle

The menstrual cycle is controlled by hormones. The cycle begins on the *first* day of menstrual bleeding and ends the day *before* menstrual bleeding begins again.

Following menstruation, eggs (ova) are usually maturing in the follicles of the ovaries. As they grow, estrogen (a hormone known as the female sex hormone) is produced in increasing amounts, and certain changes take place:

1. The lining of the uterus builds up the blood supply needed for pregnancy to occur.
2. Cervical mucus changes in character to become more hospitable to sperm so sperm can live and travel in the uterus.
3. The cervix becomes higher in the pelvis and softer as the cervical os opens to allow sperm to enter the uterus.
4. Basal body temperature (BBT) is low.

As the time of ovulation nears, some women may experience one or more of the following changes:

1. Clearer complexion and less oily hair
2. Increase in energy level
3. Vaginal aching
4. Spotting of blood
5. Pain or aching in the pelvic area
6. Breast tenderness and/or fullness

Once ovulation has occurred, there is an increase in the production of progesterone (another hormone important to the menstrual cycle and to pregnancy), and the following changes occur during the 12–16 days before menstruation begins:

1. Basal body temperature (BBT) rises
2. Mucus becomes inhospitable to sperm so they can't live and travel into the uterus

3. Cervix becomes lower, firmer, and the opening closes to prevent sperm from going into the uterus

4. Increased progesterone maintains the lining of the uterus in place for 12–16 days

As menstruation approaches, women may also experience one or more of the following changes:

1. Cramps
2. Headaches
3. Oily hair and complexion, acne or increase in acne
4. Mood changes
5. Decrease in energy level
6. Desire to eat foods with sugar and/or salt
7. Breast tenderness
8. Pelvic aching or pain
9. Low back pain; joint pain or aches

Cervical Mucus Method

Cervical mucus is produced by tiny cells in the cervix. As the ovum are maturing, the mucus will change in a special way that helps keep sperm alive and makes it easier for sperm to travel into the uterus. The mucus loses this quality within a few days after the ovum leaves the ovary. The quality or condition of the cervical mucus is an excellent indicator of the days in the menstrual cycle when the woman can become pregnant.

How to check the cervical mucus

1. Begin checking the cervical mucus when the menstrual bleeding ends or becomes light enough to let you be able to determine its presence.
2. Cervical mucus should be checked before and after urination.
3. Before checking the tissue for the presence of mucus, note mentally whether the area around the vaginal opening feels wet, moist or dry.
4. Fold a piece of toilet tissue and wipe over the vaginal opening. If the tissue slides across the vaginal opening the sensation is wet. If the tissue drags, pulls or chafes across the vaginal opening the sensation is dry. If the tissue sticks a little to the vaginal opening or if the sensation is neither wet nor dry it is a moist sensation.
5. After wiping, observe the tissue for the presence of cervical mucus. Note the color, texture and stretchiness of the mucus. The best way to observe its characteristics is to place it between two fingers and slowly open the two fingers. The woman who does not want to touch the mucus can assess its traits by holding the tissue in both hands, then pulling it apart.
6. Check sensation and for the presence of mucus each time you use the bathroom since the character of the mucus can change during the day.

MucusCheck
Artist: Glen Hawkins

How to Chart Information about the Mucus
1. A new cycle starts the first day of the menstrual bleeding, regardless of the time of the day the flow begins. Write the date that bleeding begins in the space on the natural family planning chart.
2. Record each day of bleeding with a star
3. When the period ends, if the vaginal sensation is dry, chart a dry day using the letter "D."
4. Continue to use the letter "D" each day until a moist or wet sensation is experienced. Chart a moist sensation using the letter "M" and a wet sensation by using the letter W
5. Note the color, texture and stretchiness of any mucus found or observed on toilet tissue.
6. Write an "X" through the "W" on the last day of wet vaginal sensation and/or clear, stretchy mucus. The last day of clear, stretchy mucus and/or wet sensation is called the Peak Day. This day will not be noted until the following day when the mucus will no longer be stretchy and clear and the vaginal sensation will have changed to moist or dry.

Summary of Mucus Symbols

*	D	M	W	W
menses	dry	moist	wet	Peak Day
	sensation	sensation	sensation	

Colors: yellow, white, cloudy, clear
Texture: pasty, creamy, gel, raw egg white
Stretchiness: less that ½ inch—sticky
More than ½ inch—stretchy

Always chart the most fertile sensation and the most fertile characteristics of the mucus

How to Chart Other Symptoms
1. Record intercourse by a check mark (√)
2. Record any other changes in your body, e.g., pain with ovulation, breast tenderness, etc.) in the column under "Notes. "

Natural Family Planning Chart

BASAL BODY TEMPERATURE

99.0

98.0

97.0

CYCLE DAY	1	2	3	4	5	6	7	8	9	10	11	12	13	14	15	16	17	18	19	20	21	22	23	24	25	26	27	28	29	30	31	32	33	34	35	36	37	38	39	40
DATE																																								
DAY																																								
INTERCOURSE																																								
MUCUS																																								
CERVIX																																								
NOTES:																																								

MUCUS DESCRIPTION

SENSATION

DISTURBANCES
SCHEDULE
CHANGES

3. Until you know your mucus changes well, it is helpful to write a description of your mucus in the Notes column, e.g., sticky, white.

Basal Body Temperature (BBT) Method

Basal body temperature is the temperature of the body at rest. As the ova are maturing, the temperature is low. At some time shortly before, during, or after the ovum leaves the ovary, the temperature will usually rise about 3/10ths to 1 full degree higher than it had been. This change in temperature tells you when the ovum has left the ovary; that is, that ovulation has taken place.

How to Take Basal Body Temperature

1. Begin taking temperature the first day of menstrual bleeding
2. Take temperature about the same time every day, usually in the morning when you first awake.
3. Take temperature before eating, drinking, smoking, and any physical activity.
4. The thermometer can be placed in the mouth, in the vagina, or in the rectum. Always take temperature the same way every day. Record temperature on the Natural Family Planning Chart.
5. If the temperature reading on the thermometer is between two lines, record the temperature at the lower line.

Change in Daily Events

Occasionally, a woman may become ill, drink alcoholic beverages, or change the usual time she takes her temperature. Since such events or any change in lifestyle may affect the temperature, when and if they happen, take and record the temperature anyway. In the "Notes" column on the Natural Family Planning Chart, record the possible reason for any change in the usual temperature.

To record your temperature . . .
Circle your temperature each day on the
Natural Family Planning Chart
and connect the circles with a line.

To adjust temperatures not taken at usual or base time

- pick a base time
- for every **half hour** earlier than the base time **add 1/10** of a degree to thermometer reading before it is recorded on the temperature graph
- for every **half hour** later than the base time, **subtract 1/10** of a degree from the thermometer reading before it is recorded on the temperature graph

The Cervix

After menses, the cervix is low in the vaginal canal, the opening is closed, and it feels firm or pointed, like the tip of a nose. As the ovum is developing and being released, the cervix will rise, soften and the opening will become wide. These changes help sperm travel into the uterus. Within a few days after the ovum leaves the ovary (ovulation) the cervix will lower in the vaginal canal; it will feel firm or pointed and the opening will close up. These changes help prevent sperm from traveling into the uterus. It is not necessary to check the cervix in order to use a natural method. However, observing and charting the cervical changes can give interested women additional information about their fertile and infertile days. The information can be particularly useful for the breastfeeding or premenopausal woman.

How to Check Status of the Cervix

1. Begin checking the cervix after the menstrual bleeding ends.
2. Check the cervix while in a comfortable position such as squatting or standing with one foot on a stool or chair. Use the same position each time you check the cervix.
3. Check in the evening, and at about the *same time* each day.
4. Wash your hands before placing a finger in the vagina.
5. When feeling the cervix, check for:
   - position in vagina: high (may be difficult to feel) or low (usually easy to feel)
   - softness or firmness
   - opening: open or closed
6. Chart the most fertile cervical sign of the day.

How to Chart Information About the Cervix

1. Use circles to represent the sizes of the cervical opening.
   Place the circles in different positions in the boxes on the Natural Family Planning Chart to represent the rising and lowering of the cervix.

= low and closed   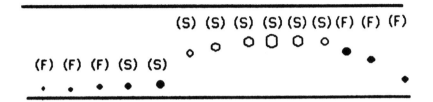 = high and open

2. You can also use the letter "F" to represent a firm cervix and the letter "S" to represent a soft cervix:

(Closed circles represent a closed cervical opening-as the, cervix opens, the circles are larger.)

3. Another way the position of the cervix can be noted is through using arrows
   a high cervix ➤
   a lowering cervix ➤
   a cervix tilted to the side = ➤ (right side) or ➤ (left side)

Symptothermal Method
Combining use of all the information described to this point.

Natural Family Planning Rules
By following the natural family planning rules, women will know on which days they are fertile and infertile during each menstrual cycle. It is important for women to check with their instructor or health care provider before following any of the rules.

OVULATION METHOD (Observing and charting cervical mucus)

To Avoid Pregnancy:

Avoid intercourse during menses

Every Other Dry Day Rule (To determine which days before ovulation are infertile). Intercourse can take place on the evening of every other dry day.

Intercourse is restricted to the evening so that the woman can observe her cervical mucus during the day undisturbed by intercourse.

It is common for some of the man's semen to be in the woman's vagina on the day after intercourse. If cervical mucus starts to be produced on that day, the presence of semen may prevent the woman from seeing or feeling the presence of mucus. This is why intercourse should not take place on consecutive evenings and why abstinence from intercourse should be followed the day after intercourse has taken place. If the day after the abstinence day is a dry day, intercourse may occur on that evening.

Dry Day	Abstinence	Dry Day	Abstinence
Intercourse in	No intercourse	Intercourse in	No intercourse
the evening	the next day	the evening	the next day

Fertitity begins when mucus is observed or the sensation changes to moist or wet.
When the fertile phase begins, the couple should not have vaginal intercourse until the fertile phase ends.

Peak Day Rule (To determine which days after ovulation are infertile)

The infertile phase after ovulation begins on the evening of the fourth day after Peak Day. This infertility lasts until the beginning of the next menses.

Remember: The Peak Day is the last day of wet sensation and/or clear, stretchy mucus.
a. Mark the Peak Day on the chart with an "X"
b. Number the days after Peak Day "1" "2" "3" "4." The sensation on these days must be moist or dry. There may be no mucus present or it may be pastry, sticky or creamy. It may cloudy, white or clear in color.

To achieve pregnancy:
Follow the every other dry day rule until the mucus sign indicates fertility. This allows the woman to accurately chart her mucus sign and to identify the start of the fertile phase.

Intercourse should occur on days identified as fertile by the cervical mucus. Particular attention should be paid to the days of wet *sensation and* clear or cloudy stretchy mucus. It is important for the couple to begin intercourse at the first signs of fertility because the fertile phase is limited in length.

BASAL BODY TEMPERATURE METHOD (observing and charting basal
body temperature)

To Avoid Pregnancy

The "6–5–0" Day Rule (To determine which days before ovulation are infertile days)

This rule cannot be used until there is a record of at least six, normal
menstrual cycles.

Shortest Past Cycle	Assume Infertile	Abstinence Begins
26 days or longer	first six days of cycle	day 7
23–25 days	first 5 days of cycle	day 6
22 days or less	0 days	day 1

21 Day Rule (To determine which days before ovulation are infertile days)

This rule can not be used until there is a record of at least six, normal
menstrual cycles.

Subtract 21 from the length of the shortest recorded cycle. The number of
days remaining equals the number of infertile days before ovulation. Intercourse can take place at any time during these days.

Example: Shortest cycle (28 days) 28–21 =7

The first 7 days of the menstrual cycle are infertile beginning with the first
day of menstrual bleeding. Abstinence begins on day 8. If a shorter cycle is
recorded, the formula needs to be recalculated.

Doering Rule (To determine which days before ovulation are infertile days)

This rule cannot be used until there is a record of at least six, normal
menstrual cycles.

Subtract 7 from the earliest recorded day of temperature rise. The number of
days remaining equals the number of infertile days before ovulation. Intercourse can take place at any time during these days.

Example: Earliest recorded day of temperature rise Day 15 15–7 = 8

The first 8 days of the menstrual cycle are infertile beginning with the first day of menstrual bleeding. Abstinence begins on day 9. If a shorter cycle is recorded, the formula needs to be recalculated.

Mean Temperature Rule (To determine which days after ovulation are infertile)

The infertile phase after ovulation begins on the evening of the fourth day of a rise in temperature on or above the line representing the mean temperature of the previous cycle.

In the previous cycle there had to be temperature readings on at least 75 % of the days and the cycle was ovulatory.

To calculate the mean temperature from the previous cycle
a. add all temperatures from the cycle
b. divide the total by the number of temperatures
c. draw a line on the new chart at the mean temperature

Four consecutive days of temperature at or above the mean temperature line-infertile phase.

Thermal Shift Rule (To determine which days after ovulation are infertile)

This rule can be used when the previous cycle was anovulatory and the Mean Temperature Rule could not be applied.

The infertile phase after ovulation begins on the evening of the third consecutive temperature that is .4° higher than the six previous temperatures.

a. Watch for the temperature rise—three temperatures in a row that are higher than the six preceding temperatures
b. Find the highest of the six temperatures immediately preceding the rise
c. Draw a line across the chart through the highest of the six temperatures immediately preceding the rise (This line is called the baseline)

The infertile phase after ovulation begins when there are 3 consecutive temperatures that are all at least .4° above the baseline

To Achieve Pregnancy

The basal body temperature pattern does not give any indication as to the start of the fertile phase. Previous charts can be reviewed to predict when a temperature rise might occur. Intercourse should occur on the days before an anticipated temperature rise.

Sympto-Thermal Method (observing and charting basal body temperature, cervical mucus, and other bodily signs)

To Postpone Pregnancy (To determine which days before ovulation are infertile days)

Use any of the following rules:

"6–5–0" Day Rule
21 Day Rule
Doering Rule
Every Other Dry Day Rule

Abstinence should begin if mucus appears at any time during the days determined infertile by the above rules.

Sympto-Thermal Rule (To determine which days after ovulation are infertile)

The infertile phase after ovulation begins on the evening of the fourth day past Peak and/or the evening of the third high reading at least .4° above the baseline whichever occurs last.

1. Mark Peak Day with an "X." Number the four days after Peak Day "1," "2," "3," "4."

Peak day is the last day of wet sensation and/or mucus with very fertile descriptions, i.e. clear, cloudy, stretchy etc. Peak Day involves cross-checking tissue and sensation.

2. Draw the Baseline.

Find three temperatures higher than six. Draw a line across the chart through the highest of the six temperatures immediately preceding the rise.

3. Circle the first three temperatures that are over the baseline and after Peak Day.

Don't circle temperatures that are above the baseline on or before peak day. Don't circle post peak temperatures that are not above the baseline.

The Sympto-Thermal Rule is fulfilled when the third circled reading is at least .4° above the baseline. If the third circled reading is not at least .4° above the baseline circle a fourth temperature above the baseline. This fourth high reading need only be above the baseline.

To Achieve Pregnancy
See corresponding section under Ovulation Method.

Web Site for NFP device: www.cyclebeads.com

For Your Information: Osteoporosis

I. Definition
Osteoporosis is characterized by decreased bone mass (loss of bone density), deterioration of bone microarchitecture, and an increase in bone fragility and risk for bone fractures (broken bones).

\II. Etiology
Humans have two types of bone—cortical and trabecular. Cortical bone is very compact; it forms the outer shell of bones and makes up 80% of the skeletons of adults. Trabecular bone, also called spongy or cancellous bone, makes up the remaining 20% and forms the interior of bones. For bones to develop properly and maintain bone mass, we need adequate calcium and phosphorus and other minerals in our diets. We also need other vitamins and adequate Vitamin D for our bodies to absorb calcium from our diets and enable the body to maintain our bones.

We reach our peak bone mass at about age 35. Estrogen seems to play a role in enabling women's bones to retain calcium and the other minerals necessary to build bone and preserve bone mass. From age 35 or so, some sources say that we lose about 2% of bone density each year. After menopause, the loss of bone mass may accelerate during the first 5 or 6 years. Thereafter, rate of loss returns to previous level. If bone mass loss becomes too great, the woman becomes very susceptible to fractures.

III. Risk Factors
The risk of developing osteoporosis is greater for women than for men (women begin with less bone mass), and increases with age. Women who have never had children, had early menopause (before age 50), are of Northern European or Asian descent, have a thin body frame, blond or red hair, fair skin and freckles, curvature of the spine (scoliosis), are unable to digest milk or dairy products, smoke, have a high alcohol intake, low calcium diet, high salt diet, not enough vitamin D, drink more than 2 or 3 cups of caffeinated beverages a day, do not exercise or exercise excessively, live in a northern climate, have little fluoride in their drinking water, and have a family history of osteoporosis are at greater risk than women with none of these risks.

IV. Prevention
We cannot change our heritage, family history, gender, our body build, hair or skin colors, the time at which we go through natural menopause, or our inability to drink milk or eat milk products. But we can exercise an appro-

priate amount, stop or never start smoking, limit alcohol intake, choose a diet with the amount of calcium we need (1200–1500 milligrams daily at ages 11–24 or when pregnant or breast feeding, 1000 milligrams between ages 25 and 49, and 1500 milligrams at age 50+), take vitamin D supplements (400–800 international units after menopause), decrease or eliminate caffeine, and decrease daily salt intake.

Calcium-rich foods include: broccoli; bok choy; collard, mustard and turnip greens; kale; and oranges. Dairy products, sardines, and salmon with bones, shrimp paste, dried anchovies, soy products (tofu, soy milk, etc.), and almonds are all high in calcium. Vitamin D (400–800 international units is the recommended daily dose) can be obtained from 5 to 10 minutes in the sun each day, drinking the equivalent of a quart of vitamin D fortified milk, or taking a vitamin D supplement. Foods rich in vitamin D include fatty fish, butter, vitamin D-fortified margarine, egg yolks, and liver.

We can help prevent osteoporosis by changing what we can change in our lifestyles and by considering hormone therapy after menopause. Hormone replacement therapy, known as HT, is not for every woman and is a decision each should make very carefully with her health care provider.

If you do not choose to use HT, in addition to all the lifestyle changes discussed above, you may also consider the use of vitamins—especially 400 units of vitamin E each day, and exploring botanicals or other homeopathic products with knowledgeable persons.

V. Treatment for Osteoporosis
If you have osteoporosis, you can prevent further loss of bone mass and, in some cases, actually restore bone mass with a regimen of exercise prescribed by a clinician specializing in osteoporosis therapy.

Calcium supplements, adequate vitamin D, hormonal and nonhormonal drug therapy, changes in lifestyle including smoking cessation, decreasing or eliminating caffeine, and lowering alcohol intake can also improve the health of your bones.

Making your home as safe as possible will help you avoid fractures. Nurses and physical therapists who specialize in working with persons with osteoporosis can help you reduce or eliminate those hazards.

From Hawkins, Roberto-Nichols, & Stanley-Haney, *Guidelines for Nurse Practitioners in Gynecologic Settings,* 8th edition, 2004, © Springer Publishing Company.

For Your Information:
Polycystic Ovary Syndrome (PCOS)

I. Definition

PCOS is a complex condition of the endocrine system (including the ovaries). It is one of the most common reproductive tract problems in women under 30 years of age. Some women, when examined with laparoscopy (a lighted scope for viewing the inside of the abdomen and pelvic area), have ovaries with a thickened capsule and multiple cysts of the follicles (which develop and release eggs). The causes of PCOS are unknown, but theories include genetic factors.

II. Signs and Symptoms (only 20–30% of women have these)
A. Menstrual cycles without ovulation
B. Infertility—inability to conceive
C. No menses (periods) or very scanty menses
D. Prolonged menses, sometimes unpredictable or irregular menses
E. Increase in body and facial hair
F. Increase in or appearance of acne
G. Loss of hair especially at the crown
H. Whitish breast discharge
I. Change in body shape—increased waist to hip ratio
J. Increase in skin pigment at nape of neck, in axillae (under arms), groin area

III. Diagnosis
A. The diagnosis is made on the basis of signs and symptoms, laboratory tests, ultrasound of the ovaries, and imaging the adrenal glands.
B. Laboratory testing can include measures of androgens (male hormones), function and hormone level tests for thyroid, adrenal, and pituitary glands.

IV. Treatment
A. Weight loss and exercise program
B. Low dose oral contraceptives to restore menstrual cycles
C. Possibly prescription drugs to reduce excessive hair growth and acne
D. Medications for type 2 (noninsulin dependent) diabetes seem to help symptoms
E. Electrolysis and/or depilatories for excessive hair
F. Medications to induce ovulation when pregnancy is desired

V. Patient Education
A. Education about PCOS and lifestyle alterations
B. Education about pharmacologic (prescription drug) interventions
C. Education about fertility
Special Notes:_____

_____

Practitioner:_____

For more information: www.pcosupport.org

From Hawkins, Roberto-Nichols, & Stanley-Haney, *Guidelines for Nurse Practitioners in Gynecologic Settings,* 8th edition, 2004, © Springer Publishing Company.

For Your Information:
Preconception Self-Care

The purpose of preconception self-care is to help you be at your healthiest as you plan a pregnancy. Advanced planning can help reduce your risk of having a low birth weight or premature baby. Working with your clinician, you can identify any medical condition or medications you are taking that need to be considered when contemplating a pregnancy. You may also wish to have a genetic consultation if you or your partner have a family history of inherited disorders such a cystic fibrosis, Tay-Sachs disease, hemophilia, or birth defects in the family. Infections such as sexually transmitted diseases and tuberculosis may affect the health of a pregnancy, or even your ability to conceive.

Good health is important for a successful pregnancy and healthy baby. A complete health history and physical examination including a Pap smear, pelvic exam, and screening for sexually transmitted diseases, as well as other communicable diseases such as hepatitis B and C and HIV prior to conception will ensure that your body is in an optimal state for a pregnancy. Having your immunizations up to date will protect you and your baby. Evaluation of your nutritional state, diet and exercise patterns, and your toxin exposure at work and at home will help you prepare your body for conception.

Smoking and using alcohol and/or street drugs can have serious consequences for the health of a pregnancy and baby. At least one month before attempting to conceive, women who smoke, drink alcohol, or use street drugs should stop. If you use prescription or over-the-counter drugs, limit them to those your clinician approves of. Also check with your clinician about use of herbals, homeopathics and vitamins.

Protect yourself from exposure to toxins as much as possible. These include pesticides, household cleaning products, gases, lead, solvents, and radiation. Modify, undertake, or continue your program of exercise. Bring your immunizations up-to-date (although some are contraindicated in pregnancy, so it is best to do this 3 months before trying to conceive).

Eat a balanced diet, paying particular attention to fresh fruits and vegetables (6–8 or more servings a day); whole-grain breads, cereals, and pasta; protein (especially fish,* poultry, legumes, and nonfat dairy products), and drink 6–8 glasses of water a day. Decrease or eliminate caffeine from your diet (including coffee and carbonated soft drinks). Begin taking 400 micrograms of folic acid a day—a prenatal vitamin that includes folic acid is fine. Increase your calcium intake to the equivalent of 1 quart of milk a day (1200 milligrams). In general, avoid food with lots of preservatives and artificial sweeteners.

---

*Follow current recommendations for pregnancy due to mercury content.

335

Avoid hot tubs and saunas as these bring your body temperature above 102 degrees, which can limit or eliminate sperm production. Avoiding such excessive heat will also protect the baby once conception has occurred.

If you are on hormonal contraceptives, stop using them at least one month before you plan to conceive to allow your body to resume cycling. Several months are advised, as it often takes that long to resume ovulatory (fertile) cycles. You can use spermicides and condoms until you wish to try to conceive.

In order to maximize the health of their sperm, men planning to father children should stop smoking and using street drugs, drink only in moderation (1/day) and avoid toxin exposure at least 3 months before attempting conception. They should also have their infectious disease status checked through a sexually transmitted disease screen and hepatitis B and C and HIV testing. One-half of the baby's genetic material comes from the father, so he needs to be in good health.

Discuss with your partner your feelings about parenting, your expectations of him or her, and what parenting means to you. How do you expect your life to change? How will having a child change your relationship, the way your household functions, your work schedule, your expectations, and those of your partner? Who will be the primary parent? Will one or both of you have maternity/parenting leave? How will your finances be affected by having a child? How do you plan to integrate a new baby into the household with other children, extended family and other members of the household?

Planning for a pregnancy will help you be at your best when you conceive. It will also help you consider the changes pregnancy and a baby will have on your life and the lives of those close to you.

For resources on genetic counseling, nutrition, prenatal care, and prenatal classes, as well as information on conception and pregnancy, ask your clinician and check your community library, your local bookstore, and on line such as:

March of Dimes Birth Defects Foundation: http://www.modimes.org

Ask NOAH about: Pregnancy: http:/Avww.noah.cuny.edu/pregnancy/Pregnancy.html

From Hawkins, Roberto-Nichols, & Stanley-Haney, *Guidelines for Nurse Practitioners in Gynecologic Settings,* 8th edition, 2004, © Springer Publishing Company.

For Your Information:
Premenstrual Syndrome (PMS)

I. Definition
The premenstrual syndrome consists of a group of behavioral and cognitive dysfunctions and physical symptoms associated with the menstrual cycle.

II. Signs and Symptoms
Usually appear one week prior to menses but may also appear up to two weeks or just several days before menses, and include:
A. Mood fluctuations—anxiety, crying, persistent anger
B. Depression, feeling hopeless
C. Fatigue, lethargy; joint or muscle pain
D. Weight gain
E. Headache
F. Irritability
G. Breast tenderness
H. Increased appetite, craving for sweets and/or salt
I. Insomnia/sleep disturbance
J. Inability to concentrate, reduced interest in usual activities
K. Constipation
L. Palpitations
M. Hot flashes
N. Abdominal bloating
O. Acne
P. Changes in sex drive

If you are bothered by these changes, make an appointment with your health care provider for a consultation. A complete history will be taken and a diet and exercise regimen suggested. You may be asked to document your temperature and symptoms daily in a journal. You will also be scheduled for a complete physical.

III. Treatment
Treatment consists of alleviating the signs and symptoms described above with a diet and exercise plan and/or medication.
A. Diet recommendation
    2. Limit your salt intake to 3 gm or less per day, i.e., avoid using the saltshaker
    3. Limit your intake of alcohol

4. Avoid caffeine, i.e., coffee, tea, chocolate, soft drinks
5. Increase your intake of complex carbohydrates, i.e., fresh fruit, vegetables, whole grains, pasta, rice, potatoes
6. Consume moderate protein and fat. Limit your red meat consumption to 2 x weekly.

B. Exercise recommendations
   Exercise 3 times per week for 30–40 minutes. Examples: brisk walking, jogging, aerobic dancing, swimming.

C. Medication
   Vitamins, calcium supplements and other medications as prescribed or recommended by your clinician.

D. Consider complementary therapies such as meditation, botanicals, aroma or muscle therapy, energy healing, acupuncture. Talk with your health care provider about these.
   You may be evaluated monthly x 3 months to determine the effects of diet, exercise, vitamins, and your symptoms. If there is no improvement at that time, a more extensive work-up may be done with possible referral.

From Hawkins, Roberto-Nichols, & Stanley-Haney, *Guidelines for Nurse Practitioners in Gynecologic Settings,* 8th edition, 2004, © Springer Publishing Company.

For Your Information: Scabies

I. Definition
Scabies is a highly contagious skin rash whose chief symptom is itching. Scabies is caused by the scabies mite (Sarcoptes scabiei), which burrows into the skin and deposits its eggs along the tunnel it has made. The eggs hatch in 3–5 days and gather around hair follicles. Newly hatched females burrow into the skin, mature in 10–19 days, then mate and start a new cycle.

II. Transmission
A. Scabies among adults may be sexually transmitted.
B. Persons living in close proximity with others, in dormitories, and in crowded living spaces are more likely to incur scabies if one person amongst them becomes infested with the mite. Persons sharing clothing or towels are at increased risk.

III. Signs and Symptoms
A. May appear 4–6 weeks after contact with scabies from another person because it takes several weeks for sensitization to develop. In persons previously infected, symptoms may appear 1–4 days after repeat exposure to the scabies mite.
B. Itching, becoming worse at night or at times when the body temperature is raised such as after exercise. Itching begins first, before other signs and symptoms.
C. Lesions are usually on the webs between fingers, the inner aspects of the wrists and elbows, areas surrounding the surrounding the nipples, umbilicus (belly button), belt line, lower abdomen, genitalia, and cleft between the buttocks; can be all over the body. These lesions look like little burrows about 1/2 to 3/4 inch in length ending in a raised red area (papule) or a raised area filled with fluid (vesicle). These lesions can become scaly and become crusted over. When scratched, the areas become raw looking and become infected.

III. Diagnosis
A. Diagnosis is made through examination of lesions and of those areas of the body most frequently involved.
B. Linear burrows can be seen in the affected area.
C. Scaling, crustation lesions, furuncles (boils), and/or scratches may be visible with secondary infection.

D. When scrapings from the lesions are examined under low power with a microscope, the mites can sometimes be seen.

IV. Treatment

A. Treatments to kill mites
1. Elimite® applied to all areas of the body from the neck down and washed off after 8–14 hours OR
2. Kwell® or Scabene® (Lindane), 1 ounce of lotion or 30 grams of cream applied in a thin layer to the entire body from the neck down, left on for 8 hours, and washed off thoroughly. These applications should not be used immediately after a shower or bath and should not be in excess of these recommendations to avoid the possibility of damage to the nervous system from absorption through the skin. These medications should not be used for women who are pregnant or breast feeding or on children under 2 years of age or in persons with extensive skin rash or sores (dermatitis) OR
3. An oral medication once and then repeated in 2 weeks (but not for children less than 33 lbs.).

B. Treatments to relieve symptoms. Antihistamines may be taken to relieve itching. (These do not kill the mites but may make you feel better)

C. General measures to decrease risk of reinfestation
1. Clothing, towels, and bed linens should be laundered (hot cycle) and dried on heat cycle or dry cleaned on day of treatment with medication.
2. If clothing items can't be washed or dry cleaned, separate them from the cleaned clothes and do not wear for at least 72 hours. Mites cannot exist for more than 2–3 days away from the body. You can decontaminate mattresses, sofas, rugs with over-the-counter sprays or powders.
3. Sexual partner and close personal or household contacts within the past month should be informed and referred to a health care provider for examination and treatment.

V. Patient Education

A. Follow the treatment regimen carefully.

B. Itching may persist for several weeks. If you do not respond to therapy and itching persists after one week, contact your health care provider to decide if further therapy is necessary.

C. Call health care provider if the infested areas bleed, do not seem to be healing, are swollen or warm to the touch or have drainage that looks like pus. You may have a secondary infection and need additional treatment.

D. Discontinue treatment and call your health care provider if you develop a rash after using medication.

VI. Follow-up

A. Call your health care provider if
   1. Lesions do not begin to resolve with treatment or you are getting new lesions.
   2. The treatment has brought out another skin condition, one you had previously, such as eczema or psoriasis.
   3. Lesions appear to be spreading and increasing in size.
   4. Lesions appear crusted.
B. Return to your health care provider if symptoms persist or new symptoms occur.
C. Return to your health care provider for evaluation of the success of the treatment, the need for retreatment.

From Hawkins, Roberto-Nichols, & Stanley-Haney, *Guidelines for Nurse Practitioners in Gynecologic Settings,* 8th edition, 2004, © Springer Publishing Company.

For Your Information: Stop Smoking

Smoking is the leading cause of preventable illness and early death in the United States. If you stop you can expect an increase in your life expectancy and improvement in your health.

Smokers are at greater risk for
- Strokes
- Oral cancers—tongue, lip, gum
- Chronic obstructive pul-monary disease
- Possibly breast cancer
- Cancer of the larynx
- Lung disease
- Heart disease and heart attacks
- Cervical cancer

Smokers also develop other smoking-related problems
- Pregnancy complications and losses
- Sinus infections
- Cataracts
- Impotence and infertility
- Abnormal Papanicolaou smears (dysplasia)
- Osteoporosis and bone density problems
- Premature skin wrinkling
- Gum disease and dental cavities
- Stained teeth and bad breath
- Poor circulation
- Poor tolerance for exercise
- High blood pressure

Family members are at greater risk for:
- lung cancer and heart disease
- children of smokers have higher incidences of sudden death syndrome, asthma and other lung problems, ear infections, colds, learning delays

The rewards of quitting are experienced quickly and long-term.

Within several weeks:
- Blood pressure drops
- Circulation improves
- Lung function improves
- Coughing, sinus infections, fatigue, and shortness of breath improve
- Number of colds decreases
- Energy level improves

After 1 year:
Excess risk of heart disease improves to half that of a smoker

After 5 years:
Lung cancer death rate decreases by almost half
Risk of cancer of the mouth, throat and esophagus is half that of a smoker

After 5–15 years:
Stroke risk is reduced to that of a nonsmoker

After 10 years:
Lung cancer death rate is similar to that of a nonsmoker

After 15 years:
The risk of coronary heart disease is that of a nonsmoker

Do you think you have a dependence on nicotine? Ask yourself the following questions:
• Do you smoke a cigarette first thing in the morning?
• Do you wake up to smoke a cigarette during the night?
• Do you smoke 5 or more cigarettes a day?
• Do you find it hard to not smoke in places where it is forbidden? Do you leave such places to smoke?
• Do you smoke more cigarettes in hours after you wake up than during the rest of the day?
• Do you smoke when you are ill?
If you answer yes to any of these questions you can consider yourself as having a nicotine problem

Want to quit? The following suggestions may help:
   Make the decision to stop smoking
   Think about why you want to stop smoking. Make a list of those reasons and the rewards associated with quitting. Keep this list with you and review it when you feel the urge to smoke
   Talk to your friends and family; ask for their support and encouragement
   Keep a journal. You can start it when you are making the decision to quit. Record each cigarette smoked, the time, the place, and the intensity of the craving and the reward of the cigarette. Think about the social cues associated with smoking and about how you will deal with these after you stop smoking. Record your thoughts and feelings. Doing this can help you identify your smoking "triggers" and assist you in adapting strategies and skills to get past those triggers. Continue recording your feelings in the journal after you have quit smoking

Avoid drinking alcohol. Alcohol will weaken your resolve

Clean your clothes, car, drapes and furniture to rid them of the smell of smoke

Throw out all cigarettes, ashtrays and smoking paraphernalia

Avoid being around other smokers

If possible, establish living space as "no smoking"

Increase exercise level (walking, weight lifting, yoga, Tai Chi). This assists in weight management, stress reduction, and general sense of well-being

Change your daily routine to avoid smoking triggers

Keep oral substitutes handy. Use low calorie vegetables and fruits; sugarless gum; toothpicks

Engage in activities that make smoking difficult, such as exercising, gardening, washing the car

Spend time in places where smoking is prohibited

Join a support group. Such groups are offered by Nicotine Anonymous, American Cancer Society, the American Lung Association and your local hospital or health care center.

Make an appointment with your health care provider and talk with her/him about your desire to stop smoking. Your provider can help you choose the most appropriate method to assist in breaking your habit. Choices available include:

- Nicotine replacements: gum, transdermal patches, nasal sprays, inhaler
- Zyban or Wellbutrin SR—a nonnicotine oral medication for smoking cessation treatment

Good luck in your journey to a smoke-free life. Remember, if you have a relapse and start smoking again, you can quit again. Many people need to try several times before they are successful. If this happens to you, don't be too hard on yourself. Review the above suggestions and begin again!

From Hawkins, Roberto-Nichols, & Stanley-Haney, *Guidelines for Nurse Practitioners in Gynecologic Settings,* 8th edition, 2004, © Springer Publishing Company.

For Your Information:
Stress or Urge Incontinence (Loss of Urine)

Stress and urge incontinence are caused by relaxation of the muscles and ligaments of the pelvic floor, that is, the muscles and ligaments that support the bladder, uterus, urethra (tube leading from the bladder to the outside), lower bowel, and vagina. Due to this relaxation, which is commonly the result of stretching due to childbirth and normal loss of muscle elasticity with aging, any stress such as laughing, coughing, or sneezing can cause involuntary loss of urine or the need to urinate urgently.

Urine can be irritating to the skin, so it is important to wash it off as soon as possible. The ammonia odor from urine leakage may be distressing also. Cotton underwear, the use of nondeodorized, unscented pantyliners, and use of prewetted wipes especially designed for the vaginal area will all help to prevent irritation, rashes, and cracking of skin. Skin cracking, irritation, and rashes will often increase the possibility of bacterial infection, especially in the warm, moist, genital area. Dusting with cornstarch will protect the skin from irritation. Only mild unperfumed soaps should be used, and used sparingly, as soap can be drying to skin. Perfumes (which are alcohol based) can increase the drying effect also and may cause an allergic reaction or chemical irritation to sensitive skin. Avoid bubble baths, vaginal hygiene products, and perfumed powders and talcums for the same reasons. Also avoid caffeine and smoking—both are bladder irritants.

Diary of Incontinence

Code numbers for WHEN
1. coughing/sneezing
2. laughing/crying
3. blowing nose
4. climbing stairs
5. bending over
6. sitting or resting
7. washing hands or dishes
8. other times

Code letters for AMOUNT
a. a drop or two
b. a teaspoonful
c. a tablespoonful
d. more than a tablespoonful
e. unable to estimate

Log of Times of Urine Loss, Circumstances of Loss, and Amount

	S	M	T	W	T	F	S
Week 1							
Week 2							
Week 3							
Week 4							

Kegel (Pelvic Floor Muscle Strengthening) Exercises

Practice contracting, holding, and relaxing each time you urinate until you can stop the flow completely and start and stop at will. Then proceed to this exercise program.

Day One
Repeated contracting, holding, and relaxing of pubococcygeus muscle (muscle band of perineal area) 4 times this day, 10 contractions and 10 relaxations each time).

Day Two
Increase to 20 contractions and 20 relaxations, 4 times this day.

Day Three
Increase to 30 contractions and 30 relaxations, 4 times this day.

Day Four
Increase to 40 contractions and 40 relaxations, 4 times this day.

Day Five
Increase to 70 contractions and 70 relaxations, 4 times this day.
Continue with Day Five regimen, so you are now doing the exercise 4 times
each day, contracting and relaxing 70 times at each of the 4 exercise periods.

Log for Pelvic Floor Exercise
(Place a checkmark in box for each exercise period each day)

	S	M	T	W	T	F	S
Week 1							
Week 2							
Week 3							
Week 4							

You may want to ask your clinician about vaginal cones to help you practice.
Graduated weighted cones are available to assist in Kegel exercises; a cone
is inserted in the vagina and Kegels are performed using the cones' feedback;
when weight of one cone can be maintained 15 minutes when walking or
standing, move to next weight. http://incontinent.com/home.htm

For Your Information:
Surgical Afterabortion Care

1. Someone should accompany you to the facility and wait there to take you home.
2. Normal physical activities may be resumed as soon as you feel ready.
3. You may be given some medication (methergine or ergotrate and/or an antibiotic) to take after your abortion. The first two medications will help your uterus return to its normal size and decrease bleeding. Antibiotics will help prevent infection. Follow the directions on how to take the pills. You may experience some uterine cramping (similar to menstrual cramps) with or without the methergine or ergotrate. It is okay to take acetaminophen (Tylenol, Datril, Tempra, Valadol, Valorin, Acephen) for cramps, or ibuprofen (Motrin, Advil).
4. Because of the risk of infection, it is important not to have intercourse or to insert anything into the vagina for 2–3 weeks. Other forms of sexual activity or orgasm will not be harmful to your body. Do not douche at all and do not use tampons for 2–3 weeks after the procedure, or until you stop bleeding. You may also be given 3 to 5 days of antibiotics to help prevent infection. Be sure to complete this medication.
5. Bleeding will probably cease after 3–4 days, but may last up to 3 weeks. There may be no bleeding at all. If bleeding exceeds two sanitary pads an hour or if you have a fever, call your health care provider or the facility where the procedure was performed.
6. Menstruation (period) should resume in 4–6 weeks but may take as long as 8 weeks and as short as 2 weeks.
7. You will be given an appointment with a clinician 2–3 weeks after your abortion. The clinician will check to see that your body is back to normal and will provide you with your desired form of contraception or schedule an appointment for a diaphragm or cap fitting 6 weeks after the abortion. An IUD can be inserted immediately after or within 3 weeks of a first trimester miscarriage or abortion. Depo-Provera® may be given the day of the abortion or within 5 days of the procedure. This appointment will also give you an opportunity to discuss your feelings. A friend or partner is welcome to see the practitioner with you if you wish.
8. If you have chosen to use a hormonal contraceptive method, begin on the Sunday following the abortion procedure. If not, be sure to use another form of contraception such as spermicide and condoms when you resume sexual relations. Remember, you will probably ovulate before you resume menses; you can become pregnant any time after your abortion. If

you received Depo-Provera after your abortion, it is still important to return for your after-abortion check-up 2 to 3 weeks after the procedure. You can then schedule your next Depo-Provera shot.

9. If you have a problem or concern, call the clinic or office at:

From Hawkins, Roberto-Nichols, & Stanley-Haney, *Guidelines for Nurse Practitioners in Gynecologic Settings,* 8th edition, 2004, © Springer Publishing Company.

For Your Information: Syphilis

I. Definition
Syphilis is a sexually transmitted disease that can affect any organ in the body such as the bones, brain or heart. It is spread by sexual contact and can also be passed on from mother to unborn baby. It is caused by the organism Treponema pallidum (T. pallidum).

II. Important Information
A. Any sexually active person can get infected with syphilis. An untreated person can spread syphilis for one year after being infected.
B. Symptoms can occur 10–90 days after sexual contact; average is 21 days.

III. Usual Signs and Symptoms. What You May Experience
A. *Primary Syphilis.* The first sign of syphilis is a painless chancre (sore) at the site of entry of the syphilis organism. The chancre may occur on the vulva, labia, opening to vagina, clitoris, cervix, nipple, lip, roof of mouth, opening to the urethra on the head of the penis, the shaft of the penis, the anal area, or the scrotum. You may notice painful and/or swollen glands in your groin area, on your neck or under your arms. The chancre will last 1–5 weeks and will go away even if not treated. If you are not diagnosed and treated you will progress to secondary syphilis.
B. *Secondary Syphilis.* In 2–8 weeks or as long as 6 months after the chancre appears (average is 6 weeks), you will notice a rash on any part of your body. It can even appear on the palms of your hands or the soles of your feet. You may also have some hair loss so that your head has a "moth eaten" look and you may lose part of your eyebrows. You may notice swollen glands in any part of your body, have a low-grade fever, a sore throat, headache, feel tired, have loss of appetite, and your joints may feel sore. This will last about 6 weeks and go away without treatment. If you are not diagnosed and treated you will progress to latent syphilis.
C. *Latent Syphilis.* You will have no symptoms, although 25% of persons may have a chancre again. During primary and secondary syphilis and early latency you are infectious to sexual partners. After 12 months have passed from the date of the initial infection, you are no longer infectious but the organism is in your blood. If you are not diagnosed and treated, you may remain in the latent stage for the rest of your life.
D. *Tertiary Syphilis.* One-third of persons infected with syphilis and not treated will go into the tertiary stage. In this stage your bones, skin, heart,

or nervous system including your brain, can be affected. Persons with tertiary syphilis can become unable to work or care for themselves and have a shortened life.

V. Diagnosis
A. History of sexual contact with a known infected person.
B. Blood tests and examination of material from a chancre under a special microscope to see the syphilis organism.

VI. Treatment
The treatment of choice is penicillin given by injection. For those allergic to penicillin, other antibiotics can be used. The amount and treatment will depend on the stage of the syphilis.

VII. Complications
A. Progression of the disease to tertiary stage.
B. Transmission of syphilis from a woman to her unborn baby causing congenital syphilis in the baby. Congenital means "present at birth." Congenital syphilis can cause permanent damage to the baby.

VIII. Patient Education
A. Follow-up for second dose of medications as instructed by health care provider.
B. Use barrier contraception (condom) each time you have sexual intercourse.
C. Look at your partner before having sex. If you see a sore (chancre), rash, swelling or discharge, consider a check up for both of you before having sex.
D. If you think you may have contracted syphilis or any other sexually transmitted disease (STD), avoid having sex and visit a local STD clinic.
E. If you are diagnosed with syphilis, report any sexual partners to your health care provider so they can be notified and treated, or notify them to seek treatment.
F. Return for testing after treatment for primary or secondary syphilis at 6 and 12 months; for latent syphilis, at 6, 12, and 24 months.
G. There is no immunity to syphilis, so you can be reinfected by an infected partner. Return for treatment if you believe you have been infected again.

Special Notes: _____

_____

Practitioner: _____

For more information for yourself or friends:
CDC (Centers for Disease Control) STD Hotline 1-800-227-8922; on line: http://www.cdc.gov
For phone numbers of free (or almost free) STD clinics see the "Community Service Numbers" in the government pages of your local phone book.

From Hawkins, Roberto-Nichols, & Stanley-Haney, *Guidelines for Nurse Practitioners in Gynecologic Settings,* 8th edition, 2004, © Springer Publishing Company.

For Your Information:
Trichomoniasis ("Trich")

I. Definition
Trichomoniasis is a parasitic infection occurring in the female vagina or urethra, or male urethra and prostate. The infection is believed to be sexually transmitted although it has been identified in non-sexually active women.

II. Signs and Symptoms
A. May appear 5–30 days after contact
B. In the female, symptoms include
   1. Odorous, greenish-yellow, frothy vaginal discharge (often fishy)
   2. Painful intercourse or urination
   3. Discomfort on tampon insertion
   4. Itchiness, redness, and irritation of the vulva and upper thigh
   5. Papanicolaou smear may be abnormal
   6. Some patients may not have any symptoms
C. In the male, symptoms include:
   1. Mild itch or discomfort in penis
   2. Moisture at tip of penis disappearing spontaneously
   3. Slight early morning discharge from penis before first urination
D. Untreated symptoms in the female or male can progress to infection of neighboring urinary and reproductive organs

III. Diagnosis
A. Female evaluation may include
   1. Vaginal examination to check for trichomoniasis and to rule out yeast infections and bacterial infections such as gonorrhea or bacterial vaginosis
   2. Blood test to rule out syphilis
B. Male evaluation may include
   1. Examination for gonorrhea or urinary tract infection
   2. Blood test for syphilis

IV. Treatment
The male should seek treatment after exposure to a partner with the infection. He may have no symptoms but could harbor the parasite in his urethra or prostate.

It is very important to report any medical conditions you have (especially seizure disorder) or medication you take regularly *before taking any treatment.*

V. Patient Education
A. *Take* no alcohol *during the 48 hours after treatment (medication)*
B. For minor side effects of medication (nausea, dizziness, or metallic taste), take medication with some food or milk
C. Advise sexual contact(s) to seek simultaneous treatment
D. Use condoms until all partners are treated

VI. Follow-up
Return to clinic if symptoms persist or new symptoms occur.
Special notes: _____
_____

Practitioner: _____

For more information, call: CDC STD Hotline: 1-800-227-8922: Phone numbers of free (or almost free) STD clinics are listed in the "Community Service Numbers" in the government pages of your local phone book. http://www.cdc.gov

From Hawkins, Roberto-Nichols, & Stanley-Haney, *Guidelines for Nurse Practitioners in Gynecologic Settings,* 8th edition, 2004, © Springer Publishing Company.

For Your Information: Vaginal Discharge

All women have a normal vaginal discharge called *leukorrhea;* the amount and consistency varies with each individual. This discharge is generally of a mucus-like consistency and tends to increase during the menstrual cycle up to two weeks before menstruation. A normal vaginal discharge may vary slightly in color, although it is usually clear or white, has no unpleasant odor, and is not itchy or irritating to the skin. Occasionally, a women may notice a fishy- or musty-smelling discharge if she has recently had intercourse. This may be due to dead sperm being cleansed from the vagina. If it occurs persistently, don't confuse it with a bacterial infection; have it checked. Some methods of birth control may affect the amount of normal vaginal discharge.

Hints for Prevention of Vaginal Infection

1. Even under the best conditions, vaginal infections sometimes occur. Don't panic if you discover that you have such an infection. Treat it with common sense—cleanliness, pelvic rest (no intercourse), and prescribed medications, and wear sensible clothing (cotton panties, no panty hose under slacks, no underwear to bed).
2. Cleanliness and personal hygiene are very important. Keep clean by bathing (shower or tub, but be sure you disinfect the tub before and after use) with soap and water. Vaginal deodorants can be irritating and are worthless in treating or preventing an infection. Avoid all use of feminine hygiene sprays and deodorants as well as deodorant or scented tampons, pads, panty liners, and toilet paper since these products tend to alter the natural environment of the vagina and make it more susceptible to irritation and/or infection.
3. *Douching is not recommended.* It can be harmful if done when an infection is already present. For example, the pressure of the douche solution may cause the infection to spread into the womb (uterus) and become even worse. Also, the douche solution removes the natural cleansing secretions of the vagina that normally help to maintain an environment that prevents infections. Indiscriminate douching with various commercial products may aggravate existing conditions, set up a chemical vaginitis, or contribute to a pelvic infection.
4. To prevent both vaginal and bladder infections from occurring, wear cotton underwear and no underwear while sleeping; change tampons or sanitary napkins after each urination or bowel movement; wipe yourself in the front first and then the back after going to the bathroom; urinate after intercourse and/or genital stimulation; and drink lots of fluids—at

355

least 6 glasses of water a day; cranberry juice may be helpful in avoiding infection.

Rules to Follow if You Have A Vaginal Infection
1. Take the entire course of medication exactly as prescribed. If you do not, the infection may "go underground" temporarily and then return and be more troublesome than before.
2. If you are treating an infection with vaginal cream or suppositories, remain lying down in bed for at least 15 minutes after insertion to allow the medication to spread deeply around the cervix, where it is needed. Standing up may cause the medicine to seep outward toward the vaginal opening.
3. Do not use tampons for protection because they will absorb the medication and reduce its effectiveness. Instead, use unscented external pads or small "minipads" to prevent staining underwear.
4. If you have a vaginal infection and use a diaphragm, soak diaphragm for 30 minutes with Betadine® scrub (not solution) or 70% rubbing alcohol, after using prescribed medication for 2 days and again when medication is completed. Use alcohol for your cervical cap.
5. Sexual relations should be avoided for at least one week, and preferably throughout the entire course of treatment. Intercourse can be very irritating to the inflamed vagina and cervix during an infection and can slow down the healing process. Also, the germs that cause your infection might spread to your partner; if the partner is male, he should use a condom during the entire treatment period.
6. Insufficient lubrication prior to intercourse may contribute significantly to vaginal infections (and bladder infections). Water-soluble jelly can be used for lubrication. There are also vaginal lubricants and moisturizers especially for peri- and postmenopausal women.

From Hawkins, Roberto-Nichols, & Stanley-Haney, *Guidelines for Nurse Practitioners in Gynecologic Settings,* 8th edition, 2004, © Springer Publishing Company.

Appendix B

Health History Form

Please fill out this confidential form so that the nurse practitioner, nurse midwife, physician assistant, and/or doctor can best help you meet your well woman and/or contraceptive needs.

Date ___/___/___

Name _____ Date of birth ___/___/___ Age _____

Address _____

Where can we contact you? _____

School status and major(if applicable) _____

Occupation _____

Do you have health insurance? _____ Which? _____

How did you find out about us? _____

1. Reason for appointment _____

2. Are you having any of the following now?

Frequent headaches ____   Allergies ____
Shortness of breath ____   Constipation ____
Breast lumps, discharge ____   Diarrhea ____
Seizures or fits ____   Yellow skin or eyes ____
Coughing spells ____   Crying spells ____
Dizzy spells ____   Fatigue ____
Loss of urine ____   Depression ____
Pain or swelling in legs ____   Varicose veins ____

Trouble with eyes, blurred vision, double vision ____

Weight changes-under or overweight ____

Phlebitis or clots in veins ____

Difficulty starting urination ____

School or social problems ____

Concern about sexually transmitted disease, HIV/AIDS ____

Do you smoke cigarettes? How many a day? ____

When did you start? _____

Do you drink alcohol? How many drinks daily? ____

How many drinks weekly? ____ Do you use street drugs? ____

If yes, which and how often? _____

3. If you have ever had or still have any of the following, please describe, including date of onset, treatment, etc. Please place a check mark on the line on the *extreme left side* if your answer is yes.

	Date of Onset,
Yes	*Treatment, Other Details*

___ rheumatic fever/frequent strep throats _____

___ heart murmur _____

___ feeling of depression or anxiety _____

___ German measles (Rubella) _____

___ cancer _____

___ high blood pressure _____

___ thyroid trouble _____

___ epilepsy _____

___ aspirin sensitivity _____

___ asthma _____

___ ulcer/gastrointestinal disease _____

___ glaucoma/eye problem _____

___ diabetes _____

___ sickle cell anemia or trait _____

___ hepatitis or liver problems _____

___ infectious mononucleosis _____

___ pelvic inflammatory disease or
       ovary/uterus problem _____

___ hyperlipidemia (high cholesterol) _____

___ arthritis or Lupus Erythematosus _____

___ migraine headaches _____

___ constipation _____

___ urinary tract infection or
       pain and burning on urination _____

___ vaginal infection, discharge, or sores _____

___ abnormal Pap smear _____

___ sexually transmitted disease
       including warts (HPV), AIDS (HIV) _____

___ any other illness not listed _____

4. List all the medications (prescription and non-prescription including vitamins and botanicals) you are now taking regularly _____

_____

Are you allergic to any medication, food, other substance?
____ If yes, what? _____

5. Have you ever been a patient in a hospital? ____ If yes, when and for what reasons? _____

6. Family History
   Circle if any of the members of your family have:

anxiety, depression	high blood pressure	diabetes
migraine headaches	sickle cell disease	cancer (type)
breast disease	varicose veins	phlebitis (blood clots)
(cancer)	hyperlipidemia	hepatitis
heart disease	(high cholesterol)	stroke
(heart attack)	lung disease/asthma	thyroid
stomach/bowel/gall	seizures (fits)	problems
bladder problems	birth defects	

7. Did your mother or you ever take DES (diethylstilbestrol) or any other medicine when pregnant (with you)? _____ Please explain: _____
   _____

8. *Menstrual History*
   Last period began on _ Age when had first period
   Do you have cramps with your period? ____ what treatment do you use for your cramps? _____
   How often do your periods occur? _____ How long does your period last? ____ days. On the heaviest day of your period how many pads or tampons do you use? ____ Do you spot or bleed between your periods? ____ Have you missed a period recently? ____ Have there been any changes in your periods over the last year? ____ Do you have premenstrual symptoms? ____ including: depression ____, fatigue ____, weight gain ____, headache ____, irritability ____, breast tenderness ____, increased appetite ____, other ____

9. Date of last pelvic (internal) exam _____ Never had exam _____
   Date of last Pap test _____ Never had test _____
   Results _____

10. Have you in the past or are you currently using:
    douches ____ deodorant ____ tampons ____ feminine ____ hygiene sprays
    ____

11. *Sexual Activity and Birth Control*
    Are you having sexual relations now? ____ How often? ____
    Have you been sexually active in the past? ____
    Age at first intercourse ____ Your sexual preference: male ____ female ____ both ____ Do you have pain during or after sexual relations? ____ bleeding? ____ any other problems? ____ If you have a male partner, are you using any birth control method? ____ If yes, which one(s) and for how long? ____ Does your partner use condoms? ____ If yes, how often? ____ Are you satisfied with your present method? ____ Have you ever had a problem, including pregnancy, with a birth control method? ____ If yes, explain _____

List in order of use

Method	Dates of Use	Problems or Comments
1.		
2.		
3.		

12. *Pregnancy History*
    Have you ever been pregnant? _____ How many children born alive? _____
    Dates of miscarriages (abortion, stillbirth) _____ Number of Cesarean sections _____ When did your last pregnancy end? _____ Did you have any problems during or after your pregnancies? _____

13. Do you plan to have children in the future? _____

14. Have you ever been sexually molested/assaulted/harassed or been a victim of incest? _____

15. Is there violence in any of your relationships? _____

16. Are you afraid of a partner or someone else? _____

From Hawkins, Roberto-Nichols, & Stanley-Haney, *Guidelines for Nurse Practitioners in Gynecologic Settings,* 8th edition, 2004, © Springer Publishing Company.

Appendix C

Gynecological Annual Exam Form

ACCT#_____   NAME:_____   MARITAL STATUS: M SEP S W D

DATE:_____   G___ P___ ___ ___ ___   AGE:____   SMOKER: Y / N PKPD___   LAST TETANUS BOOSTER:_____

BRCA ASSESSMENT: _____ 5 YEAR _____ LIFETIME   PMD_____

S: MENSES: R IRR DAYS____ IMB: Y / N

MEDICAL PROBLEMS:_____

_____

_____

_____

O: LMP:_____ CONTRACEPTION:_____ ALLERGIES_____

LATEX ALLERGY: Y / N

LAST PAP:_____ MEDS:_____

VITAMINS_____ HERBS_____

SUPPLEMENTS_____

LAST MAMM:_____ BONE DENSITY:_____

HT_____ WT_____ BP_____ URINE_____ HGB_____

GENERAL	N	ABN
APPEARANCE		
SKIN		
HEENT		
THYROID		
LYMPH NODES		
HEART		
LUNGS		
EXTREMITIES		
VARICOSITIES		
MUSCLE SKELETAL		
NEUROLOGICAL		
ABDOMEN		
BREASTS		
EXT GENITALIA		
VAGINA		
CERVIX		
UTERUS		
ADNEXA		
RECTUM (HEMORRHOIDS)		

FAMILY HX:

BREAST CA	Y	N
COLON CA	Y	N
OSTEOPOROSIS	Y	N
CARDIOVASCULAR	Y	N

A: DIAGNOSIS / SUMMARY:_____

_____

P: 1. EDUCATION: REVIEWED: SBE___   BENEFIT OF CALCIUM SUPPLEMENT_____

RISK /BENEFIT OF:_____

SMOKING CESSATION____   DIET & EXERCISE___

2. TREATMENT: PAP SMEAR_____

3. RECOMMEND: COLON CA SCREEN_____   MAMMOGRAM_____   BMD____ U/S____ SPECIALTY / PMD_____

_____

_____

4. NEXT APPT:_____

SIGNATURE:_____

MD/NP

From Ellington Ob/Gyn Associates. Used with permission 2002.

Appendix D

Informed Consent Forms

(Includes Patient Information)

Oral Contraceptives
Injectable Contraception
Diaphragm
IUD
Emergency Contraception

Informed Consent for Oral Contraceptives

(May also be used as informational handout)

I. Mechanism of Action
An oral, systemic method of preventing conception which acts by
A. Suppressing ovulation
B. Producing changes in the endometrium that make it unreceptive to implantation
C. Producing a thickened cervical mucus

II. Benefits of the Method
A. Highly effective: 99.66% for combination pill (0.1 pregnancy/year); 97% for progestin only
B. Sexual spontaneity
C. Regulated menstrual flow
D. Lighter flow and less cramping
E. Decreased incidence of uterine and ovarian cancers
F. Relief of symptoms associated with peri-menopause

III. Risk of Method
A. Minor side effects (these are rare and usually subside after several months of pill use; may be alleviated by changing type of pill or discontinuing pill). Listed are a few more common, although rare, side effects:
   1. Nausea (try taking pill with a meal or with milk; with severe nausea/vomiting, use back-up method of birth control such as condoms)
   2. Spotting
   3. Decreased menstrual flow and sometimes missed periods
   4. May have more problems with yeast infections or vaginal discharges
   5. Depression or mood changes
   6. Acne or increase in acne
   7. Headaches (not severe)
B. Major side effects (rare in women under 40 who are nonsmokers)
   1. Blood clots in legs, lungs; stroke
   2. Hypertension (high blood pressure)
   3. Gallbladder disease
   4. Heart attack (smokers age 35 and older))
   5. Smoking doubles risk factors associated with pill use. These side effects are characterized by the following danger signals (if they occur, seek medical care *IMMEDIATELY*): pain, redness or swelling of the legs or a localized tender red spot warm to the touch may indicate a blood clot in a vein; persistent and severe headaches; chest pain and/

or difficulty breathing; blurred vision, flashing vision; blindness; abdominal pain.

IV. Contraindications (reasons you may not be able to take the pill)

Woman with a history of any of the following conditions may not be able to use oral contraceptives

A. Thromboembolic disorders (blood clot) in leg, lungs
B. Impaired liver function at present time; liver problems
C. Cancer of breast or reproductive system
D. Hypertension (high blood pressure); uncontrolled, or smoking and high blood pressure
E. Hyperlipidemia (high cholesterol)
F. Stroke
G. Coronary artery disease
H. Major surgery on legs or with prolonged immobility
I. 35 years or older and currently a smoker
J. Pregnancy—known or suspected
K. Undiagnosed genital bleeding
L. Taking certain prescription drugs
M. Diabetes with vascular (blood vessel) disease
N. Headaches, migraines with neurological symptoms

V. Alternate Methods of Birth Control

A. Abstinence
B. Sterilization; natural family planning
C. Condom used with contraceptive cream, jelly or foam, contraceptive suppositories or tablets, vaginal film, contraceptive gel
D. Intrauterine device (IUD)
E. Diaphragm with contraceptive cream or jelly, FemCap
F. Cervical cap
G. Female condom
H. Depo-Provera®
I. Contraceptive patch, ring

VI. Inquiries are encouraged

Please ask us questions; a change in decision does not create a problem

VII. Explanation of method

A. Way in which oral contraceptives are prescribed
   1. A complete physical examination is done, including blood pressure, weight, urinalysis, gynecologic examination with Papanicolaou smear (unless one was done within the past year)

2. Review side effects and dangers of use; review packet
3. If requested to do so by your health care provider, review and sign an informed consent for oral contraceptives
4. You may transfer your records from another clinic or health care professional's office
B. Way in which pill is taken
   1. Start taking your first package of pills as directed by your nurse practitioner
   2. Oral contraceptive pills are *always* started initially at the same time as your period; you begin the Sunday of the week your period starts even if you are still bleeding
   3. Swallow one pill at the *same time* daily
   4. A second form of contraception is recommended for the first 7 days after starting the pill (unless specified differently)
   5. Some medications can decrease effectiveness or cause other pill-related problems (e.g., spotting). Always mention to your health care provider and pharmacist that you are on oral contraceptives prior to starting any other medication. Also tell us if you are on any medications prior to starting oral contraceptives. Use a back-up method of birth control if you have any doubts about the possibility of a drug interaction.
   6. If you are taking prescribed antibiotics for an illness, you should continue your pill but use a back-up method.
   7. Breakthrough bleeding (spotting) is common during the first few months a woman is on an oral contraceptive; do not be alarmed if you experience this.
      a. If you experience spotting after several months of pill use, make sure you are taking the pill correctly, as directed below. But make sure you discuss this at the time of your first pill check.
      b. If the pill is taken improperly, breakthrough bleeding may occur. You must make every effort to take your pill at the same time *every day.*
         1) If you take your pill more than 6 hours late, take the pill when you remember it; you are also advised to use a second method of birth control for the next 7 days.
         2) If you miss one pill: take the pill when you remember and then take the scheduled pill at the regular time. A second method of birth control is recommended for 7 days.
         3) If you miss 2 pills in the first 2 weeks of a pill pack: take two pills at the regular time and then take two pills at the regular time the next day, and use a second method of birth control for 7 days.
         4) If you miss 2 pills in the third week, or if you miss 3 or more pills at any time, and you start packets on Sunday, take a pill

each day until Sunday, then discard the remainder of that pack and start a new pack immediately, omitting the hormone-free week. (If you don't start a new pack on Sundays, throw away rest of pill pack and start a new pack that day.) **A back-up method of birth control should be used for the first 7 days of this new pill pack.**

5) If you miss 1 or more pills and used no back-up method and have no period, call to discuss possible pregnancy test.

6) If you aren't sure what to do about missed pills, use a back-up method any time you have sex and keep taking a birth control pill (hormone pill) each day until you can talk with your health care provider.

C. Occasionally, withdrawal bleeding (your period) does not occur during the week of non-hormone pills (placebos).

1. If this happens to you and all pills have been taken properly, continue with next pill cycle. If you miss two periods, start your third pill cycle but call your clinician for advice.

2. If this happens to you and you have taken your pill late or forgotten to take it, and did not use a second birth control method, start your next pill packet but call your clinician for advice

D. If you experience severe vomiting and/or diarrhea, use a back-up method of birth control since the pill may not have been absorbed properly.

I have read the above material; it has been fully explained. I have been given the opportunity to ask questions and I understand the information. I have chosen to use an oral contraceptive.

Signed _____ Date _____

Witness _____ Date _____

Danger Signals Associated with Pill Use
Abdominal pain (severe)
Chest pain (severe) or shortness of breath
Headaches (severe)
Eye problems such as blurred vision or loss of vision
Severe leg pain (calf or thigh)
Contact us at ( ) _____ if you develop any of the above problems.

NOTE: Birth control pills can be used as emergency contraception. Ask your health care provider; check directions in pill packet; call 1-888-NOT-2-LATE; http://not-2-late.com

From Hawkins, Roberto-Nichols, & Stanley-Haney, *Guidelines for Nurse Practitioners in Gynecologic Settings,* 8th edition, 2004, © Springer Publishing Company.

Consent Form for Injectable Contraception (Depo-Provera®)

(May also be used as an informational handout)

Definition
Depo-Provera® is a hormonal substance that prevents ovulation from occurring. It is injected intramuscularly every 12 weeks into the muscle of the upper arm or buttocks.

How It Works
The hormones in the injection suppress ovulation (egg production), for 12 weeks.

How Effective Is It?
Failure rate is less than one pregnancy per 100 women per year when women return for injections every 12 weeks (Depo) and when injection is done in the first 5 days of menses (bleeding).

Why Choose This Method?
A. Consider use of other methods and whether their side effects make you prefer this method
B. Desire for long-term contraceptive—12-week
C. Desire for reversible method (ability to stop injections)
D. Desire for method disconnected from intercourse—nothing to take or put in

Why You Might Not Be a Candidate
A. Known or suspected pregnancy
B. Unexplained abnormal vaginal bleeding
C. Known breast cancer
D. Known sensitivity to Depo-Provera® or any of its ingredients (have you ever had an allergic reaction to local anesthetic at the dentist?)

Things to Consider Before Choosing Depo-Provera®
A. Depression
B. Abnormal mammogram
C. Kidney disease
D. Hypertension (high blood pressure)
E. Planned pregnancy in near future

F. Gallbladder disease

G. Mild cirrhosis (liver disease)

H. Do you regularly use any prescription drugs or herbals—we need to check possible interactions with Depo-Provera®

Side Effects You Might Experience

A. Weight gain or loss; change in appetite

B. Menstrual irregularity—possibly no periods by second or third shot

C. Headaches

D. Abdominal bloating

E. Breast tenderness

F. Tiredness, weakness

G. Dizziness

H. Depression, nervousness

I. Nausea

J. No hair growth or loss or thinning of hair; increased hair growth on face or body

K. Skin rash or increased acne

L. Increased or decreased sex drive

Explanation of Method and Assessment

Depo-Provera® is injected intramuscularly in one 150 milligram dose every 12 weeks for as long as contraceptive effect is desired. It is injected in the first 5 days of the menstrual cycle (after onset of menses), within 5 days postpartum.

Use of This Method and Warning Signs

1. Drug interactions are possible when using Depo-Provera® with other prescription drugs. Always check with your physician or nurse practitioner and pharmacist for such possible interactions before taking any other prescription drug; Depo-Provera® is a medication and you need to list it in your health history.

2. Warning signs to report to your health care provider (physician or nurse practitioner):

   Sharp chest pain, coughing of blood, sudden shortness of breath

   Sudden severe headache, vomiting, dizziness, or fainting

   Visual disturbance (double vision, blurred vision, spots before your eyes or speech disturbance (slurred, unable to speak)

   Weakness or numbness in arm or leg

   Severe pain or swelling in calf or leg

Unusually heavy vaginal bleeding (unlike usual periods)
Severe pain or tenderness in lower abdomen, pelvis
Persistent pain, pus, or bleeding at injection site

Follow-up Care of Yourself

A. Visit your health care provider every 12 weeks for injection of Depo-Provera
B. The first visit should take place during first 5 days of your menses (period)
C. Review any side effects or danger signs with your health care provider
D. Review your menstrual cycles with health care provider
E. Have a Pap smear every year along with a complete physical examination including pelvic and breast examinations
F. Depo-Provera® provides no protection against sexually transmitted diseases (including AIDS) or vaginal infections, so consider using condoms to protect yourself.

I have read the above and have been given a copy of this consent form and the manufacturer's information, and I agree to have Depo-Provera®

Patient's signature _____ Date _____

Witness's signature _____ Date _____

Informed Consent for a Diaphragm

(May also be used as an informational handout)

I. Mechanism of Action

A contraceptive diaphragm is a shallow rubber cup with a flexible rim which is placed in the vagina so as to cover the cervix. It functions as both a mechanical barrier and a receptacle for spermicidal cream or jelly which must be used to ensure effectiveness.

II. Benefits of the Method

A. Effectiveness rate ranges from 80–95%: theoretically, 95%. 80–85% use effectiveness (due to user failure)
B. No chemicals are taken internally

III. Risks of the Method

A. Allergic response to the rubber and/or spermicidal agent
B. Foul-smelling discharge from leaving diaphragm in place too long (diaphragm should not be left in place longer than 24 hours)
C. Toxic shock syndrome has been reported in association with diaphragm use during menses. To avoid this, do not leave your diaphragm in place for more than 24 hours and follow use precautions at the end of these instructions

IV. Contraindications (reasons for not using diaphragm)

A. Inability to achieve satisfactory fitting
B. You are unable to learn correct insertion technique
C. Allergy to rubber or spermicidal agent
D. Inconvenience of method (e.g., lack of sexual spontaneity, timing, messiness, etc.)
E. Repeated bladder infections (cystitis)
F. Chronic constipation (causes discomfort for some users)

V. Alternative Birth Control Methods

A. Abstinence
B. Sterilization
C. Oral contraceptives (birth control pills, mini pills)
D. Intrauterine device
E. Condom used with contraceptive cream, foam, gel, suppositories or vaginal film
F. Cervical cap, FemCap
G. Natural family planning

H. Female condom
I. Depo-Provera®
J. Contraceptive patch, ring

VI. Explanation of the Method

A. How a diaphragm is prescribed
  1. A complete physical examination including Papanicolaou smear is necessary unless one has been done within the past year. A pelvic examination (bimanual) will be done at the time the diaphragm is fitted
  2. If required by your health provider, review and sign an informed consent similar to this one prior to your initial prescription
B. How a diaphragm is used
  1. How it works
    a. Inserted prior to intercourse to fit snugly in vagina
    b. Holds spermicidal cream or jelly or vaginal film against cervix and kills sperm
    c. Diaphragm is to be left in place for 8 hours after last intercourse
    d. No douching for 8 hours after intercourse
    e. Prior to repeated intercourse, additional jelly or cream should be applied with applicator to outside of diaphragm or another vaginal film should be inserted
    f. Effective immediately upon insertion and up to 4 hours without adding more cream or jelly or film, or for one intercourse (Some sources suggest 6 hours for c., d., and f.)
  2. Technique for use
    a. Empty your bladder, wash your hands carefully whenever you insert or remove your diaphragm
    b. Apply approximately 1 tablespoon spermicidal cream or jelly into the dome of the diaphragm and spread around the dome; cream or jelly need not be spread on the rim or outside of diaphragm
    c. Fold in half and insert into vagina like a tampon
    d. With index finger check rim at pubic arch and make sure cervix is covered
    e. To remove (at proper time), hook finger around rim and pull diaphragm out
  3. Care of diaphragm
    a. Wash with warm water and mild soap after removal
    b. Dry thoroughly
    c. Store in dry place (allowing it to dry thoroughly before putting it in a case keeps rubber in better condition longer and prevents odor; powder lightly with cornstarch)

    d. Soak in rubbing alcohol (70%) for 30 minutes after use following treatment for vaginal infection

VII. Diaphragm Check

A. We encourage you to return to the office one week after fitting for diaphragm check
B. If you lose or gain 10–15 pounds (or if diaphragm fit seems to change)
C. If you have a miscarriage, abortion, or a baby
D. If you have any kind of pelvic surgery
E. If you experience problems urinating or trouble moving your bowels with diaphragm in place

VIII. Inquiries are Encouraged

Please feel free to ask us questions at any time!

You may change your mind about a birth control method at any time.

I have read the above material; it has been explained fully. I have been given the opportunity to ask questions and I understand the information. I have chosen to use the diaphragm.

Patient's signature _____ Date _____

Witness's signature _____ Date _____

Toxic Shock Syndrome

Toxic shock syndrome has been reported in association with diaphragm use during menses. It is recommended that if you use your diaphragm during menses, you observe handwashing recommendations carefully, use tampons only during heaviest days (not super-absorbent type—see tampon package labeling) and monitor yourself carefully for any signs of toxic shock syndrome.

Danger Signals Associated with Possible Toxic Shock Syndrome
    Fever (temperature 100° F and above)
    Diarrhea
    Vomiting
    Muscle ache
    Rash (sunburn-like)

Contact us at ( )_____ if you develop any of the above problems (and don't use your diaphragm—remove at once)

If your diaphragm slips out of place or comes out, you can call 1-888-NOT-2-LATE for information on emergency contraception.

From Hawkins, Roberto-Nichols & Stanley-Haney, *Guidelines for Nurse Practitioners in Gynecological Settings,* 8th edition, 2004, © Springer Publishing Company.

Informed Consent for an Intrauterine Device (IUD)

(May also be used as informational handout)

I. Definition/Mechanism of Action

An intrauterine device consists of a sterile body placed in the uterus to prevent fertilization. This is accomplished through several mechanisms of action, depending on the type of device:

A. A local sterile inflammatory response to the foreign body (the IUD) causes a change in the cellular makeup of the uterine lining

B. A possible increase in the local production of prostaglandins may increase endometrial activity

C. Alteration in uterine and tubal transport of egg

D. Change in cervical mucus causing barrier to sperm penetration

E. Mirena® may stop release of an egg but this is not the primary way it works

II. Benefits of the Method

A. Encourages sexual spontaneity

B. Effectiveness rate, theoretically, 97–99%

C. Semi-permanent (depending on the type of device); replacement time varies but all devices are effective for at least one year; one device lasts 10 years

III. Risks of Method

A. Major risks
   1. Involuntary expulsion (approximately 6%)
   2. Pelvic inflammatory disease
   3. Ectopic pregnancy (outside of the uterus)
   4. Uterine perforation
   5. Pregnancy

B. Minor risks
   1. Increased menstrual flow
   2. Increased dysmenorrhea (cramps)
   3. String may cause some discomfort to partner

IV. Reasons for Not Using an Intrauterine Device (IUD)

   1. Active pelvic infection (acute or subacute) including known or suspected gonorrhea or chlamydia
   2. Known or suspected pregnancy
   3. Recent or recurrent pelvic infection

4. Purulent cervicitis, untreated acute cervicitis, or vaginosis
5. Undiagnosed genital bleeding
6. Uterine cavity not suitable for IUD insertion
7. History of ectopic pregnancy (pregnancy outside uterus)
8. Diabetes mellitus—can use ParaGard® IUD
9. Allergy to copper (known or suspected) or diagnosed Wilson's Disease—can use Mirena® IUD
10. Abnormal Pap; cervical or uterine cancer, precancer
11. Impaired response to infection (diabetes, steroid treatment, immunocompromised patients such as those with HIV/AIDS)
12. Presence of previously inserted IUD
13. Genital actinomycosis—chronic infection of genital area

V. Reasons IUD May Not Be Best Choice or Require Careful Monitoring With Health Care Provider

1. Multiple sexual partners or partner has multiple partners
2. In very rural areas, emergency treatment difficult to obtain
3. Cervical opening resistant to inserting IUD
4. Impaired blood clotting response
5. Uterine cavity too small, too large
6. Endometriosis
7. Fibroids in uterus
8. Polyps in uterine lining (endometrium)
9. Severe dysmenorrhea (Mirena® IUD may help)
10. Heavy or prolonged menstrual bleeding without anemia; consider oral iron or nutritional changes to prevent anemia
11. Unable to check for IUD string
12. Concerns for future fertility
13. Postpartum or infected abortion within the past 3 months
14. History of pelvic uterine infection
15. Valvular heart disease infection

VI. Alternatives

A. Abstinence
B. Sterilization
C. Birth control pills
D. Cervical Cap
E. Natural family planning
F. Depo-Provera®
G. Female condom
H. Contraceptive ring, patch

I. Diaphragm and spermicidal cream or jelly, film, FemCap
J. Condom used with contraceptive cream, foam, suppositories, gcl, or vaginal film

VII. Explanation of the Method

A. How the intrauterine device may work (no one is quite sure), but there are several theories:
   1. Motility of the egg in fallopian tube is altered
   2. A sterile inflammatory response to the IUD causes a change in the cells of the uterine lining
   3. A change in the cervical mucus causing a barrier to sperm
B. What you should know about caring for your IUD
   1. Know the type of device you have in place
   2. Know when your device should be replaced
   3. Learn how to check the string which extends from the center of the cervix into the vaginal canal
   4. Check the string frequently the first few months and then after each period
   5. Do not let your partner pull on the string
   6. Never try to remove IUD yourself
   7. Obtain your 6–week check-up after insertion of the device
   8. Get a check-up every year including a Pap smear
   9. Depending on your normal menstrual cycle, if you miss a period, consult your care provider for possible pregnancy
C. What to expect
   1. Possible increase in menstrual flow, menstrual cramping
      Remember: if this condition becomes intolerable, you have the option of having your IUD removed by a clinician
D. Side effects to be reported *immediately*
   1. Late period or absence of period
   2. Abdominal or pelvic pain (severe)
   3. Elevated temperature, chills (not due to illness)
   4. Unpleasant vaginal discharge (smelly, foul, bloody, or greenish color)
   5. Unusual vaginal bleeding (heavy period, clotting)
E. Insertion
   1. IUDs usually inserted within 7 days of menses
   2. Should have negative gonococcus and Chlamydia cultures prior to insertion (within 30 days); consider culture for Strep. Group B
   3. Must have recent (within the year) normal Pap smear
   4. May have some discomfort and dizziness with insertion
   5. May have spotting for several months after insertion

6. Although the IUD is effective immediately, it is recommended that intercourse not take place for 24 hours

VII. Inquiries are encouraged! Ask us questions at any time.

I have read the above material; it has been explained fully. I have been given the opportunity to ask questions and I understand the information. I have chosen to use the IUD _____ type

Signed _____ Witness _____
Date _____

Danger Signals Associated with the Use of the IUD

    Late period or absence of period
    Abdominal pain (severe)
    Elevated temperature, chills (not due to illness, e.g., flu)
    Unpleasant vaginal discharge (smelly, foul, bloody, or greenish color)
    Unusual vaginal bleeding (heavy period, clotting)

Contact us or a care provider immediately if above danger signs develop!

From Hawkins, Roberto-Nichols, & Stanley-Haney, *Guidelines for Nurse Practitioners in Gynecologic Settings,* 8th edition, 2004, © Springer Publishing Company.

Informed Consent and Information Handout for Emergency Contraception (EC)

Definition
Emergency contraception (EC), often known as the "morning after pill," is the use of birth control pills to prevent pregnancy after a contraceptive method has failed or because there was no contraception. There are now 2 products just for EC: Preven (equivalent to combination oral contraceptives) and Plan B (progestin only).

How It Works
If used within the first 72 hours after unprotected sexual intercourse, EC probably works because of one or more of the following reasons:
- Progestational hormones in the pills interfere with the sperms' ability to travel up through the uterus and into the fallopian tube to fertilize the egg; also they affect the growth of the ovary's follicles
- Estrogen hormones in the pills are thought to interfere with or disrupt ovulation (release of an egg by the ovary)

How Effective Is It?
If used within 72* hours after sex without birth control protection, EC is greater than 90% effective.

Benefits
- Pregnancy prevention
- Inexpensive
- Relatively noninvasive

Disadvantages
- May not be appropriate for women with certain medical conditions
- Pregnancy may occur due to:
  1. Fertilized egg already implanted in the uterus
  2. Too much time between unprotected sex and taking EC
  3. Failure of the emergency contraception
  4. Must be used within 72* hours of unprotected sex

Risks and Side Effects
- Nausea and/or vomiting
- Breast tenderness

---

*May be up to 120 hours—check with clinician.

- Irregular bleeding
- Headache

You May Not Be Able to Take EC if You Have:
- An active liver disease
- Unexplained bleeding from the vagina
- An already established pregnancy
- History of blood clots, inflammation in the veins, or cancer of the breast, uterus or ovaries

Alternative EC
- Progestin-only oral contraceptives used as EC
- Insertion of a copper-releasing device IUD

How EC is Prescribed
- Pelvic examination as appropriate (to be determined by you and your health care provider)
- If rape or sexual assault occurred, specimens can be collected if desired by you and your health care provider
- Pregnancy test
- Testing for sexually transmitted diseases (STDs) if desired, or if recommended by health care provider
- Blood pressure

Ways in which EC is taken
1. Take 2 Preven® tablets within 72 hours of unprotected intercourse and follow directions in 4–7. Take second pills 12 hours later.
2. Take one Plan B pill within 72 hours of unprotected intercourse and follow directions 4–7. Take second pill 12 hours later.
3. Take _____ birth control pills within 72 hours of unprotected intercourse. Do not take the pills on a empty stomach—eat a snack such as juice or milk and crackers and take the pills 20 minutes later. Take _____ birth control pills 12 hours after the first dose.
4. If you vomit within an hour after taking the birth control pills, follow the instructions your health care provider gives you.
5. Talk with your provider about methods of contraception you might be interested in for ongoing protection. Emergency contraception is just that— for emergencies—and is not recommended for routine use. Some birth control methods can be started immediately or the day after using EC. Methods vary in how soon they become effective.

6. Report any of the warning signs listed below to your health care provider at once.
7. After using EC, return to your health care provider as directed for a checkup, particularly if you have not had a normal menstrual period.

I have read the above material. I have been given the opportunity to ask questions and I fully understand the information. I have chosen to use emergency contraception.

Signed _____ Date _____

Witness _____ Date _____

Danger Signals Associated with EC:
Abdominal pain (severe)
Chest pain (severe), arm pain, or shortness of breath
Headaches (severe)
Eye problems such as blurred or double vision, loss of vision
Severe leg pain (calf or thigh)
Contact us at (   )_____ if you develop any of the above danger signals.
Emergency Contraception hotline: 800-584-9911, 888-NOT-2-LATE; websites http://not-2–late.com
www.go2planB.com

From Hawkins, Roberto-Nichols, & Stanley-Haney, *Guidelines for Nurse Practitioners in Gynecologic Settings,* 8th edition, 2004, © Springer Publishing Company.

Appendix E
Danger Assessment

Several risk factors have been asociated with homicides (murder) of both batterers and battered women in research that has been conducted after the killings have taken place. We cannot predict what will happen in your case, but we would like you to be aware of the danger of homicide in situations of severe battering and for you to see how many of the risk factors apply to your situation. (The "he" in the questions refer to your husband, partner, ex-husband, ex-partner or whoever is currently physically hurting you).

Please check **YES** or **NO** for each question below.

YES NO

___ ___ 1. Has the physical violence increased in frequency over the past year?

___ ___ 2. Has the physical violence increased in severity over the past year and/or has a weapon or threat with a weapon been used?

___ ___ 3. Does he ever try to choke you?

___ ___ 4. Is there a gun in the house?

___ ___ 5. Has he ever forced you into sex when you did not wish to do so?

___ ___ 6. Does he use drugs? By drugs I mean "uppers" or amphetamines, speed, angel dust, cocaine, "crack," or street drugs, heroin, or mixtures.

___ ___ 7. Does he threaten to kill you and/or do you believe he is capable of killing you?

___ ___ 8. Is he drunk every day or almost every day? (In terms of quantity of alcohol.)

___ ___ 9. Does he control almost all of your daily activities? For instance, does he tell you whom you can be friends with, how much money you can take with you shopping or when you can take the car?
(If he tries, but you do not let him, check here _____.)

___ ___ 10. Have you ever been beaten by him while you were pregnant?
(If never pregnant by him, check here _____.)

___ ___ 11. Is he violently and constantly jealous of you?
(For instance, does he say, "If I can't have you, no one can?")

___ ___ 12. Have you ever threatened or tried to commit suicide?

___ ___ 13. Has he ever threatened or tried to commit suicide?
___ ___ 14. Is he violent outside of the home?
___   TOTAL YES ANSWERS

THANK YOU. PLEASE TALK TO YOUR NURSE, ADVOCATE OR COUNSELOR ABOUT WHAT THE RESULTS OF THE DANGER ASSESSMENT MEAN IN TERMS OF YOUR SITUATION.

Note: Adapted from Campbell, J. (1986). Nursing assessment for risk of homicide with battered women. *Advances in Nursing Science, 8*(4), 36–51. Used with permission.

Appendix F
Self-Assessment of AIDS (HIV) Risk*

1. Do you use injectable drugs? Does your sexual partner(s)? Do you or your partner(s) have a partner(s) who uses injectable drugs? How about in the past?
2. If you or your partner(s) use injectable drugs, do you ever share needles or syringes? How about in the past? Have you ever used intranasal drugs (snorted)?
3. Did you or your partner(s) have a blood transfusion between 1975 and 1985 or have sexual exposure to partners who did?
4. Do you have or have you had a hemophiliac partner(s) who received blood or blood products between 1975 and 1985?
5. Do you or your partner(s) use latex condoms/female condoms whenever you have vaginal or anal sex?
6. Do you ever let your partner(s) ejaculate (cum) in your mouth? Do you ever have oral sex with a female partner during menses?
7. Have you ever had unprotected sex with a man who has had sex with another man?
8. Do you ever share sex toys (such as a vibrator)?
9. If you are a health-care provider, have you ever experienced a needle stick, exposure to a patient's blood, or exposure to amniotic fluid on your unprotected hands or face?
10. Are you and your partner mutually monogamous? How long have you been so?
11. Have you ever traded sex for money, shelter, food or drugs?
12. Have you ever had unwanted or forced (non-consensual) sex?

If your answer to any of the questions except 5 and 10 is yes, you may be at risk and might consider being tested.

From Hawkins, Roberto-Nichols, & Stanley-Haney, *Guidelines for Nurse Practitioners in Gynecologic Settings,* 8th edition, 2004, © Springer Publishing Company.

---

*Richard S. Ferri, Ph.D., ANP, ACRN, FAAN, provided invaluable input for this tool.

Appendix G
Vulvar Self-Examination*

How to Perform VSE...
Where To Look

POSITION. Find a comfortable, well-lighted place to sit such as a bed or a carpet. Hold a mirror in one hand. Then, expose the parts of the vulva surrounding the opening of the vagina. Once you have a good viewing position examine the main parts of the vulva as follows:

1. Check the "mons pubis" (the area above the vagina around the pubic bone where the pubic hair is located). Look carefully for any bumps, warts, ulcers, or changes in skin color (pigmentation, especially newly developed white, red or dark areas). Then, use the finger tips to check any visible change and to sense any bump just below the surface you might feel but not see.

2. Next, check the "clitoris" and surrounding area (directly above the vagina) by looking and by touch.

Parts of the Vulva
(External Female Genitals)

3. Next, examine the "labia minora" (the smaller folds of skin just to the right and left of the vaginal opening). Look and touch by holding the skin between thumb and fingers.

4. Then look closely at the "labia majora" (the larger folds of skin just next to the labia minora). Examine both right and left just as you did the labia minora.

5. Move down to the "perineum" (the area between the vagina and the anus). Check thoroughly.

6. Finally, examine the area surrounding the anal opening...as before by looking and by touch.

IMPORTANT NOTE: Every woman should know the parts of the vulva. (See the "Anatomy of the Vulva" drawing below.) You should also talk about VSE with your physician who can note what is "normal" for your individual anatomy. This is a good time to ask questions.

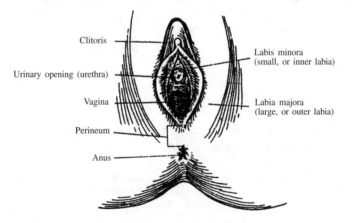

Clitoris

Urinary opening (urethra)

Vagina

Perineum

Anus

Labis minora
(small, or inner labia)

Labia majora
(large, or outer labia)

REMEMBER THE BASIC RULE: Vulvar diseases are most easily, safely, and successfully treated when discovered early. Now you know ... and now you have yet another good way to help protect your own health ... the monthly vulvar self-examination.

---

*From Lawhead, R., Alan, Jr., M.D., "What Every Woman Should Know: Your Guide to the Benefits of Vulvar Self-Examination," 1988, 1990, 1993, 1998, 2001. Used with permission.

Appendix H

Women and Heart Disease
Risk Factor Assessment*

Nonmodifiable

1. Age: postmenopausally, the risk for women increases dramatically; mortality is high for ages 35–44 and 75–84
2. Race or ethnicity: black women have a higher rate of death than white women; 5-year survival rate is lower and black women younger than 55 have >2x the death rate of white women; rates of diabetes and hypertension in black women are higher than those in white women
3. Family history of the disease especially heart attack < 50
4. Gender: attenuating advantage of being a woman especially premenopausally (premenopausally, women's risk is lower than men's)
5. Socioeconomic status: inverse association with morbidity and mortality

Modifiable

1. Lifestyle
   a. Exercise: aerobic exercise can increase HDLs (brisk walking; jogging) > 30 minutes daily or most days; sedentary life increases risk for heart disease, diabetes, obesity, high blood pressure
   b. Nutrition: cholesterol levels, lipid profile (HDL vs. LDL); high fat vs. low fat diet; < 30% fat < 70% saturated; sodium 2.4 g/day and maintain body mass index between 18.5–24.9, modifying effects of antioxidants (6–9 servings vegetables, fruits/day)
   c. Cigarette smoking
      1) Smoking and OC use increases rate of atherosclerosis
      2) Women (under 40 years old) who have MIs are mainly smokers
      3) Older women who smoke have a 50% greater chance to experience sudden death than older nonsmokers
      4) Acts synergistically with hyperlipidemia
2. Internal and external environmental factors
   a. Comorbidities: hypertension, diabetes, obesity; poor management of these chronic diseases increases risk while good management decreases risk. Blood pressure**—maintain at < 120/80

---

*Adapted from Rankin, S.H. (1997). Heart and soul: Evaluation of women with coronary artery disease. *Clinical Excellence for Nurse Practitioners, 1*(4), 231–239. See also Bibliography.
**See new guidelines www. nhlbi.nih.gov/guidelines/index.htm

b. Psychosocial concerns: stress and social support; high stress and low social support increase morbidity and mortality

c. Access to health care: unequal access appears to be a factor in morbidity and mortality

American Heart Association: www.Americanheart.org

Appendix I
General Women's Health Web Sites

The National Women's Health Information Center
www.4woman.org

Society for Women's Health Research
www.womens-health.org

Women's Health Interactive
www.womens-health.com

Appendix J
Body Mass Index Table

Body Mass Index Table

BMI	19	20	21	22	23	24	25	26	27	28	29	30	31	32	33	34	35
Height (inches)							Body Weight (pounds)										
58	91	96	100	105	110	115	119	124	129	134	138	143	148	153	158	162	167
59	94	99	104	109	114	119	124	128	133	138	143	148	153	158	163	168	173
60	97	102	107	112	118	123	128	133	138	143	148	153	158	163	168	174	179
61	100	106	111	116	122	127	132	137	143	148	153	158	164	169	174	180	185
62	104	109	115	120	126	131	136	142	147	153	158	164	169	175	180	186	191
63	107	113	118	124	130	135	141	146	152	158	163	169	175	180	186	191	197
64	110	116	122	128	134	140	145	151	157	163	169	174	180	186	192	197	204
65	114	120	126	132	138	144	150	156	162	168	174	180	186	192	198	204	210
66	118	124	130	136	142	148	155	161	167	173	179	186	192	198	204	210	216
67	121	127	134	140	146	153	159	166	172	178	185	191	198	204	211	217	223
68	125	131	138	144	151	158	164	171	177	184	190	197	203	210	216	223	230
69	128	135	142	149	155	162	169	176	182	189	196	203	209	216	223	230	236
70	132	139	146	153	160	167	174	181	188	195	202	209	216	222	229	236	243
71	136	143	150	157	165	172	179	186	193	200	208	215	222	229	236	243	250
72	140	147	154	162	169	177	184	191	199	206	213	221	228	235	242	250	258
73	144	151	159	166	174	182	189	197	204	212	219	227	235	242	250	257	265
74	148	155	163	171	179	186	194	202	210	218	225	233	241	249	256	264	272
75	152	160	168	176	184	192	200	208	216	224	232	240	248	256	264	272	279
76	156	164	172	180	189	197	205	213	221	230	238	246	254	263	271	279	287

BMI	36	37	38	39	40	41	42	43	44	45	46	47	48	49	50	51	52	53	54
Height (inches)									Body Weight (pounds)										
58	172	177	181	186	191	196	201	205	210	215	220	224	229	234	239	244	248	253	258
59	178	183	188	193	198	203	208	212	217	222	227	232	237	242	247	252	257	262	267
60	184	189	194	199	204	209	215	220	225	230	235	240	245	250	255	261	266	271	276
61	190	195	201	206	211	217	222	227	232	238	243	248	254	259	264	269	275	280	285
62	196	202	207	213	218	224	229	235	240	246	251	256	262	267	273	278	284	289	295
63	203	208	214	220	225	231	237	242	248	254	259	265	270	278	282	287	293	299	304
64	209	215	221	227	232	238	244	250	256	262	267	273	279	285	291	296	302	308	314
65	216	222	228	234	240	246	252	258	264	270	276	282	288	294	300	306	312	318	324
66	223	229	235	241	247	253	260	266	272	278	284	291	297	303	309	315	322	328	334
67	230	236	242	249	255	261	268	274	280	287	293	299	306	312	319	325	331	338	344
68	236	243	249	256	262	269	276	282	289	295	302	308	315	322	328	335	341	348	354
69	243	250	257	263	270	277	284	291	297	304	311	318	324	331	338	345	351	358	365
70	250	257	264	271	278	285	292	299	306	313	320	327	334	341	348	355	362	369	376
71	257	265	272	279	286	293	301	308	315	322	329	338	343	351	358	365	372	379	386
72	265	272	279	287	294	302	309	316	324	331	338	346	353	361	368	375	383	390	397
73	272	280	288	295	302	310	318	325	333	340	348	355	363	371	378	386	393	401	408
74	280	287	295	303	311	319	326	334	342	350	358	365	373	381	389	396	404	412	420
75	287	295	303	311	319	327	335	343	351	359	367	375	383	391	399	407	415	423	431
76	295	304	312	320	328	336	344	353	361	369	377	385	394	402	410	418	426	435	443

Source: NHLBI Obesity Education Initiative, U.S. Department of Health and Human Services, Public Health Service, National Institutes of Health, National Heart, Lung and Blood Institute. 2000 NIH Pub#00-408.

Bibliographies

Abdominal and Pelvic Pain

Ansari, A., & Bekker, G. (2002). Diagnosing uterine leiomyomas. *Women's Health in Primary Care, 2* (5), 279.

Ankum, W. M. (2000). Diagnosing suspected ectopic pregnancy. *British Medical Journal, 321,* 1235–1236.

Carter, J. F. S. (2000a). Chronic pelvic pain: Are you overlooking its nongynecologic causes? *Women's Health in Primary Care, 3*(9), 649–661.

Carter, J. F. S. (2000b). Diagnosing and treating nongynecologic chronic pelvic pain. *Women's Health in Primary Care, 3*(10), 708–725.

Chung-Park, M. (2002). A look at colorectal cancer screening in women. *Nurse Practitioner, 27*(6), 43–48.

Clark, A. (2002). Ectopic pregnancy: New developments in diagnosis and treatment. *Clinician Reviews, 12*(4), 65–70.

Eddy, L. L. H., J. (2001). Introduction to differential diagnosis in management of abdominal pain across the life span. *The American Journal for Nurse Practitioners, 5*(3), 10–28.

Grabo, T. N., & Nataupsky, L. G. (1999). Uterine myomas: Treatment options. *Journal of Obstetric, Gynecologic, and Neonatal Nursing, 28*(1), 23–31.

Krivak, T., & Propst, A. (2001). Tubo-ovarian abscess. *Female Patient, 26,* 43.

Lipscomb, G. H., Stovall, T. G., & Ling, F. W. (2000). Nonsurgical treatment of ectopic pregnancy. *New England Journal of Medicine, 343*(18), 1325–1329.

Olson, S., Mipone, L., Caputo, T., Barakat, R., & Harlap, B. (2001). Symptoms of ovarian cancer. *Obstetrics & Gynecology, 98,* 212.

Tay, J. I., Moore, J., & Walker, J. J. (2000). Ectopic pregnancy. *British Medical Journal, 320*(7239), 916–919.

Vissers, R. J., & Call, J. H. (2002, May). Systemic disease causes of abdominal pain. *The Clinical Advisor,* 58–74.

van Zandt, S. (2000). Pelvic pain in women. *Clinician Reviews, 10*(9), 51–65.

Abortion

Annas, G. J. (2001). "Partial-birth abortion" and the Supreme Court. *New England Journal of Medicine, 344*(2), 152–156.

Angulo, V., & Guendelman, S. (2002). Crossing the border for abortion services: The Tijuana-San Diego connection. *Health Care for Women International, 23*(6–7), 642–653.

Christin-Maitre, S., Bouchard, P., & Spitz, I. M. (2000). Drug therapy: Medical termination of pregnancy. *New England Journal of Medicine, 342*(13), 946–956.

Fielding, S. L., Lee, S. S., & Schaff, E. A. (2001). Professional consideration for providing mifepristone-induced abortion. *Nurse Practitioner, 26*(11), 44–54.

391

Ginty, M. M. (2001). What you need to know about RU-486. *MS., March,* 72–79.

Goldberg, A. B., Greenberg, M. B., & Darney, P. D. (2001). Misoprostol and pregnancy. *New England Journal of Medicine, 344*(1), 38–47.

Goss, G. L. (2002). Pregnancy termination. *AWHONN Lifelines, 6*(1), 46–50.

Grimes, D. A. (1999). A 26-year-old woman seeking an abortion. *Journal of the American Medical Association, 282*(12), 1169–1175.

Harvey, S. M., Beckman, L. J., & Branch, M. R. (2002). The relationship of contextual factors to women's perceptions of medical abortion. *Health Care for Women International, 23*(6–7), 654–665.

Kaplan, C. P., Erickson, P. I., Stewart, S. L., & Crane, L. A. (2001). Young Latinas and abortion: The role of cultural factors, reproductive behavior, and alternative roles to motherhood. *Health Care for Women International, 22*(7), 667–689.

Kishida, Y. (2001). Anxiety in Japanese women after elective abortion. *Journal of Obstetric, Gynecologic, and Neonatal Nursing, 30*(5), 490–495.

Kruse, B., Poppema, S., Greinin, M. D., & Paul, M. (2000). Management of side effects and complications in medical abortion. *American Journal of Obstetrics and Gynecology, 183*(2), S65–S75.

Levin, P. B., Staiger, D., Kane, T. J., & Zimmerman, D. J. (1999). Roe vs. Wade and American fertility. *American Journal of Public Health, 89*(20), 199–203.

Robinson, D. L., Dollins, A., & McConlogue-O'Shaughnessy, L. (2000). Care of the woman before and after an elective abortion. *The American Journal for Nurse Practitioners, 4*(3), 17–29.

Schaff, E. A., Fielding, S. L., Westhoff, C., Ellertson, C., Eisinger, S. H., Stadalius, L. S., & Fuller, L. (2000). Vaginal misoprostol administered 1,2,or 3 days after mifepristone for early medical abortion. *Journal of the American Medical Association, 284*(15), 1948–1953.

Simonds, W., Ellertson, C., Springer, K., & Winikoff, B. (1998). Abortion, revised: Participants in the U. S. clinical trials evaluate mifepristone. *Social Science & Medicine, 46*(10), 1313–1323.

Williams, G. B. (2001). Short-term grief after an elective abortion. *Journal of Obstetric, Gynecologic, and Neonatal Nursing, 30*(2), 174–183.

Breast Conditions

ACOG endorses tamoxifen—with caution. (2000). *Women's Health in Primary Care, 3*(5), 361–362.

Allen, J. D., Stoddard, A. M., Mays, J., & Sorensen, G. (2001). Promoting breast and cervical cancer screening at the workplace: Results from the woman to woman study. *American Journal of Public Health, 91*(4), 584–590.

Andsager, J. L., Hust, S. J. T., & Powers, A. (2000). Patient-blaming and representation of risk factors in breast cancer images. *Women & Health, 31*(2/3), 57–79.

Armstrong, K., Eisen, A., & Weber, B. (2000). Primary care: Assessing the risk of breast cancer. *New England Journal of Medicine, 342*(8), 564–571.

Arthur, B. J., P. A. (2000). Silicone breast implants. *AWHONN Lifelines, 4*(5), 28–32.

Bernhardt, B. A., Geller, G., Doksum, T., & Metz, S. A. (2000). Evaluation of nurses and genetic counselors as providers of education about breast cancer susceptibility testing. *Oncology Nursing Forum, 27*(1), 33–39.

Berry, J. A. (2001). Breast pain: All that hurts is not cancer. *The American Journal for Nurse Practitioners, 5*(4), 9–18.

Clemons, M. G., P. (2001). Estrogen and the risk of breast cancer. *New England Journal of Medicine, 344*(4), 276–285.

Coleman, E. A., Coon, S. K., Fitzgerald, A. J., & Cantrell, M. J. (2001). Breast cancer screening education: Comparing outcome skills of nurse practitioner students and medical residents. *Clinical Excellence for Nurse Practitioners, 5*(2), 102–107.

Coleman, E. A. (2001). Clinical breast examination: An illustrated educational review and update. *Clinical Excellence for Nurse Practitioners, 5*(4), 197–204.

Cummings, S. (2001). Weighing the risks: Genetic counseling for hereditary breast and ovarian cancer. *AWHONN Lifelines, 5*(3), 42–47.

Dinkel, H., Gassel, A. M., Muller, T., Lourens, S., Rominger, M., & Tschammler, A. (2001). Galactography and exfoliative cytology in women with abnormal nipple discharge. *Obstetrics and Gynecology, 97*(4), 625–629.

Duffy, S. H., Tabar, L., & Smith, R. A. (2002). The mammographic screening trials: Commentary on the recent work by Olsen and Gotzsche. *CA A Cancer Journal for Clinicians, 52*(2), 68–71.

Farley, M., Minkoff, J. R., & Bakan, H. (2001). Breast cancer screening and trauma history. *Women & Health, 34*(2), 15–27.

Finney, L. J. I., R. J. (2001). The impact of family history of breast cancer on women's health beliefs, salience of breast cancer family history, and degree of involvement in breast cancer issues. *Women & Health, 33*(3/4), 15–28.

Grabrick, D. M., Hartmann, L. C., Cerhan, J. R., Vierkant, R. A., Therneau, T. M., Vachon, C. M., Olson, J. E., Couch, F. J., Anderson, K. E., Pankratz, V. S., & Sellers, T. A. (2000). Risk of breast cancer with oral contraceptive use in women with a family history of breast cancer. *Journal of the American Medical Association, 284*(14), 1791–1798.

Haber, D. (2000). Roads leading to breast cancer. *New England Journal of Medicine, 343*(21), 1566–1568.

Hailey, B. J., Carter, C. L., & Burnett, D. R. (2000). Breast cancer attitudes, knowledge, and screening behavior in women with and without a family history of breast cancer. *Health Care for Women International, 21*(8), 701–715.

Janowsky, E. C., Kupper, L. L, & Hulka, B. S. (2000). Meta-analyses of the relation between silicone breast implants and the risk of connective-tissue diseases. *New England Journal of Medicine, 342*(11), 781–790.

Kerlikowske, K., Salzmann, P., Phillips, K. A., Cauley, J. A., & Cummings, S. R. (1999). Continiuing screening mammography in women aged 70 to 79 years. *Journal of the American Medical Association, 282*(22), 2156–2163.

Kinney, A. Y., Emery, G., Dudley, W. N., & Croyle, R. T. (2002). Screening behaviors among African American women at high risk for breast cancer. *Oncology Nursing Forum, 29*(5), 835–844.

Liu, Y., Wang, J. L., Chang, H., Barsky, S. H., & Nguyen, M. (2000). Breast-cancer diagnosis with nipple fluid bFGF. *The Lancet, 356,* 567.

Logothetis, M. L. (1995). Women's report of breast implant problems and silicon-related illness. *Journal of Obstetric, Gyencologic, and Neonatal Nursing, 24*(7), 609–616.

Machia, J. (2001). Breast cancer: Risk, prevention, & tamoxifen. *American Journal of Nursing, 101*(4), 26–35.

Marbella, A. M., Layde, P. M. (2001). Racial trends in age-specific breast cancer mortality rates in US women. *American Journal of Public Health, 91*(1), 118–121.

Marchbanks, P. A., McDonald, J. A., Wilson, H. G., Folger, S. G., Mandel, M. G., Daling, J. R., Bernstein, L., Malone, K. E., Ursin, G., Strom, B. L., Norman, S. A., Wingo, P. A., Burkman, R. T., Berlin, J. A., Simon, M. S., Spirtas, R., & Weiss, L. K. (2002). Oral contraceptives and the risk of breast cancer. *New England Journal of Medicine, 26,* 2025–2032.

Meijers-Heijboer, E. J., Verhoog, L. C., Brekelmans, C. T. M., Seynaeve, C., Tilanus-Linthorst, M. M. A., Wagner, A., Dukel, L., Devilee, P., van den Ouweland, A. W. W., van Geel, A. N., & Klijn, J. G. M. (2000). Presymptomatic DNA testing and prophylactic surgery in families with a BRCA1 or BRCA2 mutation. *The Lancet, 355,* 2015–2020.

Morris, K. T. P., R. (2000). Minimizing your risk of misdiagnosing breast cancer. *Contemporary Nurse Practitioner, fall,* 22–27.

Narod, S. A., Brunet, J., Ghadirian, P., Robson, M., Heimdal, K., Neuhausen, S. L., Stoppa-Lyonnet, D., Lerman, C., Pasini, B., de los Rios, P., Weber, B., Lynch, H. for the Hereditary Breast Cancer Clinical Study Group. (2000). Tamoxifen and risk of contralateral breast cancer in BRCA1 and BRCA2 mutation carriers: A case-control study. *The Lancet, 356,* 1876–1881.

O'Malley, M. S., Earp, J. L., Hawley, S. T., Schell, M. J., Mathews, H. F., & Mitchell, J. (2001). The association of race/ethnicity, socioeconomic status, and physician recommendation for mammography: Who gets the message about breast cancer screening? *American Journal of Public Health, 91*(1), 49–54.

Owen, C., Deslee, J., & Robbe, M. D. V. (2002). Barriers to cancer screening amongst women with mental health problems. *Health Care for Women International, 23*(6–7), 561–566.

Padgett, D. K., Yedidia, M. J., Kerner, J., & Mandelblatt, J. (2001). The emotional consequences of false positive mammography: African-American women's reactions in their own words. *Women & Health, 33*(3/4), 1–14.

Phillips, J. M., Cohen, M. Z., & Tarzian, A. J. (2001). African American women's experiences with breast cancer screening. *Journal of Nursing Scholarship, 33*(2), 135–140.

Rutter, C. M., Mandelson, M. T., Laya, M. B., Seger, D. J., & Taplin, S. (2001). Changes in breast density associated with initiation, discontinuation, and continuing use of hormone replacement therapy. *Journal of the American Medical Association, 285*(2), 171–176.

Senior, K. (2000). Hi-tech breast-cancer screening: Will it deliver? *The Lancet, 355,*

1796. Smith-Warner, S. A., Spiegelman, D., Yaun, S., Adami, H., Beeson, W. L., van den Brandt, P. A., Folson, A. R., Fraser, G. E., Freudenheim, J. L., Goldbohm. R. A., Graham, S., Miller, A. B., Potter, J. D., Rohan, T. E., Speizer, F. E., Toniolo, P., Willett, W. C., Wolk, A., Zeleniuch-Ja. (2001). Intake of fruits and vegetables and risk of breast cancer. *Journal of the American Medical Association, 285*(6), 769–776.

Tan-Chiu, E. W., D. L. (2000). Who should take tamoxifen? *Women's Health in Primary Care, 3*(9), 675–680.

Wee, C., McCarthy, E. P., Davis, R. B., & Phillips, R. S. (2000). Screening for cervical and breast cancer: Is obesity an unrecognized barrier to preventive care? *Annals of Internal Medicine, 132*(9), 697–704.

Zimmerman, V. L. (2002). BRCA gene mutations and cancer. *American Journal of Nursing 102*(8), 28–36.

Cervix, Papanicolaou Smears, HPV

Agency for Health Care Policy and Research. (1999). *Evaluation of cervical pathology.* Bethesda, MD: US Department of Health and Human Services.

Allen, J. D., Stoddard, A. M., Mays, J., & Sorensen, G. (2001). Promoting breast and cervical cancer screening at the workplace: Results from the woman to woman study. *American Journal of Public Health, 91*(4), 584–590.

American Society of Cytopathology Executive Board. (2001). Procedures used in the creation of the American Society of Cytopathology cervical cytology practice guideline. *Journal of Lower Genital Tract Disease, 5*(3), 159–184.

Anderson, P. S., & Runowicz, C. D. (2001). Beyond the Pap test: New techniques for cervical cancer screening. *Women's Health in Primary Care, 4*(12), 753–758.

Audisio, T., Pigini, T., de Riutort, S., Schindler, L., Ozan, M., Tocalli, C., & Bertolotto, P. (2002). Validity of the Papanicolaou smear in the diagnosis of candida, trichomonas vaginalis, and bacterial vaginosis. *Journal of Lower Genital Tract Disease, 5*(4), 223–225.

Baer, A., Kiviat, N. B., Kulasingam, S., Mao, C., Kuypers, J., & Koutsky, L. A. (2002). Liquid-based Papanicolaou smears without a transformation zone component: Should clinicians worry? *Obstetrics and Gynecology, 99*(6), 1053–1059.

Boyer, L. E., Williams, M., Calliser, L. C., & Marshall, E. S. (2001). Hispanic women's perceptions regarding cervical cancer screening. *Journal of Obstetric, Gynecologic, and Neonatal Nursing, 30*(2), 240–245.

Castellsague, X., Bosch, F. X., Munoz, N., Meijer, C. J. L. M., Shah, K. V., de Sanjose, S., Eluf-Neto, J., Ngelangel, C. A., Chichareon, S., Smith, J. S., Herrero, R., & Franceschi, S. for the International Agency for Research on Cancer Multicenter Cervical Cancer Study Group. (2002). Male circumcision, penile human papillomavirus infection, and cervical cancer in female partners. *New England Journal of Medicine, 346*(15), 1105–1112.

Castle, P. E., Zemlo, T. R., Burk, R. D., Scott, D. R., Sherman, M. E., Lorincz, A. T., Kurman, R. J., Glass, A. G., Rush, B. B., Liaw, K-L., & Schiffman, M. (2001).

Cervical HPV DNA detection as a predictor of a recurrent SIL diagnosis among untreated women. *Journal of Lower Genital Tract Disease, 5*(3), 138–143.

Cervical cancer screening: Which women aren't having Pap tests? (2000), *Women's Health in Primary Care, 3*(5), 309.

Cervical cancer screening: New strategies for finding high-risk women. (2001). *Women's Health in Primary Care, 4*(5), 355–356.

Cothran, M. M., & White, J. P. (2002). Adolescent behavior and sexually transmitted diseases: The dilemma of human papillomavirus. *Health Care for Women International, 23*(3), 306–319.

Dickman, E. D., Doll, T. J., Chiu, C. K., & Ferris, D. G. (2001). Identification of cervical neoplasia using a simulation of human vision. *Journal of Lower Genital Tract Disease, 5*(3), 144–152.

Dunn, T. S., Bajaj, J. E., Stamm, C. A., & Beaty, B. (2001). Management of minimally abnormal Papanicolaou smear in pregnancy. *Journal of Lower Genital Tract Disease, 5*(3), 133–137.

Gibson, C. A., Trask, C. E., House, P., Smith, S. F., Foley, M., & Nichols, C. (2001). Endocervical samplings: A comparison of endocervical brush, endocervical curette, and combined brush with curette techniques. *Journal of Lower Genital Tract Disease, 5*(1), 1–6.

Halcon, L. L., Lifson, A. R., Shew, M., Joseph, M., Hannan, P. J., & Hayman, C. R. (2002 Pap test results among low-income youth: Prevalence of dysplasia and practice implications. *Journal of Obstetric, Gynecologic, & Neonatal Nursing, 31*(3), 294–304.

Heard, I., Tassie, J., Schmitz, V., Mandelbrot, L., Kazatchkine, M. D., & Orth, G. (2000). Increased risk of cervical disease among human immunodeficiency virus-infected women with severe immunosuppression and high human papillomavirus load. *Obstetrics & Gynecology, 96*(3), 403–408.

Hewitt, M., Devesa, S., & Breen, N. (2002). Papanicolaou test among reproductive-age women at high risk for cervical cancer: Analyses of the 1995 National Survey of Family Growth. *American Journal of Public Health, 92*(4), 666–669.

Jacobson, R. G., Lapinski, R. H., & Kalir, T. (2002). The clinical importance of atypical glandular cells of undetermined significance on the cytologic smear. *Primary Care Update for OB/GYNS, 7*(6), 250–252.

Jin, X. W., Cash, J., & Kennedy, A. W. (1999). Human papillomavirus typing and the reduction of cervical cancer risk. *Cleveland Clinic Journal of Medicine, 66*(9), 533–529.

Josefsson, A. M., Magnusson, P. K. E., Ylitalo, N., Sorensen, P., Qwarforth-Tubbin, P., Andersen, P. K., Melbye, M., Adami, H., & Gyllensten, U. B. (2000). Viral load of human papilloma virus 16 as a determinant for development of cervical carcinoma in situ: A nested case-control study. *The Lancet, 355*, 2189–2193.

Managing cervical cytologic abnormalities: 2001 consensus guidelines. (2002*) Women's Health in Primary Care, 5*(6), 377.

Mandelblatt, J. S., Lawrence, W. F., Womack, S. M., Jacobson, D., Yi, B., Hwang, Y., Gold, K., Barter, J., & Shah, K. (2002). Benefits and costs of using HPV testing to screen for cervical cancer. *Journal of the American Medical Association, 287*(18), 2372–2381.

Massad, L. S., Schneider, M., Watts, H., Darragh, T., Abulafia, O., Salzer, E., Muderspach, L. I., Sidawy, M., & Melnick, S. (2002). Correlating Papanicolaou smear, colposcopic impression, biopsy: Results from the women's interagency HIV study. *Journal of Lower Genital Tract Disease, 5*(4), 212–218.

Moreno, V., Bosch, F. X., Munoz, N., Meijer, C. J. L. M., Shah, K. V., Walboomers, J. M. M., Herrero, R., Franceschi, S. for the International Agency for Research on Cancer (IARC) Multicentric Cervical Cancer Study Group. (2002). Effect of oral contraceptives on risk of cervical cancer in women with human papillomavirus infection: The IARC multicentric case-control study. *Lancet, 359,* 1085–1092.

Moscicki, A., Hills, N., Shiboski, S., Powell, K., Jay, N., Hanson, E., Miller, S., Clayton, L., Farhat, S., Broering, J., Darragh, T., & Palefsky, J. (2001). Risks for incident human papillomavirus infection and low-grade squamous intraepithelial lesion development in young females. *Journal of the American Medical Association, 285*(23), 2995–3002.

Munoz, N., Franceschi, S., Bosetti, C., Moreno, V., Herrero, R., Smith, J. S., Shah, K. V., Meijer, C. J. L. M., Bosch, F. X. for the International Agency for Research on Cancer (IARC) Multicentric Cervical Cancer Study Group. (2002). Role of parity and human papillomavirus in cervical cancer: The IARC multicentric case-controlled study. *Lancet, 359,* 1093–1101.

Nobbenhuis, M. A. E., Helmerhorst, T. J. M., van den Brule, A. J. C., Rozendaal, L., Voorhorst, F. J., Bezemer, P. D., Verheijen, R. H. M., & Meijer, C. J. L. M. (2001). Cytological regression and clearance of high-risk human papillomavirus in women with an abnormal cervical smear. *Lancet, 358,* 1782–1783.

Reid, J. (2001). Women's knowledge of pap smears, risk factors for cervical cancer, and cervical cancer. *Journal of Obstetric, Gynecologic, and Neonatal Nursing, 30*(3), 299–305.

Rubin, M. (1999, February 17–19). *New technologies for cervical screening: Can we afford not to use them?* Presentation at the 23rd Annual Postgraduate Seminar for Nurse Practitioners in Women's Health Care. Philadelphia, PA.

Rubin, M. M., & Lauver, D. (1990). Assessment and management of cervical intraepithelial neoplasia. *Nurse Practitioner, 15*(10), 23–24, 26–28, 30–31.

Saw, H.-S., Lee, J-K., Lee, H-L., Jee, H-J., & Hyun, J-J. (2001). Natural history of low-grade squamous intraepithelial lesion. *Journal of Lower Genital Tract Disease, 5*(3), 153–158.

Schaffer, S. D., & Philput, C. B. (1992). Predictors of abnormal cervical cytology: Statistical analysis of human papillomavirus and cofactors. *The Nurse Practitioner, 17*(3), 46–48, 50.

Schiffman, M., Herrero, R., Hildesheim, A., Sherman, M. E., Bratti, M., Wacholder, S., Alfaro, M., Hutchinson, M., Morales, J., Greenberg, M. D., & Lorincz, A. T. (2000). HPV DNA testing in cervical cancer screening. *Journal of the American Medical Association, 283*(1), 87–93.

Schlecht, N. F., Kulga, S., Robitaille, J., Ferreira, S., Santos, M., Miyamura, R. A.,

Duate-Franco, E., Rohan, T. E., Ferenczy, A., Villa, L. L., & Franco, E. L. (2001). Persistent human papillomavirus infection as a predictor of cervical intraepithelial neoplasia. *Journal of the American Medical Association, 286*(24), 3106–3114.

Sellors, J. W., Jeronimo, J., Sankaranarayanan, R., Wright, T. C., Howard, M., & Blumenthal, P. D. (2002). Assessment of the cervix after acetic acid wash: Interrater agreement using photographs. *Obstetrics and Gynecology, 99*(4), 635–640.

Solomon, D., Davey, D., Kurman, R., Moriarty, A., O'Connor, D., Prey, M., Raab, S., Sherman, M., Wilbur, D., Wright, T., Young, N. for the Forum Group Members and the Bethesda 2001 workshop. (2002). The 2001 Bethesda system. *Journal of the American Medical Association, 287*(16), 2114–2119.

Stoler, M., Guffikin, K., & Blumenthal, P. (2000). Cervical cancer screening in developing countries. *Primary Care Update for Ob/Gyns, 7,* 118–123.

Stoler, M. H. (2002). New Bethesda terminology and evidence-based management guidelines for cervical cytology findings. *Journal of the American Medical Association, 287*(16), 2140–2141.

Thompson, L. C., O'Connor, P., & Gibbs, R. S. (2001). A randomized controlled trial of metronidazole vaginal cream in the treatment of papanicolaou smears showing atypical squamous cells of undertermined significance (ASCUS). *Journal of Lower Genital Tract Disease, 5*(4), 219–232.

Walboomers, J. M. M., Jacobs, M. V., Manos, M. M., Bosch, F. X., Kummer, J. A., Shah, K. V., Snijders, P. J. F., Peto, J., Meijer, C. J. L. M., & Munoz, N. (1999). Human papillomavirus is a necessary cause of invasive cervical cancer worldwide. *Journal of Pathology, 189,* 12–19.

Which HPV 16–infected women are most likely to develop cervical cancer? (2001) *Women's Health in Primary Care, 4*(5), 374.

Woodman, C. B. J., Collins, S., Winter, H., Bailey, A., Ellis, J., Prior, P., Yates, M., Rollason, T. P., & Young, L. S. (2001). Natural history of cervical human papillomavirus infection in young women: A longitudinal cohort study. *Lancet, 357,* 1831–1836.

Wright, T. (2001). Is there a role for HPV DNA testing in routine practice? *OB GYN Management.*

Wright, T. C., Cox, J. T., Massad, L. S., Twiggs, L. B., & Wilkinson, E. J. for the 2001 ASCCP-sponsored Consensus Conference. (2002). 2001 consensus guidelines for the management of women with cervical cytological abnormalities. *Journal of the American Medical Association, 287*(16), 2120–2129.

Yitalo, N., Sorensen, P., Josefsson, A. M., Magnusson, P. K. E., Andersen, P. K., Poten, J., Adami, H., Gyllensten, U. B.,, & Melbye, M. (2000). Consistent high viral load of human papillomarvirus 16 and risk of cervical carcinoma in situ: A nested case-control study. *The Lancet, 355,* 2194–2198.

Complementary and Alternative Therapies

Adlercreutz, H. (2000). Phytoestrogens' epidemiology and a possible role in cancer protection. Washington, DC: U. S. Department of Health and Human Services, Environmental Health Perspectives.

Allaire, A. D., Moos, M-K., & Wells, S. R. (2000). Complementary and alternative medicine in pregnancy: A survey of North Carolina certified nurse-midwives. *Obstetrics & Gynecology, 95*(1), 19–23.

Balch, P. A., & Balch, J. F. (2000). *Prescription for nutritional healing.* New York: Avery.

Barron, B. A., Nicholson, B. R., & Strauss, J. E. (2002). A quick reference guide to dietary supplements. *Navy Medicine, 93* (1), 18–21.

Benjamin, S. D. (1999). Homeopathy: Can like cure like? *Patient Care for the Nurse Practitioner, 2*(12), 7–16.

Cozic, A. (2000). Alternative therapies: Tools for the new millenium. *Advance for Nurse Practitioners,* 64–66.

Cuccinelli, J. H. (1999). Magnetic field therapy. *Clinician Reviews, 9*(5), 119–122.

Dantas, S. M. (1999). Menopausal symptoms and alternative medicines. *Primary Care Update Ob/Gyn, 6*(6), 212–218.

Egan, C. D. (2002). Addressing use of herbal medicine in the primary care setting. *Journal of the American Academy of Nurse Practitioners, 14*(4), 166–171.

Elkind-Hirah, K. (2001), Effect of dietary phytoestrogens on hot flushes: Can soy-based proteins substitute for traditional estrogen replacement therapy? *Menopause, 8,* 154–156.

Ernst, E. (2000). Herbal medicines: Where is the evidence? *British Medical Journal, 321,* 395–396.

French, M. A. (1996). The mind-body-spirit connection. *ADVANCE for Nurse Practitioners, 4*(11), 38–46.

Foster, S., & Tyler, V. E. (1999). *Tyler's honest herbal.* Binghamton, NY: Haworth Herbal Press.

Fugh-Berman, A., & Awang, D. V. C. (2001). Black cohosh. *Alternative Therapies in Women's Health, 3*(11), 81–88.

Han, K. K., Soares, J. M., Haidar, M. A., de Lima, G. R., & Baracat, E. C. (2002). Benefits of soy isoflavone therapeutic regimen on menopausal symptoms. *Obstetrics and Gynecology, 99*(3), 389–394.

Hatcher, T. (2001). The proverbial herb. *American Journal of Nursing, 101*(2), 36–43.

Houston, R. F. V., W. A. (1998). Complementary and alternative therapies in perinatal populations: A selected review of the current literature. *Journal of Perinatal and Neonatal Nursing, 12*(3), 1–15.

Hudson, T. (2002). Essential fatty acids. *The Female Patient, 27*(1), 31–35.

Jonas, W., & Levin, J. S. (1999). *Essentials of complementary and alternative medicine.* New York: Lippincott, Williams, and Wilkins.

Jonas, W. B., & Chez, R. (2001). Is the complementary and alternative medicine intervention evidence-based? A user's guide to the medical literature. *Primary Care Update for Ob/Gyns, 8*(5), 179–185.

Kaler, M. M., & Ravella, P. C. (2002). Staying on the ethical high ground with complementary and alternative medicine. *Nurse Practitioner, 27*(7), 38–42.

Liberman, S. (2000). *Get off the menopause rollercoaster.* New York: Avery.

Marcus, C. L. (1999). Alternative medicine: The AMA reviews scientific evidence. *Clinician Reviews, 9*(2), 87–90.

McQuade-Crawford, A. (1996). *The herbal menopause book: Herbs, nutrition, and other natural therapies.* Freedom, CA: Crossing Press.

McAlindon, T. E. (2000). Can diet affect the risk and progression of osteoarthritis? *Women's Health in Primary Care, 3*(10), 741–747.

Meagher, E. A., Barry, O. P., Lawson, J. A., Rokach, J., & FitzGeraldn, G. A. (2001). Effects of vitamin E on lipid peroxidation in healthy persons. *Journal of the American Medical Association, 285*(9), 1178–1182.

Moylan, L. B. (2000). Alternative treatment modalities: The need for a rational response by the nursing profession. *Nursing Outlook, 48*(6), 259–261.

Murkies, A., Dalais, F., Briganti, E., Burger, H., Healy, D., Wahlquist, M., & Davis, S. (2000). Phytoestrogens and breast cancer in postmenopausal women: A case control study. *Menopause, 7*(5), 289–296.

Murray, M., & Pizzorno, J. (1998). *Encyclopedia of natural medicines.* Roseville, CA: Prima Publishing.

Nachtigall, S., Nachtigall, M., & Nachtigall, L. (1999). Nonprescription alternatives to hormone replacement therapy. *Female Patient, 24,* 14–15, 23–24.

Nachtigall, L. (2000, June). Assessing alternative approaches to menopause. *Contemporary Ob/Gyn, 3.*

Nestel, P., Pomeroy, S., Kay, S., Komesaroff, P., Behrsing, J., Cameron, J., & West, L. (1999). Isoflavones from red clover improve systemic arterial compliance but not plasma lipids in menopausal women. *The Journal of Clinical Endocrinology and Metabolism, 84,* 895–898.

Newton, K. M., Buist, D. S. M., Keenan, N. L., Anderson, L. A., & LaCroix, A. Z. (2002). Use of alternative therapies for menopause symptoms: Results of a population-based survey. *Obstetrics & Gynecology, 100*(1), 18–25.

Nicholson, S. (1999). Acupuncture. *Clinician Reviews, 9*(7), 87–91.

Pennachio, D. L. (2000). Drug-herb interactions: How vigilant should you be? *Patient Care for the Nurse Practitioner, 3*(10), 17–45.

Pettit, J. L. (2001). Soy. *Clinician Reviews, 11*(6), 119–120.

Pettit, J. L. (2001). Vitamin E. *Clinician Reviews, 11*(5), 31–34.

Pettit, J. L. (2000a). Black cohosh. *Clinician Reviews, 10*(4), 117–121.

Pettit, J. L. (2000b). Vitamin C. *Clinician Reviews, 10*(2), 105–108.

Pettit, J. L. (1999). Biofeedback. *Clinician Reviews, 9*(10), 113–116.

Pick, M. (2000). Herbal treatments for menopause. *ADVANCE for Nurse Practitioners, 8*(5), 29–30.

Ramsey, L. A., Ross, B. S., & Fischer, R. G. (2000). Efficacy, safety, reliability: Common concerns about herbal products. *ADVANCE for Nurse Practitioners, 8*(2), 31–33.

Robbers, J. E., & Tyler, V. E. (1999). *Tyler's herbs of choice.* Binghamton, NY: Haworth Herbal Press.

Saunders, C. S. (2000). Sorting out health claims about soy. *Patient Care for the Nurse Practitioner, 3*(12), 58–67.

Scheiber, M., & Rebar, W. (1999). Isoflavones and postmenopausal bone health: A viable alternative to estrogen therapy? *Menopause, 6,* 233–241.

Shinkarovsky, L. (1996). Hypnotherapy, not just hocus-pocus. *RN, 59*(6), 55–57.

Spencer, J. W., & Jacobs, J. J. (1999). *Complementary/alternative medicine: An evidence-based approach.* St. Louis, MO: Mosby.

Staley, C. A. (1999a). Feverfew and evening primrose. *Women's Health in Primary Care, 2*(9), 732–734.

Staley, C. A. (1999b). Three commonly used herbal medications: St. John's wort, echinacea, and ginkgo biloba. *Women's Health in Primary Care, 2*(5), 335–336.

Stark, M. A. (2001). Nature as complementary therapy for women. *Journal of Obstetric, Gynecologic, and Neonatal Nursing, 30*(6), 574–578.

Tedesco, P., & Cicchetti, J. (2001). Like cures like: Homeopathy. *American Journal of Nursing, 101* (9), 43–48.

Upmalis, D., Lobo, R., Bradley, L., Warren, M., Cone, F., & Lamia, C. (2000). Vasomotor symptom relief by soy isoflavone extract tablets in post menopausal women: A multicenter double-blind, randomized, placebo-controlled study. *Menopause, 7,* 236–242.

Van Sell, S. L. (1996). Reiki: An ancient touch therapy. *RN, 59*(2), 57–59.

Washburn, S., Burke, G., Morgan, T., & Anthony, M. (1999). Effect of soy protein supplementation on serum lipoproteins, blood pressure, and menopausal symptoms in perimenopausal women. *Menopause, 6*(1), 7–13.

Webb, D. (2001). Vitamin and mineral supplements. *ADVANCE for Nurse Practitioners, 9*(6), 77–82.

Wysocki, S. J. (1997). Unconventional and conventional medicine: Searching for common ground. *Contemporary Nurse Practitioner, 2*(4), 3–15.

Yanni, L. K., W. (2000). Alternatives to traditional hormone replacement therapy. *Women's Health in Primary Care, 3*(7), 477–489.

Youngkin, E. Q., & Thomas, D. J. (1999). Vitamins: Common supplements and therapy. *Nurse Practitioner, 24*(11), 50–70.

Contraception and Emergency Contraception

Ashraf, H. (2000). UK improves access to "morning after pill." *The Lancet, 356,* 2071.

Axcan Ltee. Department of Research and Development. (1996). *Something new in barrier contraception: The Protective® contraceptive sponge.* Mont-St-Hilaire, Quebec, Canada: Axcan Ltee.

Brown, H. P. (2001). Emergency contraceptive pills. *The Female Patient, 26*(2), 36–40.

Churchill, D., Allen, J., Pringle, M., Hippisley-Cox, J., Ebdon, D., Macpherson, M., & Bradley, S. (2000). Consultation patterns and provision of contraception in general practice before teenage pregnancy: Case-control study. *British Medical Journal, 321,* 486–489.

Davis, A. J. (2001). Should you prescribe OCs to ill teenagers? *Contemporary Nurse Practitioner, Spring-Summer,* 5–9.

Farmer, R. D. T., Williams, T. J., Simpson, E. D., & Nightingale, A. L. (2000). Effect of 1995 pill scare on rates of venous thromboembolism among women taking combined oral contraceptives: Analysis of general practice research database. *British Medical Journal, 321,* 477–482.

Fonte, D. R. (1997). The basics of natural family planning. *ADVANCE for Nurse Practitioners, 5*(3), 37–38, 41–42.

Frezieres, R. G., Walsh, T. L., Nelson, A. L., Clark, V. A., & Coulson, A. H. (1998). Breakage and acceptability of a polyurethane condom: A randomized, controlled group study. *Family Planning Perspectives, 30*(2), 73–78.

Geier, W. S. (1995). An overview of consumer-driven ambulatory surgery: Operative laparoscopy. *Nurse Practitioner, 20*(11), 36, 46–51.

Gilliam, M., Lehman, R., & Furniss, K. (2001). The benefits of low-dose oral contraceptives. *Clinician Reviews*(supplement, November), 4–13.

Gillum, L. A., Mamidipudi, S. K., & Johnston, S. C. (2000). Ischemic stroke risk with oral contraceptives: A meta-analysis. *Journal of the American Medical Association, 284*(1), 72–78.

Grimes, D. A. (2000). Intrauterine device and upper-genital-tract infection. *The Lancet, 356,* 1013–1019.

Grimes, D. A. J., K. P. (2001). *A clinician's guide to levonorgestrel intrauterine contraception.* Washington, DC: Association of Reproductive Health Professionals.

Hatcher, R. A., Trussell, J., Stewart, F., Cates, W., Stewart, G. K., Guest, F., & Kowal, D. (1998). *Contraceptive technology* (17th ed.). New York: Ardent Media.

Holt, V. L., Cushing-Haugen, K. L., & Daling, J. R. (2002). Body weight and risk of oral contraceptive failure. *Obstetrics and Gynecology, 99*(5), 820–827.

Hubacher, D., Lara-Ricalde, R., Taylor, D. J., Guerra-Infante, F., & Guzman-Rodriguez, R. (2001). Use of copper intrauterine devices and the risk of tubal infertility among nulligravid women. *New England Journal of Medicine, 345*(8), 561–567.

Jick, H., Kaye, J. A., Vasilakis-Scaramozza, C., & Jick, S. S. (2000). Risk of venous thromboembolism among users of third generation oral contraceptives compared with users of oral contraceptives with levonorgestrel before and after 1995: Cohort and case-control analysis. *British Medical Journal, 321,* 1190–1195.

Kaler, A. (2001). "It's some kind of women's empowerment": The ambiguity of the female condom as a marker of female empowerment. *Social Science & Medicine, 52,* 783–796.

Kaunitz, A. M. (1999). Intrauterine devices: Safe, effective, and underutilized. Women's *Health in Primary Care, 2*(1), 39–47.

Kaunitz, A. M., Garceau, R. J., Cromie, M. A., & the Lunelle Study Group. (1999). Comparative safety, efficacy, and cycle control of Lunelle monthly contraceptive injection (medroxyprogesterone acetate and estradiol cypionate injectable suspension) and ortho-novum 7/7/7 oral contraceptive (norethindrone/ethinyl estradiol triphasic). *Contraception, 60*(4), 179–187.

Kemmeren, J. M., Algra, A., & Grobbee, D. E. (2001). Third generation oral contraceptives and risk of venous thrombosis: Meta-analysis. *British Medical Journal, 323,* 131–134.

Lethbridge, D. J., & Hanna, K. M. (1997). *Promoting effective contraceptive use.* New York: Springer.

Marciante, K. D., Gardner, J. S., Veenstra, D. L., & Sullivan, S. D. (2001). Modeling the cost and outcomes of pharmacist-prescribed emergency contraception. *American Journal of Public Health, 91*(9), 1443–1445.

Marions, L., Hultenby, K., Lindell, I., Sun, X., Stabi, B., & Danielsson, K. G. (2002). Emergency contraception with mifepristone and levonorgestrol: Mechanism of action. *Obstetrics & Gynecology, 100*(1), 65–71.

Matteson, P. S. (1995). *Advocating for self: Women's decision concerning contraception.* New York: Harrington Park Press.

Mishell, D. R. (2002). The transdermal contraceptive system. *The Female Patient, supplement* (August), 14–25.

Mulligan, J., Appleby, J., & Harrison, A. (2000). Third generation oral contraceptives. *British Medical Journal, 321,* 190–192.

Murray, T. (1996). New contraceptive sponge also protects against STDs. *The Medical Post, 32*(9), 1.

Noone, J. (2000). Cultural perspectives on contraception: A literature review. *Clinical Excellence for Nurse Practitioners, 4*(6), 336–340.

Norris, A. E., & Beaton, M. M. (2002). Who knows more about condoms? *American Journal of Maternal/Child Nursing, 27*(2), 103–108.

O'Callaghan, M. A. A., L. C. (2001). The next step for emergency contraception: Over-the-counter availability. *Clinical Excellence for Nurse Practitioners, 5*(2), 73–79.

Olphen, J., Parker, L., & Macaluso, M. (2002). Presenting the female condom to men: A dyadic analysis of effect of the woman's approach. *Women & Health, 35*(1), 37–51.

Pennachio, D. L. (2001). New approaches to emergency contraception. *Patient Care for the Nurse Practitioner, 4*(3), 44–54.

Psychoyos, A. et al. (1993). Spermicidal and antiviral properties of a new vaginal contraceptive sponge (Protectaid®), containing sodium cholate (cholic acid). *Human Reproduction, 8*(6), 866–869.

Range, C. (2000). Understanding the noncontraceptive benefits of oral contraceptives. *Physician Assistant, 24*(8), 46–53.

Raine, T., Harper, C., Leon, K., & Darney, P. (2000). Emergency contraception: Advance provision in a young, high-risk clinic population. *Obstetrics & Gynecology, 96*(1), 1–7.

Rankin-Williams, A. (2001). Post-Soviet contraceptive practices and abortion rates in St. Petersburg, Russia. *Health Care for Women International, 22*(8), 699–710.

Rawlins, S. I. C., & Smith, D. M. (2002). Innovative contraception: New options in hormonal contraception. *American Journal for Nurse Practitioners, 6*(1), 9–28.

Rawlins, S. (2001). Balancing OC dose and tolerability. *Contemporary Nurse Practitioner (fall),* 5–11.

Richmond, D. M., Sabatini, M. M., Krueger, H., & Rudy, S. J. (2001). Contraception: Myths, facts, and methods. *The American Journal for Nurse Practitioners, spring,* 20–36.

Schnare, S. M. (2000). Emergency postcoital contraception. *The American Journal for Nurse Practitioners, 4*(2), 15–22.

Simpson, K. R., Devine, K. S., & Barron, M. L. (2001). Should emergency contraception pills be available "over the counter"? *American Journal of Maternal Child Nursing, 26*(6), 294–295.

Sulak, P., Lippman, J., Siu, C., Massaro, J., & Godwin, A. (1999). Clinical comparison of triphasic norgestimate/35ug estradiol and monophasic norethindrone acetate/20ug ethinyl estradiol. *Contraception, 59,* 161–166.

Sutton, C. (2001). Hormonal contraception: A focus on the transdermal delivery system. *Contemporary Nurse Practitioner (fall),* 12–19.

Tanis, B. C., van den Bosch, M. A. A. J., Kemmeren, J. M., Cats, V. M., Helmerhorst, F. M., Algra, A., van der Graaf, Y., & Rosendaal, F. R. (2001). Oral contraceptives and the risk of myocardial infarction. *New England Journal of Medicine, 345*(25), 1787–1793.

Taylor, H. A., Hughes, G. D., & Garrison, R. J. (2002). Cardiovascular disease among women residing in rural America: Epidemiology, explanations and challenges. *American Journal of Public Health, 92*(4), 548–551.

Tinkle, M., Reifsnider, E., & Ransom, S. P. (2002). Why women quit using Depo-Provera. *AWHONN Lifelines, 5*(6), 36–41.

Trent, A. J., & Clark, K. (1997). What nurses should know about natural family planning. *Journal of Obstetric, Gynecologic, and Neonatal Nursing, 26*(6), 642–648.

World Health Organization. (1996). *Improving access to quality care in family planning: Medical eligibility criteria for contraceptive use.* Geneva, Switzerland: World Health Organization.

Wysocki, S. (1998). Improving patient success with oral contraceptives: The importance of counseling. *The Nurse Practitioner, 23*(4), 55–56, 59–60.

Wysocki, S. (2001). Lunelle: A new contraceptive alternative. *Nurse Practitioner, 26*(6), 55–59.

Wysocki, S., Freeman, S., Moore, A., & Sutton, C. (2001). *New option in hormonal contraception: Monthly combination contraceptive injection.* Dayton, Ohio: NP Communications.

Wysocki, S., & Moore, A. A. (2002). New developments in contraception: The first transdermal contraceptive system. *Women's Health Care, 1,* 9–23.

Zieman, M. (2002). Managing patients using the transdermal contraceptive system. *The Female Patient, supplement* (August), 26–32.

Zieman, M. (2002). Transdermal contraception. *The Female Patient, 27*(1), 17–18

HIV/AIDS

Boehm, D. (2001). Women and HIV/AIDS: Act local/think global. *Journal of Obstetric, Gynecologic, and Neonatal Nursing, 30*(3), 342–350.

Cabral, R. J., Galavotti, C., Armstrong, K., Morrow, B., & Fogarty, L. (2001). Reproductive and contraceptive attitudes as predictors of condom use among women in an HIV prevention intervention. *Women & Health, 33*(3/4), 117–132.

Greiger-Zanlungo, P. (2001). HIV and women. *Female Patient, 26,* 12.

Gritter, M. (1998). The latex threat. *American Journal of Nursing, 98*(9), 26–32.

Holditch-Davis, D., Miles, M. S., Burchinal, M., O'Donnell, K., McKinney, R., & Lim, W. (2001). Parental caregiving and developmental outcomes of infants of mothers with HIV. *Nursing Research, 50*(1), 5–14.

Katz, A. (2001). HIV screening in pregnancy: What women think. *Journal of Obstetric, Gynecologic, and Neonatal Nursing, 30*(2), 184–191.

Kovacs, A., Wasserman, S. S., Burns, D., Wright, D. J., Cohn, J., Landay, A., Weber, K., Cohen, M., Levine, A., Minkoff, H., Miotti, P., Palefsky, J., Young, M., Reichelderfer, P., and the DARI and WIHS Study Groups. (2001). Determinants of HIV-1 shedding in the genital tract of women. *Lancet, 358,* 1593–1601

Lansky, A., Jones, J. L., Frey, R. L., & Lindegren, M. L. (2001). Trends in HIV testing among pregnant women: United States, 1994–1999. *American Journal of Public Health, 91*(8), 1291–1293.

Lauby, J. L., Semaan, S., O'Connell, A., Person, B., & Vogel, A. (2001). Factors related to self-efficacy for use of condoms and birth control among women at risk for HIV infection. *Women & Health, 34*(3), 71–91.

Lee, M. R.-B., & Rotheram-Borus, M. J. (2001). Challenges associated with increased survival among parents living with HIV. *American Journal of Public Health, 91*(8), 1303–1309.

Morrison-Beedy, D. L., & Lewis, B. P. (2001). HIV prevention in single, urban women: Condom-use readiness. *Journal of Obstetric, Gynecologic, and Neonatal Nursing, 30*(2), 148–156.

Roberts, J. R. (2000). The complex challenge of HIV/AIDS care: A global perspective: An update from XIIIth international AIDS conference. *Clinical Excellence for Nurse Practitioners, 4*(6), 373–379.

Rosenfield, A. F., & E. (2001). Where is the M in MTCT? The broader issues in mother-to-child transmission of HIV. *American Journal of Public Health, 91*(5), 703–704.

Royce, R. A., Walter, E. B., Fernandez, M. I., Wilson, T. E., Ickovics, J. R., & Simonds, R. for the Perinatal Guidelines Evaluation Program. (2001). Barriers to universal prenatal HIV testing in 4 US locations in 1997. *American Journal of Public Health, 91*(5), 727–733.

Songwathana, P. (2001). Women and AIDS caregiving: Women's work? *Health Care for Women International, 22*(3), 263–279.

Tamari, M. (2001). A decade in HIV treatment: What is the state of the art and how did we arrive. *Clinical Excellence for Nurse Practitioners, 5*(1), 4–12.

Infertility

Baird, D. D., Weinberg, C. R. et al. (1996). Vaginal douching and reduced fertility. *American Journal of Public Health, 86*(6), 844–850.

Cheney, B. (2002). Helping couples concerned about infertility. *Women's Health Care, 1*(1), 21–23.

Hahn, S. J., & Craft-Roseberg, M. (2002). The disclosure decisions of parents who conceive children using donor eggs. *Journal of Obstetric, Gynecologic, & Neonatal Nursing, 31*(3), 283–293.

Holditch-Davis, D., Black, B. P., et al. (1994). Beyond couvade: Pregnancy symptoms in couples with a history of infertility. *Health Care for Women International, 15*(6), 537–548.

Kirkman, M. (2001). Thinking of something to say: Public and private narratives of infertility. *Health Care for Women International, 22*(6), 523–535.

Phillips, O. (2001). Infertility Part 1: Genetic causes in females. *Female Patient, 26,* 55.

Sandelowski, M. (1994). On infertility. *Journal of Obstetric, Gynecologic, and Neonatal Nursing, 23*(9), 749–752.

Sandelowski, M., Harris, B. G., & Holditch-Davis, D. (1989). Mazing: Infertile couples and the quest for a child. *Image, 21*(4), 220–226.

Sandelowski, M., & Pollock, C. (1986). Women's experiences of infertility. *Image, 18*(4), 140–147.

Seybold, D. (2002). Choosing therapies: A Senegalese woman's experience with infertility. *Health Care for Women International, 23*(6–7), 540–549.

Swank, C. O., Christianson, C. A., Prows, C. A., West, E. B., & Warren, N. S. (2001). Effectiveness of a genetics self-instructional module for nurses involved in egg donor screening. *Journal of Obstetric, Gynecologic, and Neonatal Nursing, 30*(6), 617–625.

Van, P. (2001). Breaking the silence of African American women: Healing after pregnancy loss. *Health Care for Women International, 22*(3), 229–243.

Intimate Partner Violence/Sexual Assault

Becker, K. L. Walter-Moss, B. (2001). Detecting and addressing alcohol abuse in women. *Nurse Practitioner, 26*(10), 13–23.

Boyd, C. J., & Holmes, C. (2002). Women who smoke crack and their family substance abuse problems. *Health Care for Women International, 23*(6–7), 576–586.

Campbell, J. C. (2002). Health consequences of intimate partner violence. *Lancet, 359,* 1331–1336.

Carpiano, R. M. (2002). Long roads and tall mountains: The impact of motherhood on the recovery and health of domestic abuse survivors. *Health Care for Women International, 23*(5), 442–459.

Cook, S. L. (2002). Self-reports of sexual, physical, and nonphysical abuse perpetration. *Violence Against Women, 8*(5), 541–565.

Davis, K., Taylor, B., & Furniss, D. (2001). Narrative accounts of tracking the rural domestic violence survivors' journey: A feminist approach. *Health Care for Women International, 22*(4), 333–347.

Davis, R. E. (2002). Leave-taking experiences in the lives of abused women. *Clinical Nursing Research, 11*(3), 285–305.

Davis, R. E., & Hardh, K. E. (2001). Confronting barriers to universal screening. *Journal of Professional Nursing, 17*(6), 313–320.

D'Avolio, D., Hawkins, J. W., Haggerty, L. A., Kelly, U., Barrett, R., Toscano, S. E. D., Dwyer, J., Higgins, L. P., Kearney, M., Pearce, C. W., Aber, C. S., Mahony, D., & Bell, M. (2001). Screening for abuse: Barriers and opportunities. *Health Care for Women International, 22*(4), 349–362

Dienemann, J., Campbell, J., Landenburger, K., & Curry, M. A. (2002). The domestic violence survivor assessment: A tool for counseling women in intimate partner violence relationships. *Patient Education and Counseling, 46,* 221–228.

Draucker, C. B. (2001). Learning the harsh realities of life: Sexual violence, disillusionment, and meaning. *Health Care for Women International, 22*(1–2), 67–84.

Dube, S. R., Anda, R. F., Felitti, V. J., Chapman, D. P., Williamson, D. F., & Giles, W. H. (2001). Childhood abuse, household dysfunction, and the risk of attempted suicide throughout the life span. *Journal of the American Medical Association, 286(*24), 3089–3096.

Eisikovits, Z., & Winstok, Z. (2002). Reconstructing intimate violence: The structure and content of recollections of violent events. *Qualitative Health Research, 12*(5), 685–699.

Fishwick, N. J. (1998). Assessment of women for partner abuse. *Journal of Obstetric, Gynecologic, and Neonatal Nursing, 27*(6), 661–670.

Freeman, R. C., Prillo, K. M., Collier, K., & Rysek, R. W. (2001). Child and adolescent sexual abuse history in a sample of 1,490 women sexual partners of injection drug-using men. *Women & Health, 34*(4), 31–49.

Furniss, K. K. (1993). Screening for abuse in the clinical setting. *AWHONN's Clinical Issues in Perinatal and Women's Health Nursing, 4*(3), 402–406.

Furniss, K., Lucas, V., & Sharps, P. (1998). *Universal screening for domestic violence: Presentation package* [slide show]. Washington, DC: AWHONN.

Gaffney, K. F., Wichaikhum, O., & Dawson, E. M. (2002). Smoking among female college students: A time for change. *Journal of Obstetric, Gynecologic, and Neonatal Nursing, 31*(5), 502–507.

Garcia-Moreno, C. (2002). Dilemmas and opportunities for an appropriate health-service response to violence against women. *Lancet, 359,* 1509–1514.

Glaister, J. A., & Kesling, G. (2002). A survey of practicing nurses' perspectives on interpersonal violence screening and intervention. *Nursing Outlook, 50*(4), 137–143.

Glass, N., & Campbell, J. C. (1998). Mandatory reporting of intimate partner violence by health care professionals: A policy review. *Nursing Outlook, 46,* 279–283.

Halpern, C. T., Oslak, S. G., Young, M. L., Martin, S. L., & Kupper, L. L. (2001). Partner violence among adolescents in opposite-sex romantic relationships: Findings from the national longitudinal study of adolescent health. *American Journal of Public Health, 91*(10), 1679–1685.

Hassouneh-Phillips, D. (2001). Polygamy and wife abuse: A qualitative study of Muslim women in America. *Health Care for Women International, 22*(8), 735–748.

Hassouneh-Phillips, D. (2001). American Muslim women's experiences of leaving abusive relationships. *Health Care for Women International, 22*(4), 415–432.

Hathaway, J. E., Willis, G., & Zimmer, B. (2002). Listening to survivors' voices. *Violence Against Women, 8*(6), 687–719.

Hinson, J. V., Koverola, C., & Morahan, M. (2002). An empirical investigation of the psychological sequelae of childhood sexual abuse in an adult Latina population. *Violence Against Women, 8*(7), 816–844.

Humphreys, J., Lee, K., Neylan, T., & Marmar, C. (2001). Psychological and physical distress of sheltered battered women. *Health Care for Women International, 22*(4), 401–414.

Jewkes, R. (2002). Intimate partner violence: Causes and prevention. *Lancet, 359,* 1423–1429.

Lee, R. K., Thompson, V. L. S., & Mechanic, M. B. (2002). Intimate partner violence and women of color: A call for innovations. *American Journal of Public Health, 92*(4), 530–534.

Lown, E. A., Vega, W. A. (2001). Prevalence and predictors of physical partner abuse among Mexican American women. *American Journal of Public Health, 91*(3), 441–445.

McClellan, A. C., Killeen, M. R. (2000). Attachment theory and violence toward women by male intimate partners. *Journal of Nursing Scholarship, 32*(4), 353–360.

Meadows, L. M., Thurston, W. E., & Lackner, S. (2001). Health study: Women's reports of childhood abuse. *Health Care for Women International, 22*(5), 439–454.

Parker, B., & McFarlane, J. (1991). Identifying and helping battered pregnant women. *The American Journal of Maternal/Child Health, 16*(3), 161–164.

Parker, B., & Ulrich, Y. (1990). Nursing research consortium on violence and abuse of women. A protocol of safety: Research on abuse of women. *Nursing Research, 39*(4), 248–250.

Piispa, M. (2002). Complexity of patterns of violence against women in heterosexual partnerships. *Violence Against Women, 8*(7), 873–900.

Pulido, M. L., & Gupta, D. (2002). Protecting the child and the family. *Violence Against Women, 8*(8), 917–933.

Ryan, J., & King, M. C. (1998). Scanning for violence. *AWHONN Lifelines, 2*(3), 36–41.

Salomon, A., Bassuk, S. S., & Huntington, N. (2002). The relationship between intimate partner violence and the use of addictive substances in poor and homeless single mothers. *Violence Against Women, 8*(7), 785–815.

Schafer, J., Caetano, R., & Clark, C. L. (1998). Rates of intimate partner violence in the United States. *American Journal of Public Health, 88*(11), 1702–1704.

Stuart, G. L., Ramsey, S. E., Moore, T. M., Kahler, C. W., Farrell, L. E., Recupero, P. R., & Brown, R. A. (2002). Marital violence victimization and perpetration among women substance abusers. *Violence Against Women, 8*(8), 934–952.

Wewers, M. E., & Uno, M. (2002). Clinical interventions and smoking ban methods to reduce infants' and children's exposure to environmental tobacco smoke. *Journal of Obstetric, Gynecologic, and Neonatal Nursing, 31*(5), 592–598.

Woods, S. J., & Isenberg, M. A. (2001). Adaptation as a mediator of intimate abuse and traumatic stress in battered women. *Nursing Science Quarterly, 14*(3), 215–221.

Veenema, T. G. (2001). Children's exposure to community violence. *Journal of Nursing Scholarship, 33*(2), 167–172.

Menopause, Hormone Therapy

Alexander, I. (2000, August). Transdermal estrogen replacement therapy. *Advance for Nurse Practitioners,* 60.

Allen, M., & Higginbotham, E. (2000). Impact of hormonal changes on the eye. *Female Patient, 25,* 73.

Altman, A., Kingsberg, S., & Onel, E. (2002). Strategies for enhancing midlife sexuality. *Patient Care for the Nurse Practitioner, Spring,* 4–12.

American Heart Association. (2001). HRT and cardiovascular disease: Updated AHA recommendations. *Women's Health in Primary Care, 4*(9), 601.

Andrews, W., & Wysocki, S. (2000). Hormone replacement and chronic conditions. *Female Patient, supplement,* whole issue.

Archer, D. (2000). Perimenopausal uterine bleeding. *Female Patient, 25,* 50.

Birge, S. (2002). HRT and cognitive function: What are we to believe? *Menopause, 9,* 221.

Blumenthal, S., Bachmann, G., & Reichman, W. (1999). Postmenopausal women: Screening for cognitive decline in the Ob/Gyn office. *Primary Care Update for Ob/Gyns, 6*(4), 135.

Boyack, M., Lookinland, S., & Chasson, S. (2002). Efficacy of raloxifene for treatment of menopause: A systematic review. *Journal of the American Academy of Nurse Practitioners, 14*(4), 150–165.

Breheny, M. S., C. (2001). The importance of attitudes in predicting hormone replacement therapy use by mid-aged women in a New Zealand community sample. *Women & Health, 34*(1), 29–43.

Bromberger, J. T., Meyer, P. M., Kravitz, H. M., Sommer, B., Cordal, A., Powell, L., Ganz, P. A., & Sutton-Tyrrell, K. (2001). Psychologic distress and natural menopause: A multiethnic community study. *American Journal of Public Health, 91*(9), 1435–1442.

Brucker, M. C. & Youngkin, E. (2003). What's a woman to do? *AWHONN Lifelines, 6*(5), 408–417.

Chen, F., Lee, N., Soong, Y., & Huang, K. (2001). Comparison of transdermal and oral estrogen-progestin replacement therapy: Effects on cardiovascular risk factors. *Menopause, 8,* 347–352.

Cousins, S. O., & Edwards, K. (2002). Alice in menopauseland: The jabberwocky of a medicalized middle age. *Health Care for Women International, 23*(4), 325–343.

Crawford, S., Casey, V., Avis, N., & McKinlay, S. (2000). A longitudinal study of weight and the menopause transition: Results from the Massachusetts Women's Health Study. *Menopause, 7,* 96–104.

Elliott, J., Berman, H., & Kim, S. (2002). A critical ethnography of Korean Canadian women's menopause experience. *Health Care for Women International, 23*(4), 377–388.

Ettinger, B., Pressman, A., & VanLessel, A. (2001). Low-dosage esterified estrogens opposed by progestin at 6 month intervals. *Obstetrics & Gynecology, 98,* 205.

Finkel, M., Cohen, M., & Mahoney, H. (2001). Treatment options for the menopausal woman. *Nurse Practitioner, 26*(2), 5.

Fiorica, J. V. (Ed.). (2001). Postmenopausal hormone therapy and breast health: A review for clinicians. *Women's Health in Primary Care, 4*(supplement), 3–36.

Gambrell, R. D. (1998). Overcoming the side effects of hormone replacement therapy. *Women's Health in Primary Care, 1*(2), 160–168.

Gass, M. (2000). Premature menopause. *Female Patient, 25,* 58.

Gass, M. L. S., Utian, W. H., Ettinger, B., Gallagher, J. C., Herrington, D. M., Lobo, R. A., Stampfer, M. J., Stefanick, M. L., & Woods, N. F. (2002). Report from the NAMS Advisory Panel on postmenopausal hormone therapy. Retrieved October 4, 2002 from www. nams. org.

Gavin, N., Thorp, J., & Ohsfeldt, R. (2001). Determinants of hormone replacement therapy duration among postmenopausal women with intact uteri. *Menopause, 8,* 9.

Gelfand, M. (2001). Menopause matters: Estrogen-androgen therapy. *Female Patient, 26,* 54.

George, S. A. (2002). The menopause experience: A woman's perspective. *Journal of Obstetric, Gynecologic, and Neonatal Nursing, 31*(1), 77–85.

Grady, D., Herrington, D., Bittner, V., Blumenthal, R., Davidson, M., Hlatky, M., Hsia, J., Hulley, S., Herd, A., Khan, S., Newby, K., Waters, D., Vittinghoff, E., Wenger, N., for the HERS Research Group. (2002). Cardiovascular disease outcomes during 6.8 years of hormone therapy. *Journal of the American Medical Association, 288*(1), 49–57.

Gruber, C. J., Tschugguel, W., Schneeberger, C., & Huber, J. C. (2002). Production and action of estrogens. *New England Journal of Medicine, 346*(5), 340–352.

HRT and SERMS: New guidelines for patient management. (2002). *The Female Patient, Supplement* (March), 1–38.

Hudson, T. (2001). Managing perimenopausal symptoms. *Female Patient, 26*(8), 33–39.

The human genome project and postmenopausal hormone replacement. (2001). *The Female Patient, supplement* (December), 3–32.

Katz, A. (2002). Sexuality after hysterectomy. *Journal of Obstetric, Gynecologic, & Neonatal Nursing, 31*(3), 256–262.

Kayser, J., Ettinger, B., & Pressman, A. (2001). Postmenopausal hormonal support: Discontinuation of raloxifene versus estrogen. *Menopause, 8,* 328–332.

Knobf, M. T. (2002). Carrying on: The experience of premature menopause in women with early stage breast cancer. *Nursing Research, 51*(1), 9–17.

Lange-Collett, J. (2002). Promoting health among perimenopausal women through diet and exercise. *Journal of the American Academy of Nurse Practitioners, 14*(4), 172–177.

Lewis, L., Shaver, J., Woods, N., Lentz, M., Cain, K., Hertig, V., & Heidergott, S. (2000). Resorption levels by age and menopausal status in 5,157 women. *Menopause, 7*(1), 42–52.

Manson, J. E., & Martin, K. A. (2001). Postmenopausal hormone-replacement therapy. *New England Journal of Medicine, 345*(1), 34–40.

McKeon, V. A. (2002). Exploring HRT. *AWHONN Lifelines, 6*(1), 24–31.

Newton, K. M., Buist, D. S. M., Keenan, N. L., Anderson, L. A., & LaCroix, A. Z. (2002). Use of alternative therapies for menopause symptoms: Results of a population-based survey. *Obstetrics & Gynecology, 100*(1), 18–25.

Nogawa, N., Sumino, H., Ichikawa, S., Kumalkura, H., Mizninimaw, H., & Kurabayashi, M. (2001). Effect of long-term hormone replacement therapy on angiotensin-converting enzyme activity and bradykinen in postmenopausal women with essential hypertension and normotensive postmenopausal women. *Menopause, 8,* 210–215.

North American Menopause Society. (2003). Role of progestogen in hormone therapy for postmenopausal women. *Menopause, 10,* 113–132.

Notelovitz, M., Funk, S., Nanavati, N., & Mazzeo, M. (2002). Estradiol absorption from vaginal tablets in postmenopausal women. *Obstetrics and Gynecology, 99*(4), 556–562.

Pradham, A. D., Manson, J. E., Rossouw, J. E., Siscovick, D. S., Moulton, C. P., Rifai, N., Wallace, R. B., Jackson, R. D., Pettinger, M. B., & Ridker, P. M. (2002). Inflammatory biomarkers, hormone replacement therapy, and incident coronary heart disease. *Journal of the American Medical Association, 288*(8), 980–987.

Rajki, M., & Adams, K. (2000, September). Get moving! A mantra for perimenopausal women. *Advance for Nurse Practitioners,* 53.

Reece, S. M. (2002). Weighing the cons and pros: Women's reasons for discontinuing hormone replacement therapy. *Health Care for Women International, 23*(1), 19–32.

Saunders, C. S. (2001). Decisions in prescribing HRT. *Patient Care for the Nurse Practitioner, 4*(5), 45–58.

Rodriguez, C., Patel, A. V., Calle, E. E., Jacob, E. J., & Thun, M. J. (2001). Estrogen replacement therapy and ovarian cancer mortality in a large prospective study of US women. *Journal of the American Medical Association, 285*(11), 1460–1465.

Runowicz, C. (1999). Breast cancer and HRT: Individualizing treatment. *Menopause, 6,* 17–18, 21–22.

Sampselle, C. M., Harris, V., Harlow, S. D., & Sowers, M. (2002). Midlife development and menopause in African American and caucasian women. *Health Care for Women International, 23*(4), 351–363.

Sarrel, P. M., Kaunitz, A. M., Nachtigal, L. E., & Wysocki, S. (2002). Sexual dysfunction and the menopausal woman: Overcoming atrophic vaginitis. *Patient Care for the Nurse Practitioner, spec. ed.* (January), 4–19.

Sauer, M. (1998, August). Progesterone therapy: Modern uses and treatment alternatives. *Contemporary Ob/Gyn.*

Schaier, C., Lubin, J., Troisi, R., Sturgeon, S., Brinton, L., & Hoover, R. (2000). Menopausal estrogen and estrogen-progestin replacement therapy and breast cancer risk. *Journal of the American Medical Association, 283.*

Shulman, L. P. (2001). Sexuality. *The Female Patient, Supplement* (November), 3–7.

Simon, J. A. (2001). Hormone replacement therapy. *Clinician Reviews* (supplement, November), 4–9.

Singh, P., Haddad, E., Knutson, S., & Fraser, G. (2001). The effect of menopause on the relation between weight gain and mortality among women. *Menopause, 8,* 314–320.

Speroff, L. (2000). A clinician's response to the epidemiological data linking postmenopausal estrogen-progestin therapy with an increased risk of breast cancer. *Breast Cancer, 8*(1), 1–4.

Speroff, L., Gallagher, J. C., Pinkerton, J. V., & Raisz, L. G. (2001). Menopause management: The impact of low-dose HRT. *Contemporary Ob/Gyn for the Nurse Practitioner, July* (suppl.), 4–26.

Speroff, L., Simons, J., Kempfert, N., & Rowan, J. (2000). The effect of varying low-dose combinations of norethindrone acetate and ethinyl estradiol (Femhrt) on the frequency and intensity of vasomotor symptoms. *Menopause, 7,* 383.

Stephens, C., & Ross, N. (2002). The relationship between hormone replacement therapy use and psychological symptoms: No effects found in a New Zealand sample. *Health Care for Women International, 23*(4), 408–414.

Takaniski, G. C. (2000). Drug therapies for hot flashes in breast cancer survivors. *Women's Health in Primary Care, 3*(11), 799–800.

Transdermal HRT: New trends, emerging targets. (2002). *Contemporary OB/GYN, supplement* (March), 4–21.

Turner, S. (1999, November). Somewhere inbetween: An overview of perimenopause. *ADVANCE for Nurse Practitioners,* 63.

Vesser, P. I., Foster, S. L., Evans, S. C., & Sneed, A. (2002). Today's HRT choices. *ADVANCE for Nurse Practitioners, 10*(6), 57–62, 102.

White, V., Bennett, L, Raffin, S., Emmett, K., & Coleman, M. (2000). Use of unopposed estrogen in women with uteri: Prevalence, clinical implications, and economic consequences. *Menopause, 7,* 123–128.

Zenk, S. N., Shaver, J. L. F., Peragallo, N., Fox, P., & Chavez, N. (2001). Use of herbal therapies among midlife Mexican women. *Health Care for Women International, 22*(6), 585–597.

Menstrual Cycle: Abnormal Uterine Bleeding, PMS, Amenorrhea

Cahill, C. A. (1998). Differences in cortisol, a stress hormone in women with turmoil-type premenstrual syndrome. *Nursing Research, 47*(5), 278–284.

Chandraiah, S. (1998). Premenstrual syndrome—an update. *Resident & Staff Physician,* 67–70.

Cohen, L. (2000). New trends in treating menstrual disorders. *Journal of Clinical Psychiatry, Central Nervous System Capsules, 2* (1).

Cohen, L., Miner, C., Brown, E., Freeman, E., Holbreich, U., Sundell, K., & McCray, S. (2002). Premenstrual daily fluoxetine for premenstrual dysphoric disorder: A placebo-controlled, clinical trial using computerized diaries. *Obstetrics & Gynecology, 100,* 435.

Hillard, P. (1999). Diagnosing and controlling abnormal uterine bleeding. *Contemporary Adolescent Gynecology, 4*(1).

Korzwkwa, M., & Steiner, M. (1999). Assessment and treatment of premenstrual syndromes. *Psychiatry Update, 6*(5), 153.

Labyak, S., Lava, S., Turek, F., & Zee, P. (2002). Effects of shiftwork on sleep and menstrual function in nurses. *Health Care for Women International, 23*(6–7), 703–714.

Mishell, D. R., & Kaunitz, A. M. (1998). Devices for endometrial sampling. *Journal of Reproductive Medicine, 43*(3), 180–184.

Morse, G. (1999). Positively reframing perceptions of the menstrual cycle among women with premenstrual syndrome. *Journal of Obstetric, Gynecologic, and Neonatal Nursing, 28*(2), 165–174.

Penzias, A. (1999). A basic guide to evaluating amenorrhea. *Female Patient, 24,* 57.

Woods, N., Taylor, D., et al. (1998). Perimenstrual symptoms and health-seeking behavior. *Western Journal of Nursing Research, 14,* 418–439.

Mental Health and Emotional Issues

Antai-Otong, D. (2001). Dars days: Treating major depression. *Advance for Nurse Practitioners, 9*(3), 32–43.

Bartlett, S., & Andrews, W. (2000, November). Effective counseling. *Female Patient, supplement,* 50.

Beck, C. T. (2002). Postpartum depression: A metasynthesis. *Qualitative Health Research, 12*(4), 453–472.

Beck, C. T. (2002). Revision of the postpartum depression predictors inventory. *Journal of Obstetric, Gynecologic, and Neonatal Nursing, 31*(4), 394–402.

Beck, C. T. (2001). Predictors of postpartum depression. *Nursing Research, 50*(5), 275–285.

Beck, C. T., & Gable, R. K. (2001). Comparative analysis of the performance of the postpartum depression screening scale with two other depression instruments. *Nursing Research, 50*(4), 242–250.

Beck, C. T., & Gable, R. K. (2001). Further validation of the postpartum depression screening scale. *Nursing Research, 50*(3), 155–164.

Book, S. W., & Kates, N. (1999). A form-free psychiatric evaluation. *Patient Care for Nurse Practitioners,* 17–33.

Bouchard, G. J. (1999). Office management of mania and depression. *Clinician Reviews, 9*(8), 49–71.

Bozoky, I., & Coodley, L. (2002). Postpartum depression: Voice from a historian. *Pediatric Nursing, 28*(3), 300.

Cloitre, M., Cohen, L. R., Edelman, R. E., & Han, H. (2001). Posttraumatic stress disorder and extent of trauma exposure as correlates of medical problems and perceived health among women with childhood abuse. *Women & Health, 34*(3), 1–17.

Cohen, L. S. et al. (2001). Treatment of depression in women: From acute remission to sustained recovery. *The Journal of Gender-Specific Medicine, supplement,* 2–8.

Corwin, E. J. (2002). Fatigue as a predictor of postpartum depression. *Journal of Obstetric, Gynecologic, and Neonatal Nursing, 31*(4), 436–443.

des Rivieres-Pigeon, C., Seguin, L., Goulet, L., & Descarries, F. (2001). Unravelling the complexities of the relationship between employment status and postpartum depressive symptomatology. *Women & Health, 34*(2), 61–95.

Dibble, S. S., J. M. (2000). Gender differences for the predictors of depression in young adults with genital herpes. *Public Health Nursing, 17*(3), 187–194.

Dietch, K. V., & Bunney, B. (2002). The "silent disease" Diagnosing and treating depression in women. *AWHONN Lifelines, 6*(2), 140–145.

Edebohls, L., & Ecklund, C. (2002). Postpartum depression: Practical advice from two nurse practitioners. *Pediatric Nursing, 28*(3), 298–299.

Elliott, M. (2001). Gender differences in causes of depression. *Women & Health, 33*(3/4), 163–177.

Fernstein, R. E. (2000). Personality disorder in the primary care setting: Diagnosis, management and intervention. *Resident and Staff Physician, 46*(13), 47–56.

Howland, R. H. (2000). Chronic depression: Now a treatable condition. *Patient Care,* 54–65.

Jarvells, Y., Kornstein, S. G., et al. (2001). Advances in the treatment of depression in women: Beyond clinical lore. *Resident and Staff Physician, supplement,* 3–7.

Johnson, R. M. (2000). Diagnosis and managing seasonal affective disorders. *Nurse Practitioner, 25* (8), 56–62.

Jones, C. (2001). Premenstrual dysphoric disorder. *Advance for Nurse Practitioners, 9*(3), 87–90.

Josefsson, A., Angelsioo, L., Berg, G., Ekstrom, C., Gunnervik, C., Nordin, C., & Sydsjo, G. (2002). Obstetric, somatic, and demographic risk factors for postpartum depressive symptoms. *Obstetrics and Gynecology, 99*(2), 223–228.

Martinez, R., Johnston-Robledo, I., Ulsh, H. M., & Chrisler, J. C. (2000). Singing "the baby blues": A content analysis of popular press articles about postpartum affective disturbances. *Women & Health, 31*(2/3), 37–56.

Mausner, P. (2000). Overcoming depression. *Female Patient, supplement,* 9–16.

Norton, J. W. (2001). Personality disorders in the primary care setting. *Nurse Practitioner, 25,* 40–58.

Owen, C., Deslee, J., & Robbe, M. D. V. (2002). Barriers to cancer screening amongst women with mental health problems. *Health Care for Women International, 23*(6–7), 561–566.

Rabin, C., O'Leary, A., Neighbors, C., & Whitmore, K. (2001). Pain and depression experienced by women with interstitial cystitis. *Women & Health, 31*(4), 67–81.

Sagrestano, L. M., Rodriguez, A. C., Carroll, D., Bieniarz, A., Greenberg, A., Castro, L., & Nuwayhid, B. (2002). A comparison of standardized measures of psychosocial variables with single-item screening measures used in an urban obstetric clinic. *Journal of Obstetric, Gynecologic, and Neonatal Nursing, 31*(2), 147–155.

Shell, R. C. (2001). Antidepressant prescribing practices of nurse practitioners. *Nurse Practitioner, 26*(7), 42–47.

Ugarriza, D. N. (2002). Postpartum depressed women's explanation of depression. *Journal of Nursing Scholarship, 34*(3), 227–233.

Zamorshi, M. A. (2001). Anxiety disorders: Recognition and management in the ob/gyn setting. *Female Patient, 26,* 31–36.

Osteoporosis

Andrews, W. C. (2000). Osteoporosis Part I. *ACOG Clinical Review, 5*(3), 1–15.

Andrews, W. C. (2000). Osteoporosis Part II. *ACOG Clinical Review, 5*(3), 1, 13–15.

Berga, S. (1999). A lifelong approach to osteoporosis: Emphasize prevention. *Contemporary Ob/Gyn,* supplement, 4–18.

Can inhaled glucocorticoids cause bone loss? (2001). *Women's Health in Primary Care, 4*(12), 777–778.

Consensus statement on osteoporosis: Prevention, diagnosis, and treatment. (2000). *Women's Health in Primary Care, 3*(9), 670–672.

Curry, L. C., & Hogstel, M. O. (2002). Osteoporosis. *American Journal of Nursing, 102*(1), 26–32.

Davidson, M., & DeSimone, M. E. (2002). Osteoporosis update. *Clinician Reviews, 12*(4), 76–82.

Epstein, S., & Goodman, G. (1999). Improved strategies for diagnosis and treatment of osteoporosis. *Menopause, 6*(3), 242–250.

Ettinger, B. (2000). Sequential osteoporosis treatment for women with postmenopausal osteoporosis. *Menopausal Medicine, 8*(2), 1–4.

Ettinger, B., Black, D. M., Mitlak, B. H., Knickerbocker, R. K., Nickelsen, T., Genant, H. K., Christiansen, C., Delmas, P. D., Zanchetta, J. R., Stakkesatd, J., Gluer, C. C., Krueger, K., Cohen, F. J., Eckert, S., Ensrud, K. E., Veioli, L. V., Lips, P., & Cummings, S. R. (1999). Reduction of vertebral fracture risk in postmenopausal women with osteoporosis treated with raloxifene. *Journal of the American Medical Association, 282*(7), 637–645.

Gallagher, J. (2000). Diagnosing osteoporosis: The ABCs of Z and T scores. *The Female Patient, 25,* 66, 69.

Grady, E., & Cummings, S. R. (2001). Postmenopausal hormone therapy for prevention of fractures. *Journal of the American Medical Association, 285*(22), 2909–2910.

Harris, S. T., Watts, N. B., Genant, H. K., McKeever, C. D., Hangartner, T., Keller, M., Chesnut, C. H., Brown, J., Eriksen, E. F., Hoseyni, M. S., Axelrod, D. W., & Miller, P. D. (1999). Effects of risedronate treatment on vertebral and nonvertebral fractures in women with postmenopausal osteoporosis. *Journal of the American Medical Association, 282*(14), 1344–1352.

Holm, K., Dan, A., Wilbur, J., Suling, L., & Walker, J. (2002). A longitudinal study of bone density in midlife women. *Health Care for Women International, 23*(6–7), 678–691.

Hsieh, C., Novielli, K., Diamond, J., & Cheriwa, D. (2001). Health beliefs and attitudes toward the prevention of osteoporosis in older women. *Menopause, 8,* 372.

Licata, A. A. (1999). Update on osteoporosis: Strategies for prevention and treatment. *Women's Health in Primary Care, 2*(3), 229–243.

Lindsay, R., Gallagher, J. C., Kleerekoper, M., & Pickar, J. H. (2002). Effect of lower doses of conjugated equine estrogens with and without medroxyprogesterone acetate on bone in early postmenopausal women. *Journal of the American Medical Association, 287*(20), 2668–2676.

Lindsay, R., Silverman, S. L., Cooper, C., Hanley, D. A., Barton, I., Broy, S. B., Licata, A., Benhamou, L., Geusens, P., Flowers, K., Stracke, H., & Seeman, E. (2001). Risk of new vertebral fracture in the year following a fracture. *Journal of the American Medical Association, 285*(3), 320–323.

Lyles, K. (1999). Vertebral fractures and impact on quality of life. *The Female Patient* (supplement).

Massachusetts Medical Society (publishers of the *New England Journal of Medicine* and *Journal Watch*). (1998). Raloxifene: A future alternative to estrogen. *Journal Watch. Women's Health, 3*(1), 1–2.

McClung, B. L. (1999). Using osteoporosis management to reduce fractures in elderly women. *Nurse Practitioner, 24*(3), 26–27, 32, 35–36, 38, 41–41.

McClung, M. R., Geusens, P., Miller, P. D., Zippel, H., Bensen, W. G., Roux, C., Adami, S., Fogelman, I., Diamond, T., Eastell, R., Meunier, P. J., & Reginster, J. (2001). Effect of risendronate on the risk of hip fracture in elderly women. *New England Journal of Medicine, 344*, 333–340.

Miller, B., DeSouza, M., Slade, K., & Luciano, A. (2000). Sublingual administration of micronized estradiol and progesterone with and without micronized testosterone: Effect on biochemical markers of bond metabolism and bone mineral density. *Menopause, 7*(5), 318–326.

Milner, M., Harrison, R., Gilligan, E., & Kelly, A. (2000). Bone density changes during two years treatment with tibolone or conjugated estrogens and norgestrel, compared with untreated controls in postmenopausal women. *Menopause, 7*(5), 327–333.

Reid, I. E., Brown, J. P., Burckhardt, P., Horowitz, Z., Richardson, P., Trechsel, U., Widmer, A., Devogelaer, J., Kaufman, J., Jaeger, P., Body, J., & Meunier, P. J. (2002). Intravenous zoledronic acid in postmenopausal women with low bone mineral density. *New England Journal of Medicine, 346*(9), 653–661.

Rico, H., Roca-Bstran, C., Hernandez, E. R., Paez, F., Valencia, M., & Villa, Z. (2000). The effect of supplemental copper on osteopenia induced by ovaectomized rats. *Menopause, 7* (6), 413–416.

Roberto, K. A. (2001). The meaning of osteoporosis in the lives of rural older women. *Health Care for Women International, 22*(6), 599–611.

Schusshein, D. H. S., & E. S. (1998). Osteoporosis: Update on prevention and treatment. *Women's Health in Primary Care, 1*(2), 133–140.

Stroke risk in women: Fish, bone density, and HRT. (2001). *Women's Health in Primary Care, 4*(4), 295–302.

Torgerson, D. J., & Bell-Syer, S. E. M. (2001). Hormone replacement therapy and prevention of nonvertebral fractures. *Journal of the American Medical Association, 285*(22), 2891–2897.

Polycystic Ovary Syndrome (PCOS)

Ahles, B. L. (2002). Toward a new approach: Primary and preventive care of the woman with polycystic ovarian syndrome. *Primary Care Update for OB/GYNS, 7*(6), 275–278.

Cheung, A. (2001). Ultrasound and menstrual history in predicting endometrial hyperplasia in polycystic ovary syndrome. *Obstetrics & Gynecology, 98,* 325.

Freeman, S. B. (2002). Polycystic ovary syndrome: Diagnosis and management. *Women's Health Care, 1*(4), 15–20.

Kovacs, G. T. (2000). *Polycystic ovary syndrome.* Cambridge, England: Cambridge University Press.

Preconception Care

Cnattingius, S., Signorello, L. B., Anneren, G., Clausson, B., Ekbom, A., Ljunger, E., Blot, W. J., McLaughlin, J. K., Petersson, G., Rane, A., & Granath, F. (2000). Caffeine intake and the risk of first-trimester spontaneous abortion. *New England Journal of Medicine, 343*(25), 1839–1845.

Fiore, T., & Yeo, S. (2001). Exercise during pregnancy. *Female Patient, 26,* 12.

Hasenau, S. M., & Covington, C. (2002). Neural tube defects: Prevention and folic acid. *American Journal of Maternal Child Nursing, 27*(2), 87–92.

Hilton, J. J. (2002). Folic acid intake of young women. *Journal of Obstetric, Gynecologic, and Neonatal Nursing, 31*(2), 172–177.

Jones, S. L., & Fallon, L. A. (2002). Reproductive options for individuals at risk for transmission of a genetic disorder. *Journal of Obstetric, Gynecologic, and Neonatal Nursing, 31*(2), 193–199.

Nelson, A. L., & Zieman, M. (2002). A planned production. *The Female Patient, 27*(1), 49–50.

Tinkle, M. B., & Cheek, D. J. (2002). Human genomics: Challenges and opportunities. *Journal of Obstetric, Gynecologic, and Neonatal Nursing, 31*(2), 178–187.

Wald, N. J., Law, M. R., Morris, J. K., & Wald, D. S. (2002). Quantifying the effect of folic acid. *Lancet, 358,* 2069–2073.

Sexuality

Baxer, P. M. (2001). Midlife changes in sexual response. *ADVANCE for Nurse Practitioners, 9*(3), 67–69.

Berg, J. A. (2001). Dimensions of sexuality in the perimenopausal transition: A model for practice. *Journal of Obstetric, Gynecologic, and Neonatal Nursing, 30*(4), 421–428.

Boston Women's Health Book Collective. (1998). *Our bodies, ourselves for the new century: A book by and for women.* New York: Simon & Schuster.

Buchholz, S. E. (2000). Experiences of lesbian couples during childbirth. *Nursing Outlook, 48*(6), 307–311.

Farrell, S. A. K., K. (2000). Sexuality after hysterectomy. *Obstetrics & Gynecology, 95*(6), 1045–1050.

Hitchinson, M. K., Sosa, D., & Thompson, A. C. (2001). Sexual protective strategies of late adolescent females: More than just condoms. *Journal of Obstetric, Gynecologic, and Neonatal Nursing, 30*(4), 429–438.

Hutchinson, M. K. (1999). Individual, family, and relationship predictors of young women's sexual risk perceptions. *Journal of Obstetric, Gynecologic, and Neonatal Nursing, 28*(1), 60–67.

Johnson, B. K. (1998). A correlational framework for understanding sexuality in women age 50 and older. *Health Care for Women International, 19*(6), 553–364.

Katz, A. (2000). Birds do it, bees do it, let's talk about it. *AWHONN Lifelines, 4*(5), 40–41.

Kelly, P. J. (2001). Social influences on the sexual behaviors of adolescent girls in at-risk circumstances. *Journal of Obstetric, Gynecologic, and Neonatal Nursing, 30*(5), 481–489.

Lamp, J. K., Alteneder, R. R., & Lee, C. (2000). Nurses' knowledge, attitudes, and skills related to sexuality. *Journal of Nursing Scholarship, 32*(4), 391.

McCaffrey, R., Barnett, S., & Thomas, D. J. (2001). Seeking satisfaction: Treating decreased libido in women. *AWHONN Lifelines, 5*(4), 30–35.

Peck, S. A. (2001). The importance of the sexual health history in the primary care setting. *Journal of Obstetric, Gynecologic, and Neonatal Nursing, 30*(3), 269–274.

Russell, S. T. J., K. (2001). Adolescent sexual orientation and suicide risk: Evidence from a national study. *American Journal of Public Health, 91*(8), 1276–1281.

Sexual function improves after hysterectomy. (2000). *Women's Health in Primary Care, 3*(6), 432.

Stevens, P. E. (2001). Sexuality and safer sex: The issues for lesbians and bisexual women. *Journal of Obstetric, Gynecologic, and Neonatal Nursing, 30*(4), 439–447.

Sexually Transmitted Diseases

Alexander, I. M. (1998). Viral hepatitis: Primary care diagnosis and management. *Nurse Practitioner, 23*(10), 13–14, 17–18, 20, 25–26, 28, 31–32, 37–38, 40, 43.

Baker, D. A. (2002). Management options for non-HIV viral STDs. *Women's Health in Primary Care, 5*(2), 92–102.

Bauer, G. R. (2001). Beyond assumptions of negligible risk: Sexually transmitted disease and women who have sex with women. *American Journal of Public Health, 91*(8), 1282–1286.

Benson, L. M. (1998). Viral hepatitis. *Advance for Nurse Practitioners, 6*(6), 45–47.

Bisceglie, A., et al. (1998). Hepatitis C: Uncovering an invisible epidemic. *Patient Care Nurse Practitioner,* 18–27.

Blanchard, J. F., Moses, S., Greenaway, C., Orr, P., Hammond, G. W., & Brunham, R. C. (1998). The evolving epidemiology of chlamydial and gonococcal infections in response to control programs in Winnipeg, Canada. *American Journal of Public Health, 88*(10), 1496–1502.

Centers for Disease Control and Prevention. (2002). Sexually transmitted diseases treatment guidelines 2002. *Morbidity and Mortality Weekly Report, 51,* 80.

Crosby, R., Leichliter, J. S., & Brackbill, R. (2000). Longitudinal prediction of sexually transmitted diseases among adolescents. *American Journal of Preventive Medicine, 18*(4), 312–317.

Devine, P. (1998). Extrapelvic manifestations of gonorrhea. *Primary Care Update for Ob/Gyn,* 233–237.

DiMaio, H. (2002). Chancroid infections in women. *Primary Care Update for OB/GYNS, 8*(6), 258–259.

Holzman, C., Leventhal, J. M., Qiu, H., Jones, N. M., Wang, J., and the BV study group. (2001). Factors linked to bacterial vaginosis in nonpregnant women. *American Journal of Public Health, 91*(10), 1664–1670.

Iosue, K. (2002). Chronic hepatitis C: Latest treatment options. *Nurse Practitioner, 27*(4), 32–49.

King, R. R. (1999). Hepatitis C: Past, present and future issues. *Advance for Nurse Practitioners, 5,* 1–52, 55–56.

McQuillan, G. M., Coleman, P. J., et al. (1998). Prevalence of hepatitis B virus infection in the United States: The National Health and Nutrition Examination Survey, 1976–1994. *American Journal of Public Health, 89*(1), 14–18.

Mertz, K. J., Ransom, R. L., St. Louis, M. E., Groseclose, S. L., Hadgu, A., Levine, W. C., & Hayman, C. (2001). Prevalence of genital chlamydial infection in young women entering a national job training program, 1990–1997. *American Journal of Public Health, 91*(8), 1287–1290.

Recommendations for prevention and control of hepatitis C (HCV) infection and HCV-related chronic disease. (1998). *Morbidity and Mortality Weekly Report, 47*(RR-19), 1–39.

Roddy, R. E., Zekeng, L., Ryan, K. A., Tamoufe, U., & Tweedy, K. G. (2002). Effect of nonoxynol-9 gel on urogenital gonorrhea and chlamydial infection. *Journal of the American Medical Association, 287*(9), 1117–1122.

Roe, V. A. (2002). Antibacterials in women's health. *Women's Health Care, 1*(2), 7–19

Tiller, C. M. (2002). Chlamydia during pregnancy: Implications and impact on perinatal and neonatal outcomes. *Journal of Obstetric, Gynecologic, and Neonatal Nursing, 31*(1), 93–106.

van Devanter, N., Gonzales, V., Merzel, C., Parikh, N. S., Celantano, D., & Greenberg, J. (2002). Effect of an STD/HIV behavioral intervention on women's use of the female condom. *American Journal of Public Health, 92*(1), 109–115.

Smoking Cessation

Albrecht, S. A., & Caruthers, D. (2002). Characteristics of inner-city pregnant smoking teenagers. *Journal of Obstetric, Gynecologic, and Neonatal Nursing, 31*(4), 462–469.

Bauman, K. E., Foshee, V. A., Ennett, S. T., Pemberton, M., Hicks, K. A., King, T. S., & Foch, G. G. (2001). The influence of a family program on adolescent tobacco and alcohol use. *American Journal of Public Health, 91*(4), 604–610.

Bowen, D. J., McTiernan, A., Powers, D., & Feng, Z. (2001). Recruiting women into a smoking cessation program: Who might quit? *Women & Health, 31*(4), 41–58.

Doevr, L. (2000, June). Butts out. *Advance for Nurse Practitioners,* 45.

Easton, A., Husten, C., Elon, L., Pederson, L., & Frank, E. (2001). Non-primary care physicians and smoking cessation counseling: Women physicians' health study. *Women & Health, 34*(4), 15–29.

Faucher, M. A., & Carter, S. (2001). Why girls smoke: A proposed community-based prevention program. *Journal of Obstetric, Gynecologic, and Neonatal Nursing, 30*(5), 463–471.

Gaffney, K. F., Wichaikhum, O., & Dawson, E. M. (2002). Smoking among female college students: A time for change. *Journal of Obstetric, Gynecologic, and Neonatal Nursing, 31*(5), 502–507.

Gantt, C. J. (2001). The theory of planned behavior and postpartum smoking relapse. *Journal of Nursing Scholarship, 33*(4), 337–341.

Goldenberg, R. L. D.-M., & P. (2001). Convincing pregnant patients to stop smoking. *Contemporary Nurse Practitioner (fall),* 22–27.

Gruskin, E. P., Hart, S., Gordon, N., & Ackerson, L. (2001). Patterns of cigarette smoking and alcohol use among lesbians and bisexual women enrolled in a large health maintenance organization. *American Journal of Public Health, 91*(6), 976–979.

Horta, B. L., Kramer, M. S., & Platt, R. W. (2001). Maternal smoking and the risk of early weaning: A meta-analysis. *American Journal of Public Health, 91*(2), 304–307.

Jaakkola, N., Jaakkola, M. S., Gissler, M., & Jaakkola, J. J. K. (2001). Smoking during pregnancy in Finland: Determinants and trends, 1987–1997. *American Journal of Public Health, 91,* 284–286.

MacDonald, M., & Wright, N. E. (2002). Cigarette smoking and the disenfranchisement of adolescent girls: A discourse of resistance*? Health Care for Women International, 23*(3), 281–305.

National Institutes of Health, National Heart, Lung and Blood Institute. (1993). *Nurses: Help your patients stop smoking.* Bethesda, MD: National Institutes of Health.

Nusbaum, M., Gordon, M., Nusbaum, D., McCarthy, M., & Vasilakis, D. (2000). Smoke alarm: A review of the clinical impact of smoking on women. *Primary Care Update for Ob/Gyns, 7,* 207

Penman-Aguilar, A., Hall, J., Artz, L., Crawford, M. A., Peacock, N., vanPletsch, P. K., & Morgan, S. (2002). Smoke free families: A tobacco control program for pregnant women and their families. *Journal of Obstetric, Gynecologic, and Neonatal Nursing, 31*(1), 39–47.

Rappert, R. (1999). The last smoke. *American Journal of Nursing, 99*(11), 26.

Rodriguez, I., Kilborn, M. J., Liu, X., Pezzullo, J. C., & Woosley, R. L. (2001). Drug-induced QT prolongation in women during the menstrual cycle. *Journal of the American Medical Association, 285*(10), 1322–1326.

Ryan, H., Wortley, P. M., Easton, A., Pederson, L., & Greenwood, G. (2001). Smoking among lesbians, gays, and bisexuals: A review of the literature. *American Journal of Preventive Medicine, 21*(2), 142–149.

Thorndike, A. N., Biener, L., & Rigotti, N. A. (2002). Effect on smoking cessation of switching nicotine replacement therapy to over-the-counter status. *American Journal of Public Health, 92*(3), 437–442.

Todd, S. J. T., Lasal, K. B., & Neil-Urban, S. (2001). An integrated approach to prenatal smoking cessation interventions. *American Journal of Maternal Child Nursing, 26*(4), 185–191.

Wewers, M. E., & Uno, M. (2002). Clinical interventions and smoking ban methods to reduce infants' and children's exposure to environmental tobacco smoke. *Journal of Obstetric, Gynecologic, and Neonatal Nursing, 31*(5), 592–598.

Women and smoking. The Surgeon General's Report. (2001). *Women's Health in Primary Care 4* (6), 399–400.

Urinary Tract and Urinary Incontinence

Bent, S., Nallamothu, B. K., Simel, D. L., Fihn, S. D., & Saint, S. (2002). Does this woman have an acute uncomplicated urinary tract infection? *Journal of the American Medical Association, 287*(20), 2701–2710.

Birken, S., Santoro, N., Maydelman, Y, Kovalevskaya, G., Lobo, R., Freeman, E., Warren, M., McMahon, D., & O'Connor, J. (1999). Differences in urinary excretion patterns of the hLH beta core fragment in premenopausal, perimenopausal and post menopausal women. *Menopause, 6*(4), 290–198.

Bradley, C., & Singh, G. (2000). Interstitial cystitis: Evaluation and management. *The Female Patient, 25,* 83–88.

Chan, L. C., & A. B. (1999). Unresponsive urinary tract infection. *The Clinical Advisor, February,* 32–34.

Dougherty, M. C., Dwyer, J. W., Pendergast, J. F., Boyington, A. R., Tomlinson, B. U., Coward, R. T., Duncan, R. P., & Vogel, J. N. (2002). A randomized trial of behavioral management for continence with older rural women. *Research in Nursing and Health, 25*(1), 3–13.

Fitzgerald, S. T., Palmer, M. H., Kirkland, V. L., & Robinson, L. (2002). The impact of urinary incontinence in working women: A study in a production facility. *Women & Health, 35*(1), 1–26.

Fichenscher, L. (1999). Evaluating adult hematuria. *Nurse Practitioner, 24,* 58–65.

Foldspang, A., Mommsen, S., & Djurhuus, J. C. (1999). Prevalent urinary incontinence as a correlate of pregnancy, vaginal childbirth, and obstetric techniques. *American Journal of Public Health, 89*(2), 209–212.

Gray, M., McClain, R., Peruggia, M., Patrie, J., & Steers, W. D. (2001). A model for predicting motor urge urinary incontinence. *Nursing Research, 50*(2), 116–128.

Gupta, K., Scholes, D., & Stamm, W. E. (1999). Increasing prevalence of antimicrobial resistance among uropathogens causing acute uncomplicated cystitis in women. *Journal of the American Medical Association, 281*(8), 736–738.

Kontiokari, T., Sundqvist, K., Nuutinen, M., Pokka, T., Koskela, M., & Uhari, M.

(2001). Randomised trial of cranberry-lingonberry juice and lactobacillus GG drink for the prevention of urinary tract infections in women. *British Medical Journal, 322,* 1571–1573.

Lemack, G., & Zimmern, P. (2000, June), Treatment options for urinary incontinence in women. *Resident and Staff Physician,* 35–36, 43–46.

Maloney, C. M., & Cafiero, M. (2002). Achieving bladder control. *ADVANCE for Nurse Practitioners, 10*(5), 73–78.

Manges, A. R., Johnson, J. R., Foxman, B., O'Bryan, T. T., Fullerton, K. E., & Riley, L. W. (2001). Widespread distribution of urinary tract infections caused by a multidrug-resistant escherichia coli clonal group. *New England Journal of Medicine, 345*(14), 1007–1013.

Mokrzycki, M. L., Hatangadi, S. B., Zaccardi, J. E., & Cox, S. (2001). Preexisting stress urinary incontinence: A predictor of discontinuation with pessary management. *Journal of Lower Genital Tract Disease, 5*(4), 204–207.

Moller, L. A., Lose, G., & Jorgensen, T. (2000). Risk factors for lower urinary tract symptoms in women 40 to 60 years of age. *Obstetrics & Gynecology, 96*(3), 446–451.

Newman, D. K., & Giovannini, D. (2002). The overactive bladder: A nursing perspective. *American Journal of Nursing, 102*(6), 36–45.

Newman, D. K., & Palmer, M. H. (2003). State of the science on urinary incontinence. *American Journal of Nursing,* suppl., 4–53.

Persson, J., Wolner-Hanssen, W., & Rydhstroem, H. (2000). Obstetric risk factors for stress urinary incontinence: A population-based study. *Obstetrics & Gynecology, 96*(3), 440–445.

Preston, M. R., & Adam, R. A. (2002). Urinary incontinence in primary care patients. *Women's Health in Primary Care, 5*(2), 111–126.

Rabin, J. M. (1997). The "Femassist" a new device for the treatment of female urinary incontinence. *Advance for Nurse Practitioners, 5*(4), 199.

Richard, G. A., Childs, S. J., Fowler, C. L., Pittman, W., Nicolle, L. E., & Callery-D'Amico, S. (1998). Safety and efficacy of levofloxacin versus ciprofloxacin in complicated urinary tract infections in adults. *Pharmacy and Therapeutics* (October), 534–540.

Sampselle, C. M., Burns, P. A., Dougherty, M. C., Newman, D. K., et al. (1997). Continence for women: Evidence-based practice. *Journal of Obstetric, Gynecologic, and Neonatal Nursing, 26*(4), 375–385.

Subak,, L., Quesenberry, C., Posner, S., Cuttolica, E., & Soglukian. L. (2002). The effect of behavioral therapy on urinary incontinence: A randomized controlled trial. *Obstetrics & Gynecology, 100,* 72.

Thakar, R., & Stanton, S. (2002). Management of genital prolapse. *British Medical Journal, 324,* 1258–1262.

Van Kerrebroeck, P., Kreder, K., Jonas, U., Zinner, N., & Wein, A. (2001). Tolterodine once-daily: Superior efficacy and tolerability in the treatment of the overactive bladder. *Urology, 57*(2), 414–421.

Versi, E., et al. (1998). New external urethral occlusive device for female urinary incontinence. *Obstetrics & Gynecology, 2*(2), 286–291.

Vaginitis/Vaginosis

Andrist, L. C. (2001). Vaginal health and infections. *Journal of Obstetric, Gyneco-logic, and Neonatal Nursing, 30*(3), 306–315.

Bascom, M, Desnick, L., & Elmore, J. (1999, May). Management of vaginal infections. *Clinical Advisor, 26.*

Gallagher, K., Kunic, R., Barnum, J., & Savrin, C. (2002). Vaginal lacerations. *ADVANCE for Nurse Practitioners, 10*(6), 77–79.

Holzman, C., Leventhal, J. M., Qiu, H., Jones, N. M., Wang, J., and the BV study group. (2001). Factors linked to bacterial vaginosis in nonpregnant women. *American Journal of Public Health, 91*(10), 1664–1670.

Klebaqnoff, M. A., Carey, C., Hauth, J. C., Hillier, S. L., Nugent, R. P., Thom, E. A., Ernest, J. M., Heine, P., Wapner, R. J., Trout, W., Moawad, A., Leveno, K. J. and the National Institute of Child Health and Human Develpment Network of Mater-nal-Fetal Medicine Units. (2001). Failure of metronidazole to prevent preterm delivery among pregnant women with asymptomatic trichomonas vaginalis infection. *New England Journal of Medicine, 345*(7), 487–493.

Lichtenstein, V. N., & Nansel, T. R. (2000). Women's douching practices and related attitudes: Findings from four focus groups. *Women & Health, 31*(2/3), 117–131.

Secor, R. M. C. (2001). Bacterial vaginosis. *Clinician Reviews, 11*(11), 59–68.

Sinofsky, F. (1999). Vulvovaginal candidiasis: Topical versus oral therapy. *The Female Patient, 24,* 35, 39, 40, 42, 45.

Theroux, R. (2002). Bypassing the middleman: A grounded theory of women's self-care for vaginal symptoms. *Health Care for Women International, 23*(5), 417–431.

Vulvar Conditions

Boardman, L. A. B., & L. A. (2000). Managing vulvar infections: HPV-related disease and candidiasis. *Women's Health in Primary Care, 3*(12), 857–862.

Budd, B. (2000, March). Genital herpes in adolescents. *Advance for Nurse Practitioners,* 31.

Carter, J., & Soper, D. (1998). Strategies for managing external genital warts. *Women's Health in Primary Care, 1*(4), 320.

Driver, K. A. (2002). Managing vulvar vestibulitis. *Nurse Practitioner, 27*(7), 24–35.

Foster, D. C. (2002). Vulvar disease. *Obstetrics & Gynecology, 100*(1), 145–163.

Ferris, D. G., Nyirjesy, P., Sobel, J. D., Soper, D., Pavletic, A., & Litaker, M. S. (2002). Over-the-counter antifungal drug misuse associated with patient-diag-nosed vulvovaginal candidiasis. *Obstetrics and Gynecology, 99*(3), 419–425.

Hedden, A. Z. (2002). Persistent molluscum contagiosum. *ADVANCE for Nurse Practitioners, 10*(5), 79–82.

Kreiter, C. (2000, March). Vulvar vestibulitis: Breaking the silence. *Advance for Nurse Practitioners,* 67–69.

Secor, R. M. C. (Guest Editor). (1992). Entire issue devoted to vulvar and vaginal conditions. *Nurse Practitioner Forum, 3*(3).

Secor, R. M. C., & Fertitta, L. (1992). Vulvar vestibulitis syndrome. *Nurse Practitioner Forum, 3*(3), 161–168.

Toki, T., Katoh, K., Nakayama, H., & Fujii, S. (1999). Aggressive ansiomyxoma of the vulva associated with severe infection. *Obstetrics & Gynecology, 94*(5), 863.

Wald, A., Langenberg, A. G. M., Izu, A. E., Ashley, R., Warren, T., Tyring, S., Douglas, J. M., & Corey, L. (2001). Effect of condoms on reducing the transmission of herpes simplex virus type 2 from men to women. *Journal of the American Medical Association, 285*(24), 3100–3106.

Weight Maintenance

Anderson, R. E., & Franklin, B. A. (1999). Exercise for optimum health. *Patient Care for the Nurse Practitioner,* 13–27.

Avonne, L. J., Blackburn, G. L, & Vash, P. D. (2001). Intervening in the obesity epidemic. *Patient Care for the Nurse Practitioner,* 12, 24.

Avonne, L. (1999). Weight gain during perimenopause: The case for early intervention. *Menopause Management,* 7–11.

Bray, G. (2002). Obesity: Is there effective treatment? *Consultant, 42*(8), 1014.

Davis, P., & Krauss, H. (2001). The impact of diet on chronic disease. *Patient Care for the Nurse Practitioner,* 25–26, 29, 30.

Gillman, M. W., Rifas-Shiman, S. L., Berkey, C. S., Frazier, A. L., Rockett, H. R. H., Field, A. E., & Colditz, G. A. (2001). Risk of overweight among adolescents who were breastfed as infants. *Journal of the American Medical Association, 285*(19), 2461–2467.

Kane, A. K., Schatzkin, A., Graubard, B. I., & Schairer, C. (2000). A prospective study of diet quality and mortality in women. *Journal of the American Medical Association, 283*(16), 2109–2115.

Lichtstein, A., et al. (2002). The best diet for healthy adults. *Patient Care for the Nurse Practitioner.*

National Institutes of Health. (2000). *The practice guide: Identification, evaluation, and treatment of overweight and obesity in adults.* Bethesda, MD: NIH.

Turner, J., Knosby, K., & Popkess-Vawter, S. (2002). Nurse practitioner and client partnerships in long-term holistic weight management. *American Journal of Nurse Practitioners, 6*(6), 9–18.

White, J. H. (2000). Improving outcomes for obesity. *The American Journal for Nurse Practitioners, 4*(10), 9–18.

Women and Heart Disease

Ali, N. S. (2002). Prediction of coronary heart disease preventive behaviors in women: A test of the health belief model. *Women & Health, 35*(1), 83–96.

Anderson, J. K., & Kessenich, C. R. (2001). Women and coronary heart disease. *Nurse Practitioner, 26*(8), 12–31.

Appel, S. J., Harrell, J. S., & Deng, S. (2002). Racial and socioeconomic differences in risk factors for cardiovascular disease among southern rural women. *Nursing Research, 51*(3), 140–147.

Arslanian-Engoren, C. (2002). Recognizing heart disease. *AWHONN Lifelines, 6*(2), 114–122.

Braun, L. T., & Rosensun, R. S. (2001). Assessing coronary heart disease risk and managing lipids. *Nurse Practitioner, 26*(12), 30–41.

Duvernoy, C. S. E., & et al. (2001a). Diagnosing and treating acute myocardial infarction in women. *Women's Health in Primary Care, 4*(8), 542–556.

Duvernoy, C. S. E., & et al. (2001b). Sex differences in acute myocardial infarction. *Women's Health in Primary Care, 4*(8), 558.

Funk, M., Ostfeld, A. M., Chang, V. M., & Lee, F. A. (2002). Racial differences in the use of cardiac procedures in patients with acute myocardial infarction. *Nursing Research, 51*(3), 148–157.

Jiang, W., & O'Connor, C. M. (2002). Depression and cardiac health in women: How close is the relationship? *Women's Health in Primary Care, 5*(6), 393–405.

Meischke, H., Kuniyuki, A., Yasui, Y., Bowen, D. J., Andersen, R., & Urban, N. (2002). Information women receive about heart attacks and how it affects their knowledge, beliefs, and intentions to act in a cardiac emergency. *Health Care for Women International, 23*(2), 149–162.

Pradham, A. D., Manson, J. E., Rossouw, J. E., Siscovick, D. S., Moulton, C. P., Rifai, N., Wallace, R. B., Jackson, R. D., Pettinger, M. B., & Ridker, P. M. (2002). Inflammatory biomarkers, hormone replacement therapy, and incident coronary heart disease. *Journal of the American Medical Association, 288*(8), 980–987.

Quinlivan, E. P., McPartlin, J., McNulty, H., Ward, M., Strain, J. J., Weir, D. G., & Scott, J. M. (2002). Importance of both folic acid and vitamin B12 in reduction of risk of vascular disease. *Lancet, 359,* 227–228.

Regensteiner, J. G., & Gerhard-Herman, M. (2002). Aging and vascular disease in women. *Women's Health in Primary Care, 5*(4 suppl.), 1–40.

Sparks, E. A., & Frazier, L. Q. (2002). Heritable cardiovascular disease in women. *Journal of Obstetric, Gynecologic, and Neonatal Nursing, 31*(2), 217–228.

Weiss, J. S., & L. D. (2001). Stalking the #1 killer of women . . . detecting diabetes and heart disease. *AWHONN Lifelines, 5*(5), 26–34.

Wenger, N. K. (2002). How to keep her heart healthy. *Women's Health in Primary Care, 5*(7), 432–442.

Women's Health Care, Gynecologic Care, Pelvic Examination

Douglas, J. H. (1998). Female circumcision: Persistence amid conflict. *Health Care for Women International, 19*(6), 477–479.

Ehrenreich, B., & English, D. (1973). *Complaints and disorders: The sexual politics of sickness.* Old Westbury, NY: The Feminist Press.

Ehrenreich, B., & English, D. (1973). *Witches, midwives, and nurses: A history of women healers.* Old Westbury, NY: The Feminist Press.

Gentry, S. E. (1992). Caring for lesbians in a homophobic society. *Health Care for Women International, 13*(2), 173–180.

Hern, M. J., et al. (1998). Promoting women's health via the world wide web. *Journal of Obstetric, Gynecologic, and Neonatal Nursing, 27*(6), 606–610.

Jacobs, D. R., Meyer, K. A., et al. (1999). Is whole grain intake associated with reduced total and cause-specific death rates in older women? The Iowa women's health study. *American Journal of Public Health, 89*(3), 322–329.

Kushnir, T., Rabinowitz, S., et al. (1995). Health responsibility and workplace health promotion among women: Early detection of cancer. *Health Care for Women International, 16*(4), 329–340.

Lucas, V. A. (1992). An investigation of the health care preferences of the lesbian population. *Health Care for Women International, 13*(2), 221–228.

Messing, K. (1997). Women's occupational health: A critical review and discussion of current issues. *Women & Health, 25*(4), 39–68.

Muscari, M. E. (1999). Adolescent health: The first gynecologic exam. *American Journal of Nursing, 99*(1), 66, 58.

Olsson, H. M., & Gullberg, M. T. (1991). Fundamental and situational components in a strategy for attaining a positive patient experience of the pelvic examination: A conceptual approach. *Health Care for Women International, 12*(4), 415–429.

Peterson-Sweeney, K. L., & Stevens, J. (1996). 13-year-old female with imperforate hymen. *Nurse Practitioner, 21*(8), 90–94.

Pulliam, L. W., Plowfield, L. A., & Fuess, S. (1996). Developmental care: The key to the emergence of the vital older woman. *Journal of Obstetric, Gynecologic, and Neonatal Nursing, 25*(7), 623–628.

Reichert, G. A. (1998). Female circumcision. *AWHONN Lifelines, 2*(3), 28–34.

Robertson, M. M. (1992). Lesbians as an invisible minority in the health services arena. *Health Care for Women International, 13*(2), 155–163.

Rogge, S. A. (1998). Reforming managed care: Carving out women's rights in health care. *AWHONN Lifelines, 2*(6), 17–18.

Taylor, D., & Dower, C. (1997). Toward a woman-centered health care system: Women's experiences, women's voices, women's needs. *Health Care for Women International, 18*(4), 407–422.

Williams, J. G., Park, L. I., & Kline, J. (1995). Physicians' attitudes toward a new gynecological examination gown. *Women & Health, 22*(2), 1–9.

Woods, N. F., Lentz, M., & Mitchell, E. (1993). The new woman: Health-promoting and health-damaging behaviors. *Health Care for Women International, 14*(5), 389–405.

Index

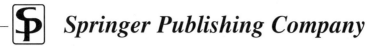
Springer Publishing Company

Annual Review of Nursing Research
Volume 19: Women's Health Research
Joyce J. Fitzpatrick, PhD, RN, FAAN, Series Editor
Diana Taylor, PhD, RN, NP, FAAN, and
Nancy Fugate Woods, PhD, RN, FAAN, Volume Editors

This book demonstrates that nurses have made an important contribution to the advancement and expansion of women's health knowledge. Selecting the health issues of most importance to women, the editors have assembled leading nurse researchers to review, summarize, and critique nursing research within each area. A general overview of the field is also provided.

Contents: Part I: Introduction
What We Know and How We Know It: Contributions from Nursing to Women's Health Research and Scholarship, *D. Taylor and N. Woods* • Conceptual Models for Women's Health Research: Reclaiming Menopause as an Exemplar of Nursing's Contributions to Feminist Scholarship, *L. C. Andrist and K. MacPherson*

Part II: Research on Women's Social Roles and Health
Women as Mothers and Grandmothers, *A. B. McBride and C. P. Shore* • Women and Employment: A Decade Review, *M. G. Killien* • Interventions for Women as Family Caregivers, *M. J. Bull*

Part III: Research on Diversity and Women's Health
Lesbian Health and Health Care, *L. A. Berhard* • Immigrant Women and Their Health, *K. Aroian*

Part IV: Research on Women's Health and Illness Issues
Women and Stress, *C. Cahill* • Sleep and Fatigue, *K. A. Lee* • Intimate Partner Violence Against Women, *J. Humphreys, B. Parker, and J. Campbell* • Health Decisions and Decision Support for Women, *M. L. Rothert and A. M. O'Connor* • Female Troubles: An Analysis of Menstrual Cycle Research in the NINR Portfolio as a Model for Science Development in Women's Health, *N. K. Reame*

2001   376pp   0-8261-1408-3   hardcover

536 Broadway, New York, NY 10012 • Telephone: 212-431-4370
Fax: 212-941-7842 • Order Toll-Free: 877-687-7476 • Order On-line: www.springerpub.com

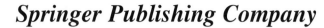

Springer Publishing Company

From the Springer Series on Social Work...

Adolescent Pregnancy
Policy and Prevention Services
Naomi Farber, PhD, MSW

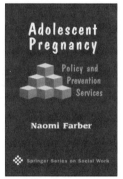

The author provides social work practitioners with research-based information necessary to develop prevention programs and policies that target young people according to their different levels of early sex, pregnancy, and parenthood experiences. The need to develop policies and services designed to reduce teenage pregnancy in ways appropriate for the social worker's specific client population is emphasized throughout.

Identifying and synthesizing the wide literature on prevention theory and practice, this book offers "best practice" applications for effective social work intervention.

Partial Contents:
* Dimensions of Adolescent Sexual Activity and Fertility
* Theories of Illegitimacy
* Contemporary Research: Sexual Risk Taking
* Conceptual Framework: A Continuum of Risk
* Approaches to Prevention of Adolescent Pregnancy
* Planning Prevention Services: An Assessment Framework
* Alcohol and Drug Use and Adolescent Pregnancy, *N. N. Brown*
* A Developmental Perspective on Adolescent Parenting *J. R. Shapiro*
* Appendix A: State Laws on Minors' Access to Abortion
* Appendix B: State Policies for Sexuality and STD/HIV Education

2003   232pp   0-8261-2372-4   hardcover

536 Broadway, New York, NY 10012 • Telephone: 212-431-4370
Fax: 212-941-7842 • Order Toll-Free: 877-687-7476 • Order On-line: www.springerpub.com

℞ *Springer Publishing Company*

Clinical Excellence for
Nurse Practitioners
The International Journal of NPACE

Joellen W. Hawkins, RNC, PhD, FAAN, Editor
Susan Daggett Bennett, MSN, RN, CS-ANP
Frances Medaglia Dwyer, PhD, RN, CS-GNP
Richard S. Ferri, PhD, ANP, ACRN, FAAN
Joyce Pulcini, PhD, RN, CS-PNP, Associate Editors

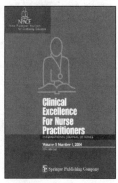

This quarterly is a peer-reviewed journal designed to facilitate communication about practice, education, and research for advanced practice nurses. Each issue presents columns on clinical practice, clinical studies, pharmacology, policy and regulatory issues, and APN education. *Clinical Excellence for Nurse Practitioners* is the official publication of NPACE (Nurse Practitioner Associates for Continuing Education). Its intent is to be global in both its content and its audience, emphasizing the practical application of policy, practice, and research findings.

Sample Contents:
Editorial
- Musings on Attitudes and Their Effects on Our Health and Well-Being: You're Only as Old as You Feel or Behave, *Joellen W. Hawkins*

Clinical Practice
- Diagnosis and Treatment of Persons With Restless Legs Syndrome, *Norma G. Cuellar*
- Breast Cancer Screening Behavior Among Low-Income and Minority Women, *Mary Kerans*

Clinical Studies
- Experiences of Adoptive Parents of Children With Fetal Alcohol Syndrome, *Joan Granitsas*
- The Incubator Model: Is It Effective Prenatal Care, *Brandy L. Worley, Linda F. C. Bullock, and Elizabeth Geden*
- The Availability and Accessibility of Gynecological and Reproductive Services for Women With Developmental Disabilities, A Nursing Perspective, *Catharine Kopac, and Joni Fritz*

ISSN 1085-2360 • Volume 8, 2004 • Published 4 times per year

---

536 Broadway, New York, NY 10012 • Telephone: 212-431-4370
Fax: 212-941-7842 • Order Toll-Free: 877-687-7476 • Order On-line: www.springerpub.com